Controversies in Thyroid Nodules and Differentiated Thyroid Cancer

Sanziana A. Roman • Wen T. Shen
Julie Ann Sosa

Editors

Controversies in Thyroid Nodules and Differentiated Thyroid Cancer

A Case-Based Approach

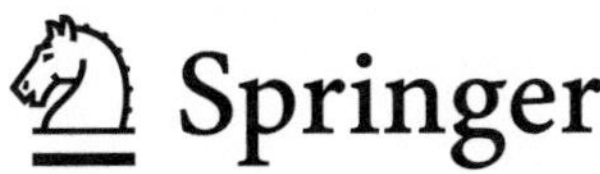 Springer

Editors
Sanziana A. Roman
Department of Surgery
University of California, San Francisco
San Francisco, CA, USA

Wen T. Shen
Department of Surgery
University of California, San Francisco
San Francisco, CA, USA

Julie Ann Sosa
Department of Surgery
University of California, San Francisco
San Francisco, CA, USA

ISBN 978-3-031-37137-0   ISBN 978-3-031-37135-6   (eBook)
https://doi.org/10.1007/978-3-031-37135-6

This Springer imprint is published by the registered company Springer Nature Switzerland AG
The registered company address is: Gewerbestrasse 11, 6330 Cham, Switzerland

Paper in this product is recyclable.

Preface

The evaluation and management of thyroid nodules and differentiated thyroid cancer (DTC) are continually evolving. Despite extensive research and multiple published comprehensive practice guidelines, numerous controversies remain within this field covering a wide range of issues, including incidence and epidemiology, radiographic evaluation, criteria for needle biopsy, cytopathologic and molecular diagnostics, active surveillance vs. operation for low-risk tumors, extent of surgery, indications for radioactive iodine treatment and external beam radiation, and optimal protocols for follow-up. In this book, we highlight and explore the most significant controversies in the diagnosis and treatment of thyroid nodules and DTC and provide practical, case-based, and evidence-guided recommendations. We feature a diverse group of authors with expertise spanning the entire spectrum of thyroid care, representing a wide range of institutions from the USA and abroad. Our goal is to help guide practitioners of all levels in their care of patients with thyroid nodules and DTC and to stimulate further inquiry and evidence-based change in knowledge and practice in this area.

We thank Sabrina Lum for invaluable administrative support, and we express our gratitude to our colleagues, families, and patients. We dedicate this book to the memory and legacy of Dr. Orlo H. Clark, a founding figure in the field of endocrine surgery and one of the most impactful thought leaders in thyroid research and care.

San Francisco, CA, USA
San Francisco, CA, USA
San Francisco, CA, USA

Sanziana A. Roman
Wen T. Shen
Julie Ann Sosa

Contents

Contents

Contributors

Mohamed Abdelgadir Adam Department of Surgery, University of California San Francisco, San Francisco, CA, USA

Noor Addasi Department of Internal Medicine, Division of Diabetes, Endocrinology, and Metabolism, University of Nebraska Medical Center, 984120 Nebraska Medical Center, Omaha, NE, USA

Cotton O'Neil Diabetes and Endocrinology, Stormont Vail Health, Topeka, KS, USA

Mariam Ali-Mucheru, MD Surgical Specialists of Atlanta, Atlanta, GA, USA

Martin Almquist Department of Surgery, Lund University, Lund, Sweden

Wilson Alobuia Department of Surgery, Stanford University, Stanford, CA, USA

Arvind K. Badhey Department of Otolaryngology, University of Cincinnati, Cincinnati, OH, USA

Lindsay A. Bischoff Department of Medicine, Vanderbilt University, Nashville, TN, USA

Iuliana Bobanga MatSu Surgical Associates, MatSu Regional Medical Center, Palmer, AK, USA

James D. Brierley Department of Radiation Oncology, University of Toronto, Toronto, ON, Canada

Department of Radiation Oncology, Princess Margaret Cancer Centre, Toronto, ON, Canada

Debbie W. Chen Department of Medicine, University of Michigan School of Medicine, Ann Arbor, MI, USA

Jessica Dahle Department of Surgery, Section of Endocrine Surgery, Duke University Medical Center, Durham, NC, USA

Endocrine and General Surgery, Ochsner Health, New Orleans, LA, USA

Clifton Davis Department of Internal Medicine, Division of Diabetes, Endocrinology, and Metabolism, University of Nebraska Medical Center, 984120 Nebraska Medical Center, Omaha, NE, USA

Priya H. Dedhia Department of Surgery, The Ohio State University Wexner Medical Center and Arthur G. James Cancer Center, Columbus, OH, USA

John A. (Drew) Ridge Department of Surgical Oncology, Fox Chase Cancer Center, Philadelphia, PA, USA

Sara H. Duffus Department of Pediatrics, University of North Carolina Chapel Hill, Chapel Hill, NC, USA

Fernanda Romero-Hernandez Department of Surgery, University of California San Francisco, San Francisco, CA, USA

Stephanie Fish Endocrinology Division, Memorial Sloan Kettering Cancer Center, New York, NY, USA

Whitney S. Goldner Department of Internal Medicine, Division of Diabetes, Endocrinology, and Metabolism, University of Nebraska Medical Center, 984120 Nebraska Medical Center, Omaha, NE, USA

Megan R. Haymart Department of Medicine, University of Michigan School of Medicine, Ann Arbor, MI, USA

Maureen V. Hill Department of Surgical Oncology, Fox Chase Cancer Center, Philadelphia, PA, USA

Hadiza S. Kazaure Department of Surgery, Section of Endocrine Surgery, Duke University Medical Center, Durham, NC, USA

Electron Kebebew Department of Surgery, Stanford University, Stanford, CA, USA

Cari M. Kitahara Radiation Epidemiology Branch, Division of Cancer Epidemiology and Genetics, National Cancer Institute, National Institutes of Health, Bethesda, MD, USA

Jennifer H. Kuo Department of Surgery, Columbia University, New York City, NY, USA

Jelena Lukovic Department of Radiation Oncology, University of Toronto, Toronto, ON, Canada

Department of Radiation Oncology, Princess Margaret Cancer Centre, Toronto, ON, Canada

Christopher R. McHenry Case Western Reserve University School of Medicine, Cleveland, OH, USA

Department of Surgery, MetroHealth Medical Center, Cleveland, OH, USA

Division of General Surgery, MetroHealth Medical Center, Cleveland, OH, USA

Julie A. Miller Department of Endocrine Surgery, Royal Melbourne Hospital, Parkville, VIC, Australia

May-Anh Nguyen Section of Endocrine Surgery, Division of General Surgery, University Health Network, University of Toronto, Toronto, ON, Canada

Jesse D. Pasternak Section of Endocrine Surgery, Division of General Surgery, University Health Network, University of Toronto, Toronto, ON, Canada

Jennifer A. Sipos Department of Internal Medicine, The Ohio State University Wexner Medical Center and Arthur G. James Cancer Center, Columbus, OH, USA

Rebecca S. Sippel, MD Department of Surgery, University of Wisconsin-Madison, Madison, WI, USA

David L. Steward Department of Otolaryngology, University of Cincinnati, Cincinnati, OH, USA

Ray Wang Department of Diabetes and Endocrinology, Royal Melbourne Hospital, Parkville, VIC, Australia

Christopher M. K. L. Yao Department of Surgical Oncology, Fox Chase Cancer Center, Philadelphia, PA, USA

Chapter 1
Incidence and Epidemiology of Differentiated Thyroid Cancer: Is Thyroid Cancer Incidence Truly Increasing, or Is It Simply a Finder Effect?

Cari M. Kitahara

Case 1

M.S. is a 60-year-old woman who finally decided to schedule an annual physical examination with her primary care physician. For years, Ms. S. avoided her primary care physician because she knew she was eligible for various cancer screenings and feared what the examinations would reveal. Her mother and her spouse had both recently died from highly aggressive cancers (breast and pancreatic cancers, respectively).

During her physical exam, Ms. S's general practitioner palpates the thyroid, finds a lump, and orders a thyroid ultrasound. The ultrasound shows three small hypoechoic nodules, each measuring under $20 \times 20 \times 20$ mm with no aggressive features. Fine-needle aspiration biopsy shows that the nodule on the left lobe is malignant, and it is preoperatively diagnosed as papillary thyroid carcinoma. Ms. S is devastated by the diagnosis and terrified that she will suffer the same fate as her mother and spouse. Despite some disagreement among her care team, Ms. S insists on the most aggressive approach to treating her cancer. She has a total thyroidectomy followed by radioactive iodine ablation.

C. M. Kitahara (✉)
Radiation Epidemiology Branch, Division of Cancer Epidemiology and Genetics, National Cancer Institute, National Institutes of Health, Bethesda, MD, USA
e-mail: kitaharac@mail.nih.gov

S. A. Roman et al. (eds.), *Controversies in Thyroid Nodules and Differentiated Thyroid Cancer*, https://doi.org/10.1007/978-3-031-37135-6_1

Overview

In 2020, thyroid cancer was the tenth most common malignancy diagnosed worldwide, accounting for 3% of all cancer diagnoses, with an age-standardized incidence rate of 6.6 per 100,000 [1]. Unlike most cancers, thyroid cancer is diagnosed more often in women than men (at a ratio of about 3:1) [1, 2] (Fig. 1.1). This sex disparity is evident starting in adolescence and peaks in middle age [3]. Thyroid cancer ranks second among cancers diagnosed in women under the age of 40 years [1]. Thyroid cancer is one of few malignancies that has risen in incidence over recent decades, a pattern observed almost globally [4]. It was previously unclear whether the rising incidence was occurring primarily in affluent countries, such as the United States, Canada, Australia, and many Western and Northern European countries, as high-quality and long-term data from other parts of the world had been limited [5]. However, recent data from India, China, Colombia, Lithuania, and Belarus have shown similar increases over time [6, 7].

True Increase or Overdiagnosis?

Some researchers have argued that the rise in thyroid cancer has been an epidemic of "overdiagnosis," rather than a real increase in disease [5, 8]. Overdiagnosis occurs when a disease is detected and diagnosed that would not otherwise have caused harm to the individual. In general, the trends in incidence have been driven

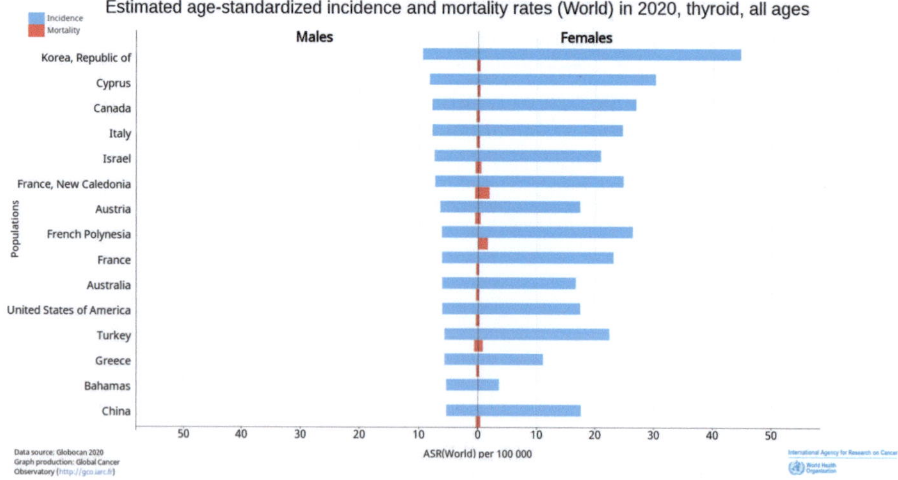

Fig. 1.1 Estimated age-standardized thyroid cancer incidence and mortality (number of cases or deaths per 100,000 annually) for males and females in selected countries, 2020. Globocan 2020. http://gco.iarc.fr

by papillary histologic types (accounting for about 90% of all thyroid cancers) [9, 10]. Papillary thyroid cancer is often indolent or slow growing and highly amenable to treatment, and the prognosis is typically excellent (99.7% 5-year relative survival in the United States [2]). Although the incidence of both early-stage and advanced papillary thyroid cancers has increased over time, the rate of increase has been greatest for small, localized papillary tumors, indicative of overdiagnosis [11]. In contrast, incidence trends for follicular, medullary, and anaplastic histologic types have been stable [9, 11]. Thyroid cancer mortality (about 0.5 deaths per 100,000 annually) is also much lower than incidence (Fig. 1.2), with little geographic variation, and stable or declining trends over time in most regions [12, 13].

The introduction and more widespread use of thyroid ultrasonography and fine-needle aspiration biopsy for detecting and diagnosing thyroid cancer were clearly major contributors to rising thyroid cancer incidence rates since the 1980s [8, 14]. These tools, in addition to the explosive growth in the use of diagnostic imaging (including computed tomography scans), have allowed for the ability to detect and diagnose increasingly smaller thyroid nodules and cancer in a population known to have a reservoir of latent disease [8, 15]. In 2006, Davies and Welch reported an increasing proportion of smaller versus larger papillary thyroid cancers diagnosed over time in the United States [8]. Prior to these developments, most thyroid cancers were either symptomatic, detected during thyroid palpation as a part of regular medical care, or identified during the follow-up of a benign thyroid condition. The prevalence of thyroid nodules in the general population has been estimated to range between 10% and 70% [16], depending on age of the patient and the level of diagnostic scrutiny or dissection of the thyroid, and about 5% of nodules undergoing diagnostic work-up are determined to be malignant [17]. Estimates at the higher end of this range generally stem from autopsy studies involving fine dissection of the thyroid gland. However, a review of radiological reports found that most thyroid

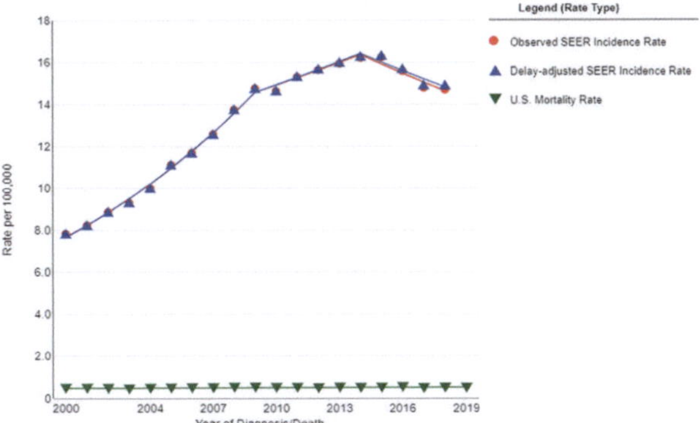

Fig. 1.2 Trends in thyroid cancer incidence (observed and delay-adjusted) and thyroid cancer mortality (number of cases or deaths per 100,000 annually) for U.S. males and females. Incidence data were provided by the SEER-21 cancer registries for the years 2000–2018. Mortality data were provided by the U.S. National Center for Health Statistics, Centers for Disease Control and Prevention, for the years 2000–2019. https://seer.cancer.gov/explorer/cancer-sites.html

nodules (especially those <1 cm) are not reported by the radiologist or referred for diagnostic follow-up, suggesting that far fewer thyroid nodules and cancer are incidentally detected from routine imaging of the thyroid gland than has been suggested from autopsy reports or dedicated radiological review [17]. Thus, there is some ambiguity over the size of the so-called subclinical reservoir of thyroid cancer in the general population, and the extent to which incidental imaging has contributed to the rising incidence of thyroid cancer after considering actual, "real life" reporting and diagnostic practices.

Researchers from the International Agency for Research on Cancer estimated the extent of thyroid cancer overdiagnosis in 26 countries, by comparing age-specific thyroid cancer incidence curves with historical age-specific incidence data collected from long-standing, high-quality cancer registries [5, 6]. By 2008–2012, they estimated that 93% of female thyroid cancer cases in South Korea, 91% in Belarus, 87% in China, 84% in Italy and Croatia, and 83% in Slovakia and France were attributable to overdiagnosis [6]. Overdiagnosis was less common in Denmark (66%), Norway (65%), Ireland (63%), the United Kingdom (58%), Japan (55%), and Thailand (44%). In general, the extent of overdiagnosis was about 10% higher in female than male patients. In India, about half of all thyroid cancers diagnosed in women are attributable to overdiagnosis, whereas no evidence for overdiagnosis was observed in men [7].

South Korea, with the world's highest incidence of thyroid cancer (about 107 per 100,000 annually in women and 21 per 100,000 annually in men during 2008–2010) and most dramatic increases in incidence over time, represents an extreme example of a region affected by thyroid cancer overdiagnosis [12]. In the late 1990s, a national cancer screening was implemented and highly encouraged by the government and by clinicians, and thyroid ultrasonography was offered as a low-cost option. Most individuals appeared to be uninformed or unconcerned about the potential harms of thyroid cancer overdiagnosis [18]. A survey administered in 2010 revealed that, in the prior 2 years, 14% of the population had undergone thyroid cancer screening [12]; 63% were women and 28% were aged between 50 and 59 years. There was also a strong correlation between regional screening and incidence, especially in women [12]. The result was a 15-fold increase in incidence between 1993 and 2001, driven entirely by papillary thyroid cancer, with no corresponding increase in mortality [10]. After 2012, the incidence declined, likely reflecting greater awareness and publicity around overdiagnosis in the country [19]. Similar recent declines resulting from awareness and actions taken against the problem of overdiagnosis have been observed in countries such as the United States [20] (Fig. 1.2).

In general, overdiagnosis appears to be a greater contributor to thyroid cancer age-specific patterns and temporal trends among women than men. U.S. cancer registry data show a threefold higher incidence of thyroid cancer in women than men overall and a more than fourfold higher incidence of small (<2 cm) localized papillary cancers [21]. The sex ratio for small localized papillary thyroid cancers also increased over time. In contrast, thyroid cancer mortality rates are nearly identical in women and men. Autopsy studies have shown that subclinical thyroid cancer is prevalent in about 14% of women and 11% of men [21]. Researchers have argued that the observed sex ratio for thyroid cancer incidence reflects greater engagement of women than men with the healthcare system and more conditioning by clinicians to look for thyroid disorders in women, thereby creating more opportunities for incidental detection of thyroid cancer [21]. Furthermore, the notion of thyroid cancer as a malignancy predominantly affecting women may inadvertently lead to delayed diagnosis and treatment for thyroid cancer in men. This phenomenon could explain the more pronounced rise in thyroid cancer mortality in U.S. men (annual percent change of 1.1% during 1983–2019) compared to women (annual percent change of 0.3% during 1988–2019) [2] (Fig. 1.3).

Thyroid cancer screening and overdiagnosis are of major public health concern for several reasons. First, individuals with a screen-detected nodule often undergo fine-needle aspiration biopsy and other diagnostic testing, which contributes to anxiety and stress around the potential cancer diagnosis [22]. Having a diagnosis of cancer, even when accompanied by an excellent prognosis, further induces stress, anxiety, and worry. Nearly all diagnosed thyroid cancers are treated, and treatments tend to be extensive, involving surgical removal of all (typically) or part of the thyroid gland, and thyroidectomy is often accompanied by radioactive iodine ablation. Side effects of surgery include permanent hypothyroidism (100% for those undergoing total thyroidectomy) and thus the need for lifelong thyroid hormone replacement and complications, including hypoparathyroidism and recurrent laryngeal nerve injury, which are reduced for patients treated by a high-volume surgeon [22]. Side effects of radioactive iodine are dose-dependent and include lacrimal gland inflammation, obstruction of lacrimal duct and epiphora, conjunctivitis, sialadenitis, nausea and vomiting, hematological abnormalities, transient ovarian or testicular insufficiency, and second primary malignancies [22]. Management of this disease can be costly, especially considering that a large proportion of thyroid cancer patients are young or middle-aged women, many of whom may not have full-time

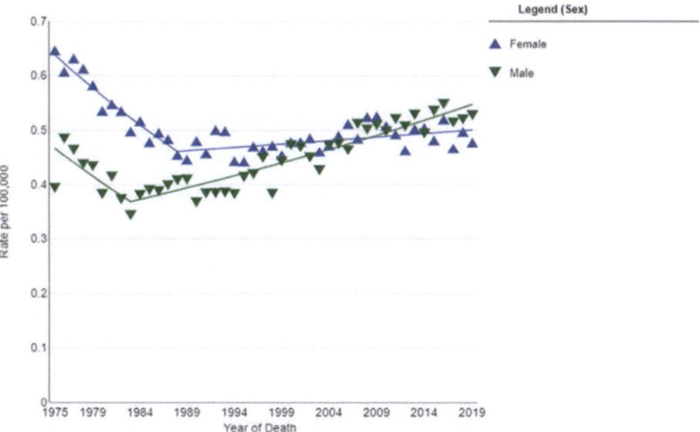

Fig. 1.3 Trends in thyroid cancer mortality (number of cases or deaths per 100,000 annually) for U.S. males and females (1975–2019). Mortality data were provided by the U.S. National Center for Health Statistics, Centers for Disease Control and Prevention. *APC* annual percent change. https://seer.cancer.gov/explorer/cancer-sites.html

or stable employment, adequate paid sick leave, or insurance coverage, and may simultaneously bear significant family and caregiving responsibilities [23]. In a study of female adolescent and young adult cancer survivors (including thyroid cancer survivors), employment disruption related to cancer diagnosis and treatment was associated with a 17% increased prevalence of financial hardship and an 8% increased prevalence of psychological distress [24]; these associations were more pronounced among women who were younger at diagnosis, Hispanic, and/or care-givers. For all these reasons, thyroid cancer survivors have been shown to have a reduced quality of life, even compared to other cancer survivors [25, 26], and these hardships are associated with younger age, female sex, lower socioeconomic status, minority race/ethnicity, and lower acculturation [27]. Thyroid cancer also has a major societal cost; in 2013, alone, thyroid cancer care was associated with $1.6 billion in the United States [28].

In response to the growing awareness of the many problems associated with overdiagnosis and overtreatment of thyroid cancer, since 2009, the American Thyroid Association (ATA) guidelines for the management of differentiated thyroid cancer have increasingly supported a more risk stratified and less intensive approach to diagnosis and treatment [29–31]. The recommendations now discourage fine-needle aspiration biopsy of most small nodules to avoid identification, diagnosis, and treatment of very low-risk papillary thyroid cancers. Also, there is a higher stage threshold for the use of radioactive iodine and support of lower administered activities (down to 30 mCi). The guidelines also now support less extensive surgery (lobectomy rather than total thyroidectomy) for small, low-risk cancers. For some very low-risk (sub-centimeter) papillary thyroid cancers, active surveillance was raised as a potentially viable option for the first time in the 2015 guidelines [30]. Likewise, in 2017, the U.S. Preventive Services Task Force gave a D recommenda-tion for screening thyroid cancer in asymptomatic individuals [32], although there remains support for thyroid cancer screening in symptomatic and high-risk groups [22]. Similar recommendations against thyroid cancer screening in healthy indi-viduals were published in 2015 by the Korean National Cancer Screening Guidelines Committee [33].

Another recent development was the 2017 recommendation by the ATA to reclas-sify the noninvasive encapsulated follicular variant of papillary thyroid cancer (non-invasive EFVPTC) from a "cancer" to an in situ "neoplasm," using the term noninvasive follicular neoplasm with papillary-like nuclear features (NIFTP) [34]. This recommendation followed evidence of highly indolent tumor behavior and a very low prevalence of adverse outcomes in these patients [35]. In addition, these tumors tend to harbor *RAS* and other mutations that are more typical of follicular adenomas, follicular thyroid carcinomas, and EVPTCs rather than classical papil-lary thyroid cancers, which are more likely to harbor *BRAF* [35]. The purpose of reclassifying these tumors as something other than "cancer" is to reduce anxiety and stigma around the diagnosis and to facilitate deescalated management (less surgery and radioactive iodine). If fully adopted by the clinical community, this nomencla-ture change is estimated to reduce the incidence of papillary thyroid cancer by about 20% [35]. By 2017, there was already evidence of a small rise in the incidence of

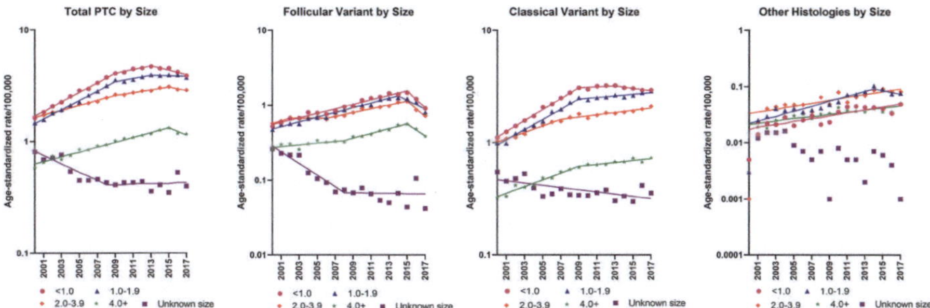

Fig. 1.4 Trends in age-adjusted incidence rates (cases per 100,000 annually) for total papillary thyroid carcinoma (PTC) and PTC subtypes, including follicular variant of PTC, classical PTC, and all other PTC variants, by tumor size at diagnosis. Figures were reproduced from Kitahara CM, et al. *J Clin Endocrinol Metab* 2020 [36]

NIFTP and a decline in incidence of FVPTCs (Fig. 1.4) from U.S. cancer registry data, likely reflecting implementation of the new thyroid cancer coding guidelines [36].

Although there is near universal agreement that overdiagnosis has been a major contributor to thyroid cancer incidence patterns worldwide and over time, the possibility has been raised of a small but real increase in thyroid cancer, resulting from increased prevalence or exposure to environmental, lifestyle-related, or hormonal risk factors. First, closer examinations of trends in papillary thyroid cancer incidence in the United States and elsewhere since the 1970s and 1980s have shown increases in tumors of all stages and sizes at diagnosis, including the larger and more advanced tumors which fall outside of the category of "overdiagnosis" [11, 37, 38]. Recent U.S. data showing a plateau (2009–2013) and subsequent downturn (after 2013) in thyroid cancer incidence have been driven by small (<1 cm) classical-type papillary thyroid cancers, which is consistent with ATA recommendations for higher tumor size thresholds for fine-needle aspiration biopsy; however, the incidence of larger classical-type papillary thyroid cancers has continued to increase at a steady pace (Fig. 1.4) [36]. Larger tumors and those that have progressed outside the thyroid gland are considered clinically significant, and require more extensive treatment (e.g., total thyroidectomy, often followed by radioactive iodine ablation or therapy) [30]. Moreover, thyroid cancer mortality has increased by about 1% per year in the United States since the mid-1980s, with a more pronounced increase in men than women (Fig. 1.3) and white individuals than other race/ethnicity groups [2]. The rise in thyroid cancer mortality has been shown to be restricted to patients initially diagnosed with papillary thyroid cancer, especially metastatic disease [11]. Slight increases in thyroid cancer mortality also have been observed in Australia and Canada since the 1990s [13].

Until recently, childhood exposure to ionizing radiation was considered the only established modifiable risk factor for thyroid cancer [39]. In the early 1980s, natural background radiation (e.g., radon) was the primary source of ionizing radiation exposure to the US general population [15]. However, by the mid-2000s, diagnostic radiological imaging contributed a nearly equal amount of effective dose, per capita, as natural background radiation [15]. Between the early-1980s and mid-2000s, the per capita effective dose to the U.S. general population nearly doubled (3.6–6.2 mSv), primarily due to a substantial increase in performance of computed tomography scans, nuclear medicine, and interventional fluoroscopy procedures, which yield much higher per-procedure doses than general radiological procedures. On the other hand, patients undergoing these imaging procedures are middle-aged or older adults, at ages when individuals are much less susceptible to the carcinogenic effects of radiation on the thyroid gland [39]. While increased performance of childhood computed tomography scans to the head and neck region could have contributed to overall increases in thyroid cancer incidence [40], the population attributable risk (proportion of new thyroid cancers diagnosed each year attributable to that exposure) is expected to be very low, considering the narrow range of susceptible ages at exposure and the modest association between low-dose radiation exposure and subsequent thyroid cancer. Higher exposures (e.g., from radiotherapy), especially in childhood, are uncommon and unlikely to have had any observable effect on population-level trends in thyroid cancer incidence.

Obesity is a direct cause of numerous chronic health conditions, including multiple cancers, and it has recently emerged as a plausible risk factor for thyroid cancer. The prevalence of overweight and obesity has increased dramatically over time across much of the world, including in the United States [41]. Data from large observational studies have also shown an association between higher body mass index (BMI) and risk of thyroid cancer. A pooled analysis of data from 22 prospective studies, totaling more than two million men and women across four continents, showed that BMI, waist circumference, and adulthood BMI gain were each positively associated with thyroid cancer incidence (except medullary thyroid cancer) and thyroid cancer mortality [42]. Other epidemiologic studies have similarly observed stronger associations of obesity with risk of papillary thyroid cancers having more aggressive features, including *BRAF^{V600E}* mutation [43]. In a U.S.-based study, it was estimated that about 15% of all papillary thyroid cancers, including about 60% of large (>4 cm) tumors, are attributable to overweight and obesity [44]. Postulated biological mechanisms include a more direct role of insulin resistance, inflammation, estrogen, and thyroid-stimulating hormone in thyroid cancer cell proliferation and disease promotion [45]. Altogether, these results suggest that maintaining a healthy weight may help to prevent the occurrence or progression of papillary thyroid cancer.

Many other environmental, hormonal, and lifestyle-related exposures have been postulated to contribute to thyroid cancer development, but very few have been evaluated across multiple well-controlled observational studies. A relatively large number of studies have been conducted on reproductive and hormonal factors, such as parity, age at menarche and menopause, ages at first and last birth, and use of exogenous hormones, in relation to thyroid cancer in women, but results have been mixed [46]. A small number of studies have shown positive associations for hysterectomy, recent childbirth, infertility medications, greater birth weight, and an inverse association for breastfeeding, although it is not clear whether these factors are simply indicators for medical surveillance (and thus incidental thyroid cancer detection) [46]. Separating true risk factors from indicators of more intense medical surveillance is a major challenge in thyroid cancer epidemiologic studies.

Interestingly, current cigarette smoking has been consistently inversely associated with thyroid cancer risk in case-control and prospective studies. While smoking may be associated with less healthy behaviors, including lower likelihood of thyroid cancer screening or other general health check-ups, these studies have shown evidence of dose response, whereby greater cumulative exposure to cigarette smoke is associated incrementally with thyroid cancer risk. Current smoking has also been more clearly associated with papillary thyroid cancers harboring the more aggressive $BRAF^{V600E}$ mutation compared to those without that mutation [47]. Cigarette smoking has been inversely associated with circulating thyroid-stimulating hormone [48], which may inhibit thyroid cancer cell growth and differentiation. Although no serious public health measures would be recommended based on these findings, they provide some clues about biological mechanisms that may contribute to the development and progression of thyroid cancer and may lead to the identification of other modifiable risk factors that could become the targets of public health interventions.

Conclusion

Overdiagnosis has been the predominant factor contributing to rising thyroid cancer incidence worldwide, and this is a problem that has extended to resource-limited countries, including China and India. Over the past 10–15 years, there has been increased effort to raise awareness of the problems associated with thyroid cancer overdiagnosis, and clinical practice recommendations have been modified to further reduce the potential for unnecessary diagnosis and treatment of patients with low-risk disease. However, there is still tremendous progress to be made to further reduce the occurrence of overdiagnosis and overtreatment.

References

1. Ferlay JEM, Lam F, Colombet M, Mery L, Piñeros M, Znaor A, Soerjomataram I, Bray F. Global cancer observatory: cancer today Lyon. France: International Agency for Research on Cancer; 2020. [Available from: https://gco.iarc.fr/today]
2. SEER*Explorer: An interactive website for SEER cancer statistics [Internet] [Internet]. Surveillance Research Program, National Cancer Institute. 2021 [cited November 10, 2021]. Available from: https://seer.cancer.gov/explorer/.
3. Vaccarella S, Lortet-Tieulent J, Colombet M, Davies L, Stiller CA, Schuz J, et al. Global patterns and trends in incidence and mortality of thyroid cancer in children and adolescents: a population-based study. Lancet Diabetes Endocrinol. 2021;9(3):144–52.

4. Kilfoy BA, Zheng T, Holford TR, Han X, Ward MH, Sjodin A, et al. International patterns and trends in thyroid cancer incidence, 1973-2002. Cancer Causes Control. 2009;20(5):525–31.

5. Vaccarella S, Franceschi S, Bray F, Wild CP, Plummer M, Dal Maso L. Worldwide thyroid-cancer epidemic? The increasing impact of overdiagnosis. N Engl J Med. 2016;375(7):614–7.

6. Li M, Dal Maso L, Vaccarella S. Global trends in thyroid cancer incidence and the impact of overdiagnosis. Lancet Diabetes Endocrinol. 2020;8(6):468–70.

7. Panato C, Vaccarella S, Dal Maso L, Basu P, Franceschi S, Serraino D, et al. Thyroid cancer incidence in India between 2006 and 2014 and impact of overdiagnosis. J Clin Endocrinol Metab. 2020;105:8.

8. Davies L, Welch HG. Increasing incidence of thyroid cancer in the United States, 1973–2002. JAMA. 2006;295(18):2164–7.

9. Miranda-Filho A, Lortet-Tieulent J, Bray F, Cao B, Franceschi S, Vaccarella S, et al. Thyroid cancer incidence trends by histology in 25 countries: a population-based study. Lancet Diabetes Endocrinol. 2021;9(4):225–34.

10. Ahn HS, Kim HJ, Welch HG. Korea's thyroid-cancer "epidemic"—screening and overdiagnosis. N Engl J Med. 2014;371(19):1765–7.

11. Lim H, Devesa SS, Sosa JA, Check D, Kitahara CM. Trends in thyroid cancer incidence and mortality in the United States, 1974-2013. JAMA. 2017;317(13):1338–48.

12. Ahn HS, Kim HJ, Kim KH, Lee YS, Han SJ, Kim Y, et al. Thyroid cancer screening in South Korea increases detection of papillary cancers with no impact on other subtypes or thyroid cancer mortality. Thyroid. 2016;26(11):1535–40.

13. Li M, Brito JP, Vaccarella S. Long-term declines of thyroid cancer mortality: an international age-period-cohort analysis. Thyroid. 2020;30(6):838–46.

14. Sosa JA, Hanna JW, Robinson KA, Lanman RB. Increases in thyroid nodule fine-needle aspirations, operations, and diagnoses of thyroid cancer in the United States. Surgery. 2013;154(6):1420–6. discussion 6-7

15. NCRP. Ionizing radiation exposure of the population of the United States. Bethesda, MD; 2009.

16. Guth S, Theune U, Aberle J, Galach A, Bamberger CM. Very high prevalence of thyroid nodules detected by high frequency (13 MHz) ultrasound examination. Eur J Clin Investig. 2009;39(8):699–706.

17. Uppal A, White MG, Nagar S, Aschebrook-Kilfoy B, Chang PJ, Angelos P, et al. Benign and malignant thyroid incidentalomas are rare in routine clinical practice: a review of 97,908 imaging studies. Cancer Epidemiol Biomark Prev. 2015;24(9):1327–31.

18. Park SH, Lee B, Lee S, Choi E, Choi EB, Yoo J, et al. A qualitative study of women's views on overdiagnosis and screening for thyroid cancer in Korea. BMC Cancer. 2015;15:858.

19. Oh CM, Lim J, Jung YS, Kim Y, Jung KW, Hong S, et al. Decreasing trends in thyroid cancer incidence in South Korea: what happened in South Korea? Cancer Med. 2021;10(12):4087–96.

20. Lee M, Powers AE, Morris LGT, Marti JL. Reversal in thyroid cancer incidence trends in the United States, 2000-2017. Thyroid. 2020;30(8):1226–7.

21. LeClair K, Bell KJL, Furuya-Kanamori L, Doi SA, Francis DO, Davies L. Evaluation of gender inequity in thyroid cancer diagnosis: differences by sex in US thyroid cancer incidence compared with a meta-analysis of subclinical thyroid cancer rates at autopsy. JAMA Intern Med. 2021;181(10):1351–8.

22. Lamartina L, Grani G, Durante C, Filetti S, Cooper DS. Screening for differentiated thyroid cancer in selected populations. Lancet Diabetes Endocrinol. 2020;8(1):81–8.

23. Mongelli MN, Giri S, Peipert BJ, Helenowski IB, Yount SE, Sturgeon C. Financial burden and quality of life among thyroid cancer survivors. Surgery. 2020;167(3):631–7.

24. Meernik C, Kirchhoff AC, Anderson C, Edwards TP, Deal AM, Baggett CD, et al. Material and psychological financial hardship related to employment disruption among female adolescent and young adult cancer survivors. Cancer. 2020;127(1):137–48.

25. Applewhite MK, James BC, Kaplan SP, Angelos P, Kaplan EL, Grogan RH, et al. Quality of life in thyroid cancer is similar to that of other cancers with worse survival. World J Surg. 2016;40(3):551–61.

26. Goldfarb M, Casillas J. Thyroid cancer-specific quality of life and health-related quality of life in young adult thyroid cancer survivors. Thyroid. 2016;26(7):923–32.
27. Chen DW, Reyes-Gastelum D, Veenstra CM, Hamilton AS, Banerjee M, Haymart MR. Financial hardship among Hispanic women with thyroid cancer. Thyroid. 2021;31(5):752–9.
28. Lubitz CC, Kong CY, McMahon PM, Daniels GH, Chen Y, Economopoulos KP, et al. Annual financial impact of well-differentiated thyroid cancer care in the United States. Cancer. 2014;120(9):1345–52.
29. American Thyroid Association Guidelines Taskforce on Thyroid N, Differentiated Thyroid C, Cooper DS, Doherty GM, Haugen BR, Kloos RT, et al. Revised American Thyroid Association management guidelines for patients with thyroid nodules and differentiated thyroid cancer. Thyroid. 2009;19(11):1167–214.
30. Haugen BR, Alexander EK, Bible KC, Doherty GM, Mandel SJ, Nikiforov YE, et al. 2015 American Thyroid Association management guidelines for adult patients with thyroid nodules and differentiated thyroid cancer: the American Thyroid Association guidelines task Force on thyroid nodules and differentiated thyroid cancer. Thyroid. 2016;26(1):1–133.
31. Haugen BR. 2015 American Thyroid Association management guidelines for adult patients with thyroid nodules and differentiated thyroid cancer: what is new and what has changed? Cancer. 2017;123(3):372–81.
32. Force USPST, Bibbins-Domingo K, Grossman DC, Curry SJ, Barry MJ, Davidson KW, et al. Screening for thyroid cancer: US Preventive Services Task Force recommendation statement. JAMA. 2017;317(18):1882–7.
33. Ahn HS, Welch HG. South Korea's thyroid-cancer "epidemic"—turning the tide. N Engl J Med. 2015;373(24):2389–90.
34. Haugen BR, Sawka AM, Alexander EK, Bible KC, Caturegli P, Doherty GM, et al. American Thyroid Association Guidelines on the Management of Thyroid Nodules and Differentiated Thyroid Cancer Task Force Review and recommendation on the proposed renaming of encapsulated follicular variant papillary thyroid carcinoma without invasion to noninvasive follicular thyroid neoplasm with papillary-like nuclear features. Thyroid. 2017;27(4):481–3.
35. Nikiforov YE, Seethala RR, Tallini G, Baloch ZW, Basolo F, Thompson LD, et al. Nomenclature revision for encapsulated follicular variant of papillary thyroid carcinoma: a paradigm shift to reduce overtreatment of indolent tumors. JAMA Oncol. 2016;2(8):1023–9.
36. Kitahara CM, Sosa JA, Shiels MS. Influence of nomenclature changes on trends in papillary thyroid cancer incidence in the United States, 2000 to 2017. J Clin Endocrinol Metab. 2020;105:12.
37. Enewold L, Zhu K, Ron E, Marrogi AJ, Stojadinovic A, Peoples GE, et al. Rising thyroid cancer incidence in the United States by demographic and tumor characteristics, 1980-2005. Cancer Epidemiol Biomark Prev. 2009;18(3):784–91.
38. Pandeya N, McLeod DS, Balasubramaniam K, Baade PD, Youl PH, Bain CJ, et al. Increasing thyroid cancer incidence in Queensland, Australia 1982-2008 - true increase or overdiagnosis? Clin Endocrinol. 2016;84(2):257–64.
39. Ron E, Lubin JH, Shore RE, Mabuchi K, Modan B, Pottern LM, et al. Thyroid cancer after exposure to external radiation: a pooled analysis of seven studies. Radiat Res. 1995;141(3):259–77.
40. Schonfeld SJ, Lee C, Berrington de Gonzalez A. Medical exposure to radiation and thyroid cancer. Clin Oncol (R Coll Radiol). 2011;23(4):244–50.
41. Hales CM, Carroll MD, Fryar CD, Ogden CL. Prevalence of obesity and severe obesity among adults: United States, 2017–2018. Hyattsville, MD; 2020.
42. Kitahara CM, McCullough ML, Franceschi S, Rinaldi S, Wolk A, Neta G, et al. Anthropometric factors and thyroid cancer risk by histological subtype: pooled analysis of 22 prospective studies. Thyroid. 2016;26(2):306–18.
43. Rahman ST, Pandeya N, Neale RE, McLeod DSA, Bain CJ, Baade PD, et al. Obesity is associated with BRAF(V600E)-mutated thyroid cancer. Thyroid. 2020;30(10):1518–27.
44. Kitahara CM, Pfeiffer RM, Sosa JA, Shiels MS. Impact of overweight and obesity on US papillary thyroid cancer incidence trends (1995-2015). J Natl Cancer Inst. 2020;112(8):810–7.

45. Pazaitou-Panayiotou K, Polyzos SA, Mantzoros CS. Obesity and thyroid cancer: epidemiologic associations and underlying mechanisms. Obes Rev. 2013;14(12):1006–22.
46. Troisi R, Bjorge T, Gissler M, Grotmol T, Kitahara CM, Myrtveit Saether SM, et al. The role of pregnancy, perinatal factors and hormones in maternal cancer risk: a review of the evidence. J Intern Med. 2018;283(5):430–45.
47. Rahman ST, Pandeya N, Neale RE, McLeod DSA, Baade PD, Youl PH, et al. Tobacco smoking and risk of thyroid cancer according to BRAF(V600E) mutational subtypes. Clin Endocrinol. 2021.
48. Belin RM, Astor BC, Powe NR, Ladenson PW. Smoke exposure is associated with a lower prevalence of serum thyroid autoantibodies and thyrotropin concentration elevation and a higher prevalence of mild thyrotropin concentration suppression in the third National Health and nutrition examination survey (NHANES III). J Clin Endocrinol Metab. 2004;89(12):6077–86.

Chapter 2
Criteria for Fine Needle Aspiration Biopsy in Thyroid Nodules

Priya H. Dedhia and Jennifer A. Sipos

Case A 30-year-old man presents for a routine physical exam and is found to have an enlarged thyroid. His past medical history is significant for astrocytoma, for which he underwent radiation to the head at the age of 10 years. His family history is significant for papillary thyroid cancer in his mother. Thyroid function tests are normal.

Thyroid ultrasound demonstrates an enlarged thyroid and a solitary 1.3 cm right thyroid nodule. The nodule is solid, hypoechoic, well-circumscribed, and wider than tall. The nodule does not have echogenic foci. The Thyroid Imaging, Reporting and Data System (TIRADS) score is 4 and ATA intermediate risk (Fig. 2.1).

Ultrasound Features and Size as Predictors of Malignancy

Ultrasound of the neck is an ideal tool for the evaluation of patients with thyroid nodules. In the hands of a skilled sonographer, ultrasound is an inexpensive, low-risk imaging modality that is highly sensitive and specific in identifying nodules and stratifying their risk of malignancy. Ultrasound of the neck should be performed in all patients suspected of having a thyroid nodule, not only to confirm the presence of a nodule but also to inform the decision to perform FNAB [1].

Thyroid nodules can be seen in up to 68% of ultrasound examinations [2, 3]. Clinical detection of nodules on physical examination, however, is far less sensitive, with only 5% of patients having a palpable nodule [4]. This large reservoir of disease detected on imaging necessitates an efficient triaging system because only 4–6.5% of all thyroid nodules harbor malignancy [5, 6].

P. H. Dedhia
Department of Surgery, The Ohio State University Wexner Medical Center and Arthur G. James Cancer Center, Columbus, OH, USA
e-mail: Priya.Dedhia@osumc.edu

J. A. Sipos (✉)
Department of Internal Medicine, The Ohio State University Wexner Medical Center and Arthur G. James Cancer Center, Columbus, OH, USA
e-mail: Jennifer.Sipos@osumc.edu

© The Author(s), under exclusive license to Springer Nature Switzerland AG 2023
S. A. Roman et al. (eds.), *Controversies in Thyroid Nodules and Differentiated Thyroid Cancer*, https://doi.org/10.1007/978-3-031-37135-6_2

Fig. 2.1 Thyroid ultrasound demonstrating 1.3 cm right thyroid nodule is solid, hypoechoic, well-circumscribed, wider than tall, and without echogenic foci (TIRADS 4)

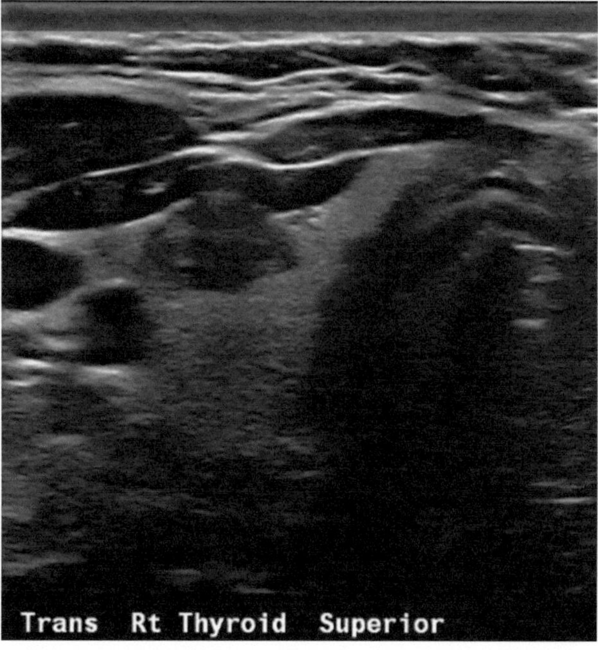

Although certain sonographic features including hypoechogenicity, taller-than-wide shape, irregular/infiltrative margins, or microcalcifications (also called punctate echogenic foci) are associated with an increased risk of malignancy, their absence does not rule out the possibility of thyroid cancer. On the other hand, other sonographic features such as predominantly cystic composition, isoechogenicity (similar echotexture to the surrounding thyroid parenchyma), or a spongiform appearance (greater than 50% of the nodule is composed of microcystic spaces) may provide reassurance that the nodule is benign.

Historically, risk of malignancy was thought to be unrelated to nodule size [7]. However, a large, more recent analysis including over 20,000 nodules revealed that increasing nodule diameter was positively correlated with risk of malignancy [8]. This discrepancy is likely due to the evolution of FNAB thresholds over time as well as earlier studies being underpowered to detect a difference in size-related malignancy risk [9]. Ultimately, this recent analysis revealed a 10–30% increase in malignancy risk for each incremental 1 cm increase in maximal nodule diameter over 1.9 cm compared to nodules measuring 1–1.9 cm [8]. These findings highlight the importance of cytologic evaluation of larger nodules.

Assessment of Sonographic Risk Stratification Systems

As outlined above, individual ultrasound features alone are insufficiently sensitive and specific to reliably predict malignancy risk in the majority of nodules. Consequently, various sonographic risk stratification systems (SRSSs) have been created to further refine the malignancy risk of thyroid nodules. The three main systems currently in use include the American Thyroid Association (ATA) SRSS [1], the American College of Radiology Thyroid Imaging Reporting and Data System (ACR-TIRADS) [10], and the Korean TIRADS (K-TIRADS) [11]. Using differing methodology, each of these SRSSs classify nodules into one of 4 or 5 categories with a corresponding malignancy risk. As the likelihood of cancer increases with each tier, the size threshold for FNA decreases (Table 2.1).

The ATA SRSS utilizes a pattern-based approach to classify nodules into one of five risk categories. In this SRSS, pattern recognition was utilized over individual features for stratification of nodules because the latter has been associated with high interobserver variability in reporting certain sonographic findings [12]. Indeed, pattern-based classification of nodules is more robust in terms of reproducibility of nodule classification among readers of differing skill levels [13–16]. Once familiarized with the varying patterns, the ATA system provides a rapid method for classification of nodules and is associated with a high sensitivity for detection of malignancy [15–17].

ATA high-suspicion nodules are hypoechoic and solid (or partially cystic with a hypoechoic solid component) with one or more high-risk ultrasound features. High-risk features in this system include microcalcifications, taller-than-wide shape, evidence of extrathyroidal extension (ETE), irregular margins, or a disrupted rim calcification with an extrusive hypoechoic soft tissue component. This pattern of

Table 2.1 Comparison of sonographic risk stratification systems by malignancy rate and size threshold for fine needle aspiration biopsy

Sonographic risk stratification systems	Category				
ATA	Benign	Very low suspicion	Low suspicion	Intermediate suspicion	High suspicion
Malignancy rate	<1%	<3%	5–10%	10–20%	70–90%
Size threshold	Not indicated	Consider ≥2.0 cm	≥1.5 cm	≥1.0 cm	≥1.0 cm
ACR-TIRADS	TR1	TR2	TR3	TR4	TR5
Malignancy rate	0%	0%	<5%	5–80%	>80%
Size threshold	Not indicated	Not indicated	≥2.5 cm	≥1.5 cm	≥1.0 cm
K-TIRADS	1	2	3	4	5
Malignancy rate	Not applicable	0%	7.8%	25.4%	79.3%
Size threshold	Not indicated	≥2.0 cm	≥1.5 cm	≥1.0 cm	≥1.0 cm

nodules is highly concerning for the presence of papillary thyroid carcinoma (PTC). The threshold for FNAB of ATA high-suspicion nodules is 1 cm.

Intermediate suspicion nodules are hypoechoic and solid but lack suspicious ultrasound features. This pattern has the highest sensitivity for detecting malignancy, but lacks specificity, as only 10–20% are malignant. The FNAB threshold for this class of nodules is 1 cm.

The ATA low-suspicion category is defined as isoechoic/hyperechoic and solid nodules or partially cystic nodules with an eccentric solid components that lack suspicious features. The risk of malignancy in this group of nodules is 5–10% and FNAB is recommended at a size threshold of 1.5 cm.

Very low-suspicion nodules are spongiform or largely cystic nodules that lack any suspicious ultrasound features. These lesions may be observed or considered for FNAB when larger than 2 cm as their risk of malignancy is less than 3%.

Simple cysts are classified as benign lesions with the ATA SRSS. As such, FNAB is not indicated for diagnostic purposes. If symptomatic, these lesions may be therapeutically aspirated to alleviate compressive symptoms.

An important limitation of the ATA SRSS is that up to 18% of nodules, especially isoechoic ones with one or more high-risk features, are non-classifiable [18]. The risk of malignancy in these non-classifiable nodules is unclear and variably reported, but is likely similar to intermediate—suspicion nodules at 20% [19–22].

The ACR-TIRADS created five classes of nodules using a point-based system. Each nodule is given a score for five sonographic features including composition, echogenicity, shape, margins, and echogenic foci. The sum of each of these scores is tallied which derives the risk class of the nodule. A size threshold is then recommended based on this TIRADS score (Table 2.2).

The main limitation of the ACR-TIRADS is the need to memorize the scores associated with each of the sonographic features. Additionally, the process of

Table 2.2 American College of Radiology TIRADS SRSS

Sonographic features with associated points									
Composition		**Echogenicity**		**Shape**		**Margin**		**Echogenic foci**	
Cystic	0	Anechoic	0	Wider than tall	0	Smooth	0	None	0
Spongiform	0	Hyper/ isoechoic	1	Taller than wide	3	Ill-defined	0	Comet-tails	0
Mixed	1	Hypoechoic	2			Lobulated/ irregular	2	Macrocalcifications	1
Solid	2	Very hypoechoic	3			ETE	3	Peripheral/rim	2
								Punctate	3

Points	0 points	2 points	3 points	4–6 points	≥ 7 points
Score	TR1	TR2	TR3	TR4	TR5
Descriptor	Benign	Not suspicious	Mildly suspicious	Moderately suspicious	Highly suspicious
FNAB	Not indicated	Not indicated	≥ 2.5 cm	≥ 1.5 cm	≥ 1.0 cm

tabulating a score for each nodule, particularly in a multinodular goiter, can be time consuming.

K-TIRADS stratifies nodules into one of four risk categories. This SRSS assesses nodule composition, echogenicity, and the presence of suspicious ultrasound features to assign malignancy risk. K-TIRADS 1 indicates no nodule. K-TIRADS 2, the lowest risk category of nodules, includes pure cysts or spongiform nodules. A mixed composition (with cystic and solid components) and isoechoic nodule without suspicious ultrasound features is represented by K-TIRADS 3, whereas a similar nodule with suspicious ultrasound features is represented by K-TIRADS 4. A solid, hypoechoic nodule with suspicious ultrasound features is categorized by K-TIRADS 5.

Although there are advantages and disadvantages to each SRSS, in general, their integration into clinical practice has reduced unnecessary FNAB and subsequent surgery [23]. Many studies have compared the performance of these SRSSs for their ability to distinguish benign and malignant nodules. The ATA and K-TIRADS systems have a high sensitivity for detecting malignancy but suffer from lower specificity. In contrast, the ACR-TIRADS has a higher specificity but lower sensitivity than ATA and K-TIRADS [23].

Generally, all three major SRSSs classify nodules similarly—the concordance rates for classifying nodules as intermediate or high suspicion with each system was very high [24]. Furthermore, when nodules were classified by ATA or K-TIRADS, but ACR-TIRADS biopsy criteria were applied, sensitivity and specificity more closely resembled that of ACR-TIRADS. The reverse was also true such that nodules classified by ACR-TIRADS but biopsied based on ATA or K-TIRADS criteria demonstrated sensitivity and specificity similar to the latter two SRSSs. The authors of this study concluded that the differences in the diagnostic performance between these three SRSS are mostly influenced by the size thresholds used to recommend FNAB [24].

Significance of Clinical History—Risk Factors, Pregnancy, and Comorbidities

Clinical history in conjunction with ultrasound findings plays an important role in the decision to perform FNAB. Risk factors predicting malignancy, such as history of radiation, family history of thyroid cancer syndrome, rapid nodule growth or immobility, hoarseness or vocal cord paralysis, or cervical lymphadenopathy must be assessed in patients presenting with thyroid nodules (Table 2.2). Patients with a higher pretest probability of thyroid cancer can be considered for FNAB at lower size cutoffs [1].

Patient age predicts thyroid nodule malignancy risk. Younger patients have a higher risk of malignancy. This risk decreases by 2.2% per year between the ages of 20–60 years and plateaus thereafter [25]. Older patients with thyroid nodules may

Table 2.3 Risk factors for thyroid cancer

Risk factors for thyroid cancer in a patient with thyroid nodule(s)
History of radiation (childhood cranial or whole body, environmental)
Family history of thyroid cancer syndrome (syndrome or ≥ 3 first deg. relatives with PTC)
Rapid nodule growth or fixation on physical examination
Hoarseness/vocal cord paralysis
Cervical lymphadenopathy
Young age (<16 years)
Male sex

have a lower risk of malignancy than younger patients, but are at increased risk for aggressive thyroid cancers, including high-risk pathologic variants, poorly differentiated cancers, or anaplastic thyroid cancers, as well as thyroid cancer-related mortality (Table 2.3) [25–27].

While FNAB is a relatively safe procedure, the potential need for surgical management, especially in the presence of comorbidities, should be considered carefully [28]. In a study of 1129 patients aged 70 years and older who underwent FNAB, only 1.5% of patients were found to have high-risk thyroid cancer, which was easily identifiable on ultrasound or FNAB [27]. Survival analysis demonstrated that thyroid cancer-related deaths occurred in only 0.9% of patients and were limited to patients with high-risk thyroid cancer. During 4 years of follow-up, 14% of patients died due to non-thyroid causes. Those patients with coronary disease or a non-thyroidal malignancy at the time of nodule evaluation had a more than a two-fold increased risk of death. The authors concluded that in patients aged above 70 years, the surgical management of thyroid cancer without high-risk features should be tempered, particularly in the setting of comorbid illness. Similarly, the ATA guidelines indicate that a conservative approach to thyroid nodules is appropriate in patients with high surgical risk and those with a short life expectancy [1]. Therefore, shared decision-making between patients and clinicians incorporating comorbidities and goals of care as well as thyroid cancer biology is essential when managing older adults with thyroid nodules.

In general, the evaluation of thyroid nodules discovered during pregnancy should be similar to the non-pregnant patient with measurement of serum TSH and ultrasonography [1]. In addition, FNAB can be performed safely during pregnancy. Because the majority of thyroid cancers are associated with an indolent growth pattern, surgery for most malignancies that are identified during pregnancy may be safely delayed until the postpartum period [1, 29]. For rare tumors with a more aggressive clinical course or more extensive tumor burden that might necessitate removal during pregnancy, the optimal time for surgical resection is during the second trimester.

Incidentally Discovered Thyroid Nodules

Thyroid nodules are incidentally identified on computed tomography (CT) and magnetic resonance imaging (MRI) in up to 16% of patients without known history of thyroid nodules [30, 31]. The malignancy rate of thyroid nodules identified on CT is 3.9–11.3% [32]. Because of the limited utility of imaging characteristics in predicting malignancy [31–33], thyroid nodules incidentally discovered on CT or MRI should be evaluated by ultrasonography to determine the need for subsequent FNAB [1].

Incidental thyroid nodules are prevalent in up to 2.3% of 18-fluorodeoxyglucose positron emission tomography (PET) and 11% of gallium-68 Dotatate (DOTA) studies [34–36]. Focal uptake is associated with malignancy in up to 34.8% of patients on PET and 21% of DOTA studies [36–38]. Because of the increased malignancy risk with focal uptake on PET or DOTA, further evaluation with ultrasonography is indicated, and FNAB can be considered for all nodules ≥1 cm, if warranted by the clinical scenario that precipitated the imaging [1].

In the setting of diffuse uptake, FNAB may be performed according to usual SSRSs, if nodules are present. In the absence of clearly defined nodules, thyroid function testing and/or antibody testing may be helpful to assess for Hashimoto's disease or other causes of diffuse thyroid disorders.

Strengths and Limitations of Fine Needle Aspiration Biopsy

Fine needle aspiration biopsy (FNAB) is the "gold standard" to identify malignancy preoperatively and can be safely and easily performed in the clinic. Furthermore, FNAB provides rapid feedback on the nature of the lesions with acceptable reproducibility [39]. The decision to perform FNAB is directed by the risk of malignancy, which necessitates evaluation of clinical history, patient demographics, nodule size, and ultrasound features.

In addition to the deliberation of malignancy risk, the potential limitations of FNAB should be considered in the decision to obtain a cytologic diagnosis. The overall accuracy of FNAB is greater than 95%; however, the risk of false diagnoses or non-diagnostic results also must be considered.

False diagnoses may be due to sampling error or cytologic misclassification. The false negative rate of FNAB, which refers to benign FNAB cytology that is later diagnosed as a malignant lesion on surgical pathology, ranges from 1.5% to 11.5% [40, 41]. Several studies have revealed that nodules with a sonographically suspicious appearance are more likely to harbor a missed malignancy compared to those nodules with a lower risk pattern, even in the setting of low-risk nodule growth on post-FNA surveillance [42, 43]. Consequently, several guidelines advocate for a repeat FNA within 6–12 months for a cytologically benign nodule with a high-risk sonographic features (ATA 2016, K-TIRADS). Larger nodule size also poses a theoretical risk for false-negative FNAB results due to sampling error; however, data to this effect are controversial. Some studies confirmed increased risk of sampling error with nodules over 3 cm in diameter, but others suggested FNAB results remained sensitive even with larger nodules [44–47]. On the other end of the size spectrum, nodules smaller than 5 mm can be challenging to biopsy and also can result in increased rates of non-diagnostic or false-negative results. Additionally, increasing cystic content in a nodule can be associated with higher non-diagnostic rates as well as cytologic misclassification [48]. Finally, the likelihood of non-diagnostic cytology is inversely related to the experience level of the person performing the FNAB [49–51]. In the context of these limitations of FNAB, caution should be exercised in recommending FNAB of nodules with a low pretest probability of malignancy.

Thyroid Nodule Management—Multiple Nodules and Surveillance

Multiple factors must be considered in the management of thyroid nodules, and special regard should be given to multiple nodules or nodule growth during surveillance. Although malignancy is more likely to be identified in patients with a single nodule, the incidence of thyroid cancer in patients with multiple nodules is the same as in patients with a solitary nodule [7]. Thus, in a patient with multinodular goiter, all nodules with suspicious features should be biopsied. If no nodules have suspicious features, then FNAB of the largest nodule can be performed [52].

For nodules that do not meet criteria for FNAB or nodules with benign cytology on FNAB, surveillance ultrasound is necessary due to the small risk of unidentified malignancy. The timing of surveillance ultrasound is dictated by sonographic features of the nodule. For suspicious nodules, ultrasound can be repeated at 6 months; whereas for low to intermediate suspicion nodules or low-risk nodules, ultrasound can be repeated at 12 months or 24 months, respectively [53]. Nodules that increase more than 50% by volume or more than 20% in two dimensions should be reassessed by FNAB due to the low risk of malignancy [54–56].

Case Conclusion The patient underwent FNAB of the right thyroid nodule, which demonstrateds atypia of undetermined significance, oncocytic cell variant (formerly Hurthle cell). The patient then choose to undergo diagnostic right thyroid lobectomy. Pathology demonstrated nodular hyperplasia and oncocytic cell (formerly Hurthle cell) follicular microadenoma.

Concluding Remarks

Thyroid nodules are common and carry a 4–6.5% risk of malignancy. The initial evaluation after identification of a thyroid nodule includes history and physical exam, evaluation of thyroid function, and ultrasonography to determine the need for

FNAB. To minimize the burden of unnecessary procedures, the decision to perform FNAB should be made in the context of thyroid biology, such as ultrasound characteristics, and patient factors.

References

1. Haugen BR, Alexander EK, Bible KC, et al. 2015 American Thyroid Association Management guidelines for adult patients with thyroid nodules and differentiated thyroid cancer: the American Thyroid Association guidelines task force on thyroid nodules and differentiated thyroid cancer. Thyroid. 2016;26(1):1–133. https://doi.org/10.1089/thy.2015.0020.
2. Dean DS, Gharib H. Epidemiology of thyroid nodules. Best Pract Res Clin Endocrinol Metab. 2008;22(6):901–11. https://doi.org/10.1016/j.beem.2008.09.019.
3. Guth S, Theune U, Aberle J, Galach A, Bamberger CM. Very high prevalence of thyroid nodules detected by high frequency (13 MHz) ultrasound examination. Eur J Clin Investig. 2009;39(8):699–706. https://doi.org/10.1111/j.1365-2362.2009.02162.x.
4. Desforges JF, Mazzaferri EL. Management of a solitary thyroid nodule. N Engl J Med. 1993;328(8):553–9. https://doi.org/10.1056/NEJM199302253280807.
5. Hegedüs L. The thyroid nodule. N Engl J Med. 2004;351(17):1764–71. https://doi.org/10.1056/NEJMcp031436.
6. Lin J-D, Chao T-C, Huang B-Y, Chen S-T, Chang H-Y, Hsueh C. Thyroid cancer in the thyroid nodules evaluated by ultrasonography and fine-needle aspiration cytology. Thyroid. 2005;15(7):708–17. https://doi.org/10.1089/thy.2005.15.708.
7. Frates MC, Benson CB, Doubilet PM, et al. Prevalence and distribution of carcinoma in patients with solitary and multiple thyroid nodules on sonography. J Clin Endocrinol Metab. 2006;91(9):3411–7. https://doi.org/10.1210/jc.2006-0690.
8. Angell TE, Maurer R, Wang Z, et al. A cohort analysis of clinical and ultrasound variables predicting cancer risk in 20,001 consecutive thyroid nodules. J Clin Endocrinol Metab. 2019;104(11):5665–72. https://doi.org/10.1210/jc.2019-00664.
9. Sipos JA. The thyroid nodule conundrum: evaluate or leave it alone? J Clin Endocrinol Metab. 2020;105(3):e885–8. https://doi.org/10.1210/clinem/dgz124.
10. Tessler FN, Middleton WD, Grant EG, et al. ACR thyroid imaging, reporting and data system (TI-RADS): white paper of the ACR TI-RADS Committee. J Am Coll Radiol. 2017;14(5):587–95. https://doi.org/10.1016/j.jacr.2017.01.046.
11. Shin JH, Baek JH, Chung J, et al. Ultrasonography diagnosis and imaging-based management of thyroid nodules: revised Korean Society of Thyroid Radiology Consensus Statement and Recommendations. Korean J Radiol. 2016;17(3):370. https://doi.org/10.3348/kjr.2016.17.3.370.
12. Liu H, Ma A-L, Zhou Y-S, et al. Variability in the interpretation of grey-scale ultrasound features in assessing thyroid nodules: a systematic review and meta-analysis. Eur J Radiol. 2020;129:109050. https://doi.org/10.1016/j.ejrad.2020.109050.
13. Russ G, Royer B, Bigorgne C, Rouxel A, Bienvenu-Perrard M, Leenhardt L. Prospective evaluation of thyroid imaging reporting and data system on 4550 nodules with and without elastography. Eur J Endocrinol. 2013;168(5):649–55. https://doi.org/10.1530/EJE-12-0936.
14. Xu T, Gu J, Ye X, et al. Thyroid nodule sizes influence the diagnostic performance of TIRADS and ultrasound patterns of 2015 ATA guidelines: a multicenter retrospective study. Sci Rep. 2017;7(1):43183. https://doi.org/10.1038/srep43183.
15. Huang BL, Ebner SA, Makkar JS, et al. A multidisciplinary head-to-head comparison of American College of Radiology Thyroid Imaging and Reporting Data System and American Thyroid Association ultrasound risk stratification systems. Oncologist. 2020;25(5):398–403. https://doi.org/10.1634/theoncologist.2019-0362.

16. Kuru B, Kefeli M, Danaci M. Comparison of five thyroid ultrasound stratification systems for differentiation of benign and malignant nodules and to avoid biopsy using histology as reference standard. Endocr Pract. Published online April. 2021:S1530891X2100570X. https://doi.org/10.1016/j.eprac.2021.04.411.
17. Valderrabano P, McGettigan MJ, Lam CA, et al. Thyroid nodules with indeterminate cytology: utility of the American Thyroid Association sonographic patterns for cancer risk stratification. Thyroid. 2018;28(8):1004–12. https://doi.org/10.1089/thy.2018.0085.
18. Lauria Pantano A, Maddaloni E, Briganti SI, et al. Differences between ATA, AACE/ACE/AME and ACR TI-RADS ultrasound classifications performance in identifying cytological high-risk thyroid nodules. Eur J Endocrinol. 2018;178(6):595–603. https://doi.org/10.1530/EJE-18-0083.
19. Ha EJ, Na DG, Moon W-J, Lee YH, Choi N. Diagnostic performance of ultrasound-based risk-stratification systems for thyroid nodules: comparison of the 2015 American Thyroid Association Guidelines with the 2016 Korean Thyroid Association/Korean Society of Thyroid Radiology and 2017 American College of Radiology Guidelines. Thyroid. 2018;28(11):1532–7. https://doi.org/10.1089/thy.2018.0094.
20. Yoon JH, Lee HS, Kim E-K, Moon HJ, Kwak JY. Malignancy risk stratification of thyroid nodules: comparison between the thyroid imaging reporting and data system and the 2014 American Thyroid Association Management Guidelines. Radiology. 2016;278(3):917–24. https://doi.org/10.1148/radiol.2015150056.
21. Peng J-Y, Pan F-S, Wang W, et al. Malignancy risk stratification and FNA recommendations for thyroid nodules: a comparison of ACR TI-RADS, AACE/ACE/AME and ATA guidelines. Am J Otolaryngol. 2020;41(6):102625. https://doi.org/10.1016/j.amjoto.2020.102625.
22. Middleton WD, Teefey SA, Reading CC, et al. Comparison of performance characteristics of American College of Radiology TI-RADS, Korean Society of Thyroid Radiology TIRADS, and American Thyroid Association Guidelines. Am J Roentgenol. 2018;210(5):1148–54. https://doi.org/10.2214/AJR.17.18822.
23. Kim PH, Suh CH, Baek JH, Chung SR, Choi YJ, Lee JH. Unnecessary thyroid nodule biopsy rates under four ultrasound risk stratification systems: a systematic review and meta-analysis. Eur Radiol. 2021;31(5):2877–85. https://doi.org/10.1007/s00330-020-07384-6.
24. Zhan J, Ding H. Application of contrast-enhanced ultrasound for evaluation of thyroid nodules. Ultrasonography. 2018;37(4):288–97. https://doi.org/10.14366/usg.18019.
25. Kwong N, Medici M, Angell TE, et al. The influence of patient age on thyroid nodule formation, multinodularity, and thyroid cancer risk. J Clin Endocrinol Metab. 2015;100(12):4434–40. https://doi.org/10.1210/jc.2015-3100.
26. Toniato A, Bernardi C, Piotto A, Rubello D, Pelizzo MR. Features of papillary thyroid carcinoma in patients older than 75 years. Updat Surg. 2011;63(2):115–8. https://doi.org/10.1007/s13304-011-0060-0.
27. Wang Z, Vyas CM, Van Benschoten O, et al. Quantitative analysis of the benefits and risk of thyroid nodule evaluation in patients ≥70 years old. Thyroid. 2018;28(4):465–71. https://doi.org/10.1089/thy.2017.0655.
28. Ospina NS, Papaleontiou M. Thyroid nodule evaluation and management in older adults: a review of practical considerations for clinical endocrinologists. Endocr Pract. 2021;27(3):261–8. https://doi.org/10.1016/j.eprac.2021.02.003.
29. Moosa M, Mazzaferri EL. Outcome of differentiated thyroid cancer diagnosed in pregnant women. J Clin Endocrinol Metab. 1997;82(9):2862–6. https://doi.org/10.1210/jcem.82.9.4247.
30. Youserm DM, Huang T, Loevner LA, Langlotz CP. Clinical and economic impact of incidental thyroid lesions found with CT and MR. AJNR Am J Neuroradiol. 1997;18(8):1423–8.
31. Yoon DY, Chang SK, Choi CS, et al. The prevalence and significance of incidental thyroid nodules identified on computed tomography. J Comput Assist Tomogr. 2008;32(5):810–5. https://doi.org/10.1097/RCT.0b013e318157fd38.

32. Shetty SK, Maher MM, Hahn PF, Halpern EF, Aquino SL. Significance of incidental thyroid lesions detected on CT: correlation among CT, sonography, and pathology. Am J Roentgenol. 2006;187(5):1349–56. https://doi.org/10.2214/AJR.05.0468.
33. Ishigaki S, Shimamoto K, Satake H, et al. Multi-slice CT of thyroid nodules: comparison with ultrasonography. Radiat Med. 2004;22(5):346–53.
34. Cohen MS, Arslan N, Dehdashti F, et al. Risk of malignancy in thyroid incidentalomas identified by fluorodeoxyglucose-positron emission tomography. Surgery. 2001;130(6):941–6. https://doi.org/10.1067/msy.2001.118265.
35. Kang KW, Kim S-K, Kang H-S, et al. Prevalence and risk of cancer of focal thyroid incidentaloma identified by [18] F-fluorodeoxyglucose positron emission tomography for metastasis evaluation and cancer screening in healthy subjects. J Clin Endocrinol Metab. 2003;88(9):4100–4. https://doi.org/10.1210/jc.2003-030465.
36. Nockel P, Millo C, Keutgen X, et al. The rate and clinical significance of incidental thyroid uptake as detected by Gallium-68 DOTATATE positron emission tomography/computed tomography. Thyroid. 2016;26(6):831–5. https://doi.org/10.1089/thy.2016.0174.
37. Are C, Hsu JF, Schoder H, Shah JP, Larson SM, Shaha AR. FDG-PET detected thyroid incidentalomas: need for further investigation? Ann Surg Oncol. 2006;14(1):239–47. https://doi.org/10.1245/s10434-006-9181-y.
38. Soelberg KK, Bonnema SJ, Brix TH, Hegedüs L. Risk of malignancy in thyroid incidentalomas detected by [18] F-fluorodeoxyglucose positron emission tomography: a systematic review. Thyroid. 2012;22(9):918–25. https://doi.org/10.1089/thy.2012.0005.
39. Cibas ES, Baloch ZW, Fellegara G, et al. A prospective assessment defining the limitations of thyroid nodule pathologic evaluation. Ann Intern Med. 2013;159(5):325. https://doi.org/10.7326/0003-4819-159-5-201309030-00006.
40. Gharib H. Fine-needle aspiration biopsy of the thyroid: an appraisal. Ann Intern Med. 1993;118(4):282. https://doi.org/10.7326/0003-4819-118-4-199302150-00007.
41. Oertel YC. Fine-needle aspiration of the thyroid: technique and terminology. Endocrinol Metab Clin N Am. 2007;36(3):737–51. https://doi.org/10.1016/j.ecl.2007.05.001.
42. Rosário PW, Calsolari MR. What is the best criterion for repetition of fine-needle aspiration in thyroid nodules with initially benign cytology? Thyroid. 2015;25(10):1115–20. https://doi.org/10.1089/thy.2015.0253.
43. Kwak JY, Koo H, Youk JH, et al. Value of US correlation of a thyroid nodule with initially benign cytologic results. Radiology. 2010;254(1):292–300. https://doi.org/10.1148/radiol.2541090460.
44. Hall TL, Layfield LJ, Philippe A, Rosenthal DL. Sources of diagnostic error in fine needle aspiration of the thyroid. Cancer. 1989;63(4):718–25. https://doi.org/10.1002/1097-0142(19890215)63:4<718::aid-cncr2820630420>3.0.co;2-n.
45. Yu X-M, Patel PN, Chen H, Sippel RS. False-negative fine-needle aspiration of thyroid nodules cannot be attributed to sampling error alone. Am J Surg. 2012;203(3):331–4. https://doi.org/10.1016/j.amjsurg.2011.09.016.
46. Shrestha M, Crothers BA, Burch HB. The impact of thyroid nodule size on the risk of malignancy and accuracy of fine-needle aspiration: a 10-year study from a single institution. Thyroid. 2012;22(12):1251–6. https://doi.org/10.1089/thy.2012.0265.
47. Zhu Y, Song Y, Xu G, Fan Z, Ren W. Causes of misdiagnoses by thyroid fine-needle aspiration cytology (FNAC): our experience and a systematic review. Diagn Pathol. 2020;15(1):1. https://doi.org/10.1186/s13000-019-0924-z.
48. Cibas ES, Ali SZ. The 2017 Bethesda system for reporting thyroid cytopathology. Thyroid. 2017;27(11):1341–6. https://doi.org/10.1089/thy.2017.0500.
49. Dhingra JK. Ultrasound-guided fine-needle biopsy of first 1000 consecutive thyroid nodules: single-surgeon experience. OTO Open. 2020;4(2):2473974X2092900. https://doi.org/10.1177/2473974X20929008.

50. McIvor NP, Freeman JL, Salem S, Elden L, Noyek AM, Bedard YC. Ultrasonography and ultrasound-guided fine-needle aspiration biopsy of head and neck lesions: a surgical perspective. Laryngoscope. 1994;104(6):669–74. https://doi.org/10.1288/00005537-199406000-00005.
51. Fernandes VT, De Santis RJ, Enepekides DJ, Higgins KM. Surgeon-performed ultrasound guided fine-needle aspirate biopsy with report of learning curve; a consecutive case-series study. J Otolaryngol Head Neck Surg. 2015;44(1):42. https://doi.org/10.1186/s40463-015-0099-x.
52. Mehanna HM, Jain A, Morton RP, Watkinson J, Shaha A. Investigating the thyroid nodule. BMJ. 2009;338(mar13 1):b733. https://doi.org/10.1136/bmj.b733.
53. Brito JP, Ito Y, Miyauchi A, Tuttle RM. A clinical framework to facilitate risk stratification when considering an active surveillance alternative to immediate biopsy and surgery in papillary microcarcinoma. Thyroid. 2016;26(1):144–9. https://doi.org/10.1089/thy.2015.0178.
54. Durante C, Costante G, Lucisano G, et al. The natural history of benign thyroid nodules. JAMA. 2015;313(9):926. https://doi.org/10.1001/jama.2015.0956.
55. Kim S-Y, Hwa Han K, Jung Moon H, Young Kwak J, Youn Chung W, Kim E-K. Thyroid nodules with benign findings at cytologic examination: results of long-term follow-up with US. Radiology. 2014;271(1):272–81. https://doi.org/10.1148/radiol.13131334.
56. Alexander EK, Hurwitz S, Heering JP, et al. Natural history of benign solid and cystic thyroid nodules. Ann Intern Med. 2003;138(4):315. https://doi.org/10.7326/0003-4819-138-4-200302180-00010.

Chapter 3
Preoperative Molecular Testing for Indeterminate Thyroid Nodules

Clifton Davis, Noor Addasi, and Whitney S. Goldner

Case

A 48-year-old healthy female presents for evaluation of a thyroid nodule. This was discovered incidentally on computed tomography (CT) of the chest done to evaluate pneumonia. Neck ultrasound shows a solitary 2.5 cm solid hypoechoic nodule in the right lobe of the thyroid. Margins are regular and do not appear to extend beyond the thyroid capsule, no calcifications are present, and no abnormal appearing lymph nodes. Sonographically, it is consistent with the American Thyroid Association (ATA) intermediate suspicion of malignancy (10–20% risk [1]) and Thyroid Imaging Reporting & Data System (TIRADS) 4 (5–80% risk [2]). She does not have a personal or family history of thyroid disease, thyroid cancer, or autoimmunity, and does not have a history of radiation exposure. She is asymptomatic and thyroid function tests are normal. She has already undergone thyroid fine needle aspiration (FNA) biopsy, and cytopathology is indeterminate, consistent with follicular neoplasm (Bethesda IV). She has read about molecular testing for thyroid nodules and would like to know if she should have it performed, and if so which test?

C Davis, N Addasi are co-first authors

C. Davis · W. S. Goldner (✉)
Department of Internal Medicine, Division of Diabetes, Endocrinology, and Metabolism, University of Nebraska Medical Center, 984120 Nebraska Medical Center, Omaha, NE, USA
e-mail: clifton.davis@unmc.edu; wgoldner@unmc.edu

N. Addasi
Department of Internal Medicine, Division of Diabetes, Endocrinology, and Metabolism, University of Nebraska Medical Center, 984120 Nebraska Medical Center, Omaha, NE, USA

Cotton O'Neil Diabetes and Endocrinology, Stormont Vail Health, Topeka, KS, USA

Background

Thyroid nodules are exceedingly common, with a reported prevalence of up to 70% of adults [3, 4]. Most of these nodules are incidentally detected on imaging for other pathologies. The standard evaluation of thyroid nodules using clinical assessment, imaging, and cytopathology yields a definitive diagnosis in about two-thirds of these nodules [3–8]. The management of the remaining 20–30% of these nodules; labeled as cytologically indeterminate (Bethesda III and IV) is challenging and has continued to evolve over the years. Prior to the development of molecular testing, patients with cytologically indeterminate thyroid nodules were offered diagnostic surgery as the next step in management. However, with a cancer prevalence of only 5–30% in cytologically indeterminate thyroid nodules [5, 7], such practice resulted in high numbers of unnecessary surgeries, especially in patients without other indications for surgery. Thyroid surgery is overall low risk, but can result in surgical complications, necessitate life-long hormone replacement, diminish the health-related quality of life, and increase the direct and indirect healthcare costs [3, 7]. Hence, there was a need to better determine appropriate indications for surgery in the evaluation of indeterminate thyroid nodules (Fig. 3.1).

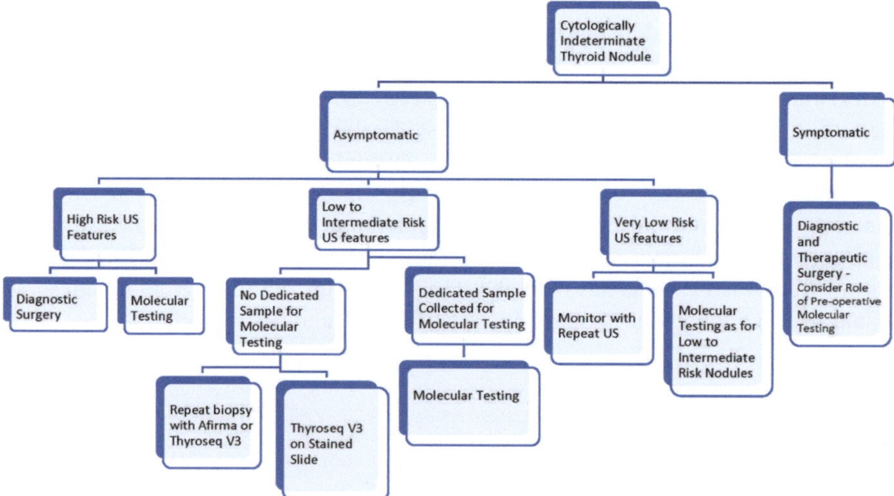

Fig. 3.1 Our Approach to a cytologically indeterminate thyroid nodule. A patient with a symptomatic nodule with indeterminate biopsy results is referred for surgical removal. Molecular analysis could be considered preoperatively, as high-risk mutations could influence the degree of surgery. An asymptomatic patient with an indeterminate thyroid nodule and high-risk ultrasound features is referred for surgical removal as well. Again, molecular analysis could be considered prior to surgery to help guide the extent of surgery. For other asymptomatic patients with indeterminate thyroid nodules, we stratify them by their ultrasound features. A very low suspicion nodule could either be monitored by repeat ultrasound or sent initially for molecular testing. For low-to-intermediate risk nodules, we recommend molecular testing. Either Afirma GSC or ThyroSeq v3 testing can be done on FNA samples, whether on repeat biopsy or a dedicated sample obtained at the time of original procedure. ThyroSeq v3 does uniquely offer analysis of stained slides with adequate cellularity if a dedicated FNA sample is not available

Over the last decade, multiple types of molecular tests have emerged to be used preoperatively for cytologically indeterminate thyroid nodules. Each test is slightly different in its approach to detect genetic alterations associated with thyroid cancer. The most common methodologies include DNA and RNA sequencing and mRNA expression. Many have proprietary algorithms and have gone through multiple generations to improve sensitivity and specificity.

Fortunately, molecular testing of cytologically indeterminate thyroid nodules has significantly reduced the need for diagnostic lobectomies/thyroidectomies [3, 5, 9], which reduces the less frequent but possible complications, including transient or permanent damage to the parathyroid glands, laryngeal nerves and the need for postoperative thyroid hormone replacement therapy. Hence, there has been a shift in guidelines for evaluation of thyroid nodules, now recommending consideration of preoperative molecular testing for indeterminate nodules rather than diagnostic lobectomy/thyroidectomy [1, 10]. However, one of the biggest challenges for clinicians is to determine when exactly to use molecular testing, and which one to use. We illustrate the clinical considerations needed when approaching a patient with a cytologically indeterminate thyroid nodule.

Approach to the Patient

The decision to perform molecular testing on a cytologically indeterminate thyroid nodule should start with a comprehensive discussion between the provider and the patient. It is not as simple as just deciding which test to use. Not all patients need molecular testing. It is important to consider all the factors that will influence the overall clinical management of an indeterminate thyroid nodule to determine if molecular testing will overall impact decision-making (Table 3.1).

First, consider the preoperative malignancy risk. The nodule discussed above has an ATA intermediate suspicion of malignancy/TIRADS 4. However, if the sonographic risk is ATA high or TIRADS 5 (risk of malignancy >70–90%, and >80%, respectively [1, 2]), it is important to consider if sonographic risk (pretest probability) will affect the patient's decision about pursuing diagnostic surgery. If molecular testing is performed and negative, will the patient proceed to surgery regardless of the molecular test result? If so, molecular testing may not impact the ultimate

Table 3.1

Factors to consider when determining whether molecular testing is indicated
Symptoms
Ultrasound characteristics of the nodule and sonographic risk of malignancy
Availability of molecular testing in the clinic or hospital where they are seen
Willingness of patient to undergo a second biopsy
Willingness to have continued ultrasound monitoring if molecular testing is negative
Overall preference of the patient
Cost

decision, and may be unnecessary. Conversely, if the sonographic risk is ATA low or very low suspicion (risk of malignancy <3%, and 5–10%, respectively [1]) or TIRADS 2–3 (risk of malignancy 0%, and <5%, respectively [2]), and the patient prefers to avoid surgery, a negative molecular test may help them avoid a diagnostic surgery. A recent study by Ahmadi et al. retrospectively evaluated patients with cytologically indeterminate thyroid nodules who ultimately underwent surgery. In their cohort, none of the patients with very low suspicion nodules/ TIRADS 1 and 2 had cancer. This is in contrast to the indeterminate nodules with high-suspicion sonographic features where 66.7% of the Bethesda III nodules with ATA high/ TIRADS 5 and 50% of the Bethesda IV ATA high suspicious/ TIRADS 5 nodules were malignant. The study was limited by small numbers, but supports using sonographic risk as an adjunct to thyroid FNA to determine whether molecular testing is indicated [11].

Second, it is important to evaluate for the presence of symptoms that impact whether the patient is planning to pursue surgery. If the patient has compressive symptoms, hoarseness secondary to posterior extension of the nodule, or cosmetic concerns about the nodule and is planning to undergo surgery regardless of the molecular result, then the addition of molecular testing to a cytologically indeterminate FNA currently may not impact decision-making or treatment.

Third, very importantly, consider patient preference and other issues that may impact decision-making. Is the patient willing to undergo a second biopsy to aid in decision-making? If the result is negative, are they willing to continue with routine ultrasound surveillance of the nodule? For how long? Are there financial considerations that need to be discussed? Will long-term monitoring after benign molecular testing cost more or less than upfront surgical removal? Is the patient already on thyroid hormone medication? If so, the long-term cost and consequence of surgical treatment are lower. Often time, clinicians do not consider these questions as strongly as the medical questions about diagnosis and treatment, however, they can play an equal, if not stronger role in influencing patient medical decision-making.

Once you have considered the above factors, and if you have decided to proceed with molecular testing, then the next step is to consider which molecular test to use. The two most common commercially available tests in the United States are Veracyte Afirma Genomic Sequencing Classifier (GSC) + Genome Atlas, and ThyroSeq version 3 (v3) [4]. For this discussion, we will focus on these two tests since they have the most data and have undergone direct comparison (Table 3.2).

Table 3.2

Performance of Afirma GSC and ThyroSeq v3 in Bethesda III and IV Indeterminate thyroid nodules

Study	Blinded validation [7] Patel et al.	Parallel randomized trial [5] Livhits et al.	Parallel randomized trial [5] Livhits et al.	Prospective blinded cohort [16] Steward et al.
Molecular test	Afirma GSC	Afirma GSC	ThyroSeq v3	ThyroSeq v3
Disease prevalence %	23.7	20	20	27.5
Sensitivity % (95%CI)	91.1 (79–98)	100 (88–100)	96.9 (83.8–100)	94.1 (86–98)
Specificity % (95%CI)	68.3 (60–76)	79.6 (71.7–86.1)	84.8 (77.0–90.7)	81.6 (75–87)
NPV % (95%CI)	96.1 (90–99)	100 (96.6–100)	99 (94.6–100)	97.3 (93–99)
PPV % (95%CI)	47.1 (36–58)	53.5 (39.9–66.7)	63.3 (48.3–76.6)	65.9 (56–75)
Benign call rate %	54	53	61	61

Molecular Tests

Afirma GSC + Genome Atlas The newest version of the Afirma molecular test (GSC) has been available commercially since 2017. GSC evaluates genomic content of thyroid nodules through RNA sequencing technology that helps evaluate more than 10,000 genes, of these 1115 are core genes that drive the prediction behavior of the model, while the remaining genes improve classifier stability. This technology includes sequencing of nuclear and mitochondrial transcript level RNA, changes in genomic copy number and loss of heterozygosity. The updated platform has multiple classifiers including a benign vs malignant classifier with additional Hurthle cell and Hurthle neoplasm cassettes, a parathyroid classifier, a medullary thyroid cancer classifier, and a BRAF V600E classifier. It can also identify RET/PTC1 and RET/PTC3 fusions if present [4, 6, 7, 9]. A GSC benign result indicates a 4% cancer probability while a GSC suspicious result indicates a 50% cancer probability [12]. In 2018, Veracyte launched the Afirma Xpression Atlas (XA) which was most recently updated in March 2020. Similar to Afirma GSC, it uses RNA sequencing to identify an additional 905 variants and 235 fusions in 593 genes. To perform molecular testing using Afirma GSC + Genoma Atlas, samples need to be collected at the time of the FNA. Veracyte recommends obtaining two additional passes at the time of FNA biopsy, and placing them in a solution provided by the company [4, 6, 7, 9]. This analysis cannot be done on stained slides at a later time after the FNA.

The initial validation study of the Afirma GSC test utilized a cohort of thyroid nodule biopsies with Bethesda III or IV that had been resected surgically. This cohort was previously utilized to validate the Genomic Expression Classifier (GEC); the first generation of the Afirma molecular test [7]. Patel et al. reported GSC sensitivity of 91% (95% CI, 79–98%), specificity of 68% (95% CI, 60–76%), a negative predictive value (NPV) of 96% (95%, CI 90–99) and a positive predictive value (PPV) of 47% (95% CI, 36–58%) at a cancer prevalence of 24% [7]. Multiple retrospective studies were followed to evaluate the real-world experience with GSC [3, 9, 13]. The benign call rate (BCR) ranged from 65.8% to 76.2% with a PPV of 50–85% of resected nodules [3, 9, 13]. A final histopathological diagnosis was not reported in all of these cohorts since most GSC benign nodules were not surgically removed, and the assumption that GSC benign nodules were truly benign resulted in a high reported sensitivity of 90.6–100%, specificity of 92.6–94% and a NPV of 96.3–100% [3, 9].

ThyroSeq v3 is DNA and RNA-based next-generation sequencing that analyzes 112 genes for point mutations, insertions, deletions, gene fusions, copy number alterations, and abnormal gene expression [14] and was validated in 2017. ThyroSeq v3 analyzes more than 120 gene fusions and includes a genomic classifier, a proprietary algorithm that analyzes all genetic alterations and results in a score to separate benign and malignant nodules into positive or negative test results [14]. A negative test represents a risk of malignancy of 3% which is equivalent to a cytologically benign result [15], while very low-grade mutations are classified as "currently negative" with probabilities of cancer of 5–10% [12]. Positive cases are assigned an individual probability of cancer according to the type and number of mutation findings ranging from 30% to 99% [12].The improved negative predictive value is valid for cancer prevalence of 10–40% for Bethesda III and IV categories [5, 14, 16]. To perform molecular testing using ThyroSeq v3, it is recommended to obtain one additional pass at the time of FNA biopsy and place it in a solution provided by the company. If the sample is not obtained at the time of FNA, cytology smear slides with adequate cellularity can be used alternatively in most cases but this is not the preferred method [17].

The initial validation study of ThyroSeq v3 included 238 surgically removed tissue samples, 175 FNA samples with indeterminate cytology (Bethesda III, IV, and V) from nodules subsequently removed, as well as 16 cell lines and 4 reference controls. The test sensitivity was 98.0% (95% CI, 92.9–99.4%), specificity was 81.8% (95% CI, 71.8–88.9%), and accuracy was 90.9% (95% CI, 85.7–94.3%) [14]. A follow-up prospective, blinded, multicenter study by Stewards et al. demonstrated a sensitivity of 94% (95% CI, 86–98%), a specificity of 82% (95% CI, 75–87%), a NPV of 97% (95% CI, 93–99%), and a PPV of 66% (95% CI, 56–75%) with a BCR of 61% in indeterminate Bethesda III and IV nodules [16].

Multiple validation and real-world experience studies report a high sensitivity, specificity, and negative predictive value of both Afirma GSC and ThyroSeq v3 molecular tests [3, 5, 7, 9, 13, 16]. Livhits et al. directly compared the two tests in a prospective study design and found no significant difference in sensitivity; Afirma GSC and ThyroSeq v3 had sensitivities of 100.0% (95% CI, 88.8–100.0%) and 96.9% (95% CI, 83.8–100.0%), respectively ($P > 0.99$), and specificity; Afirma GSC and ThyroSeq v3 were 79.6% (95% CI, 71.7–86.1%) and 84.8% (95% CI, 77.0–90.7%), respectively ($P = 0.32$). The predictive values of both tests were similar as well; PPV; Afirma GSC and ThyroSeq v3 were 53.5% (95% CI, 39.9–66.7%)

and 63.3% (95% CI, 48.3–76.6%), respectively ($P = 0.33$), and NPV; Afirma GSC and ThyroSeq v3 were 100.0% (95% CI, 96.6–100.0%), and 99.0% (95% CI 94.6–100.0%), respectively ($P = 0.49$) [5]. The study also included a sub-analysis of Hurthle cell nodules which formed about 13.7% of study nodules and were similarly present in both test cohorts. Afirma GSC had a BCR of 71.4% of Hurthle nodules [5] which is considered an improvement compared to its previous version GEC and was similarly captured in other studies [3, 9, 13]. ThyroSeq v3, on the other hand, had a BCR of 47.8%. Both tests had a 100% sensitivity, with a specificity of 83.3% for Afirma GSC vs 57.9% for ThyroSeq v3 [5]. Diagnostic thyroidectomy was avoided in 51% of patients tested with Afirma GSC and 49% of patients tested with ThyroSeq v3 without a statistically significant difference between the two tests. Both tests performed similarly well in real-world studies and reduced the need for diagnostic lobectomy.

The Role of Molecular Testing in Determining the Extent of Surgery

Both Afirma GSC + Genome Atlas and ThyroSeq v3 provide recommendations regarding possible tumor types, risk of malignancy, and predicted aggressiveness and risk of recurrence, however, studies to evaluate this are ongoing; most studies addressing the use of preoperative molecular testing to dictate extent of surgery are retrospective in nature and have shown inconsistent findings [18]. BRAFV600E mutation is present in up to 60% of papillary thyroid carcinoma [18] with some studies suggesting a more aggressive behavior of these tumors [8, 19] while others show no significant increase in risk of aggressive behavior or thyroid cancer-related mortality [20, 21]. In contrast, TERT promoter mutations were more consistently shown to predict a high risk of aggressive tumor behavior and worse prognosis and would be a stronger indication for a more aggressive surgery [8, 18, 20, 21].

There is emerging data linking particular genetic mutations to tumor aggressiveness and risk of recurrence in thyroid cancer which may be able to help guide the extent of surgical treatment in patients with thyroid nodules showing these genetic alterations and possibly the intensity of follow-up as well. In the study by Chin et al., indeterminate nodules were evaluated by ThyroSeq v2 or v3 and all of the ones with RAS-like genetic mutations that were confirmed malignant histopathologically were classified as ATA low risk of recurrence postoperatively while more patients with TERT/TP53 and BRAF-like nodules had vascular invasion and extrathyroidal extension qualifying for ATA intermediate and high risk of recurrence categories [22]. Similar findings were also noted in the Afirma XA validation study [23] and the result report would include these specific mutations identified like BRAF V600E, the predicted risk of malignancy and expected aggressiveness of behavior including extrathyroidal extension, lymph node metastasis as well as information about FDA approved targeted therapies for these mutations when available [23, 24]. However, the data are still unclear, hence more studies are needed before we can routinely use molecular tests to determine the extent of surgery.

Cost-Effectiveness

The short-term cost of molecular tests (estimated at $3000–$6000) is expensive but remains less than a diagnostic lobectomy (estimated at $9000–$12,000). However, previous studies evaluating the long-term cost-effectiveness of these tests have shown variable results and many of these studies addressed older versions of the currently available molecular tests [4, 25]. Nicholson et al. published a recent analysis utilizing data from the Centers for Medicare and Medicaid Services (CMS) to evaluate the cost-effectiveness of two currently available molecular tests in an euthyroid 40-year-old patient model with a solitary indeterminate thyroid nodule. Both molecular tests studied (Afirma GSC and ThyroSeq v3) were significantly more cost effective with an estimated cost per correct diagnosis of $14,277 for ThyroSeqv3 and $17,873 for GSC compared with $38,408 for diagnostic lobectomy [25]. However, they used a theoretical model with limited applicability to real-world patients.

In contrast, surgery was found to be more cost effective than active surveillance in an Australian cohort with papillary microcarcinoma, especially in younger patients with longer life expectancy. The annual cost of active surveillance was estimated at 756 Australian dollars vs a total cost of surgery at $10,226 (equivalent to 16.2 years of active surveillance). The cost of surveillance includes clinic visits, thyroid ultrasound, and possible repeat biopsy with or without molecular testing [26]. Since this study focused on active surveillance for a known micropapillary thyroid carcinoma, it is not the same clinical situation as ultrasound surveillance for a cytologically indeterminate thyroid nodule with negative molecular testing where the ultrasound surveillance would not be as frequent or as long as a known thyroid cancer. However, Zhu and colleagues recently reported a 6% false negative rate in cytologically indeterminate thyroid nodules with negative molecular testing during a 3-year follow-up. During median surveillance of 26.7 months, 10/83 nodules were resected, four of which were malignant [27]. This supports the recommendations for ongoing surveillance of cytologically indeterminate thyroid nodules with negative molecular testing, which adds to ongoing costs, with 12% of these nodules ultimately undergoing surgery during surveillance. The optimal duration of surveillance has not been established and needs to be evaluated further.

Back to the Case

In this patient, we recommend additional molecular testing for her Bethesda IV cytologically indeterminate thyroid nodule. With the current evidence, both of the available tests; Afirma GSC and ThyroSeq v3 are good options if planned at the time of biopsy and samples for molecular testing are collected. If the extra samples for molecular testing are not collected at the time of biopsy and the patient wants to avoid a repeat biopsy, then the prepared slides can be used for ThyroSeq v3 testing only. Her ultrasound does not show any high-risk features and her predicted risk of malignancy is approximately 30% according to the ATA criteria. She is currently asymptomatic and would like to avoid surgery. Hence, a negative molecular test result would reduce her risk of malignancy to 3–4% and she could avoid surgery at this time. If her result is positive, her risk of malignancy would be higher than her predicted sonographic risk, so would help inform the decision to pursue surgery.

However, if this patient's nodule was ATA high suspicion/ TIRADS 5 sonographically, she might opt for a diagnostic surgery knowing her risk of malignancy is >70–90% based on imaging alone. If she plans to undergo surgery regardless of the molecular result, we do not recommend molecular testing since there is no definitive evidence to influence the extent of surgery. If she wants to avoid surgery, then we recommend molecular testing. If negative or "benign," continued close follow-up is indicated to evaluate for change.

On the other end of the spectrum, if the patient's nodule has low or very low sonographic ATA suspicion/ TIRADS 2–3, benign molecular testing would help the patient avoid an unnecessary surgery, so would definitely impact treatment decisions. Given this, we recommend molecular testing in this scenario to be able to avoid surgery, however, Ahmadi et al. suggest that these nodules could be considered for ongoing surveillance rather than molecular analysis. This is compelling but requires additional investigation [11].

What if the nodule was Bethesda III rather than Bethesda IV? Guidelines [1, 10, 15] for management of adults with thyroid nodules differentiate between Bethesda III and IV nodules, suggesting consideration of a repeat FNA biopsy, molecular testing, or lobectomy for Bethesda III nodules in contrast to Bethesda IV with recommendations for molecular testing or lobectomy, but not observation or repeat biopsy without molecular testing. The risk of malignancy (ROM) is lower in Bethesda III than in Bethesda IV nodules. If including Noninvasive Follicular Thyroid Neoplasm with Papillary-Like Nuclear Features (NIFTP) in the cancer category (i.e., those requiring surgery), the ROM is 10–30% for Bethesda III and 25–40% for Bethesda IV. If excluding NIFTP from cancer category, then the ROM is 6–18% in Bethesda III, and 10–40% in Bethesda IV [24]. Hence, if the overall ROM is lower based on FNA Bethesda categorization, then FNA ROM could be combined with sonographic risk to determine the overall clinical suspicion.

Conclusion

The decision to perform molecular testing on a cytologically indeterminate thyroid nodule should not be reflexive for every cytologically indeterminate thyroid nodule, but should include multiple factors including sonographic suspicion, Bethesda category, patient preference, financial considerations, and availability of different tests at different centers. The current available molecular tests have high sensitivity, specificity, and negative predictive value. Currently, head-to-head trials of the two most common commercially available tests in the United States show equivalency when predicting malignancy and reduction in surgical rates. More studies are needed to establish the role of molecular testing to determine overall aggressiveness and behavior of specific tumors and extent of surgery.

References

1. Haugen BR, Alexander EK, Bible KC, Doherty GM, Mandel SJ, Nikiforov YE, et al. 2015 American Thyroid Association management guidelines for adult patients with thyroid nodules and differentiated thyroid cancer: the American Thyroid Association guidelines task force on thyroid nodules and differentiated thyroid cancer. Thyroid. 2016;26(1):1–133.
2. Kwak JY, Han KH, Yoon JH, Moon HJ, Son EJ, Park SH, et al. Thyroid imaging reporting and data system for US features of nodules: a step in establishing better stratification of cancer risk. Radiology. 2011;260(3):892–9.
3. San Martin VT, Lawrence L, Bena J, Madhun NZ, Berber E, Elsheikh TM, et al. Real-world comparison of Afirma GEC and GSC for the assessment of cytologically indeterminate thyroid nodules. J Clin Endocrinol Metabol. 2020;105(3):e428–e35.
4. Khan TM, Zeiger MA. Thyroid nodule molecular testing: is it ready for prime time? Front Endocrinol. 2020;11:590128.
5. Livhits MJ, Zhu CY, Kuo EJ, Nguyen DT, Kim J, Tseng CH, et al. Effectiveness of molecular testing techniques for diagnosis of indeterminate thyroid nodules: A randomized clinical trial. JAMA Oncol. 2021;7(1):70–7. https://doi.org/10.1001/jamaoncol.2020.5935. PMID: 33300952; PMCID: PMC7729582.
6. Hao Y, Choi Y, Babiarz JE, Kloos RT, Kennedy GC, Huang J, et al. Analytical verification performance of afirma genomic sequencing classifier in the diagnosis of cytologically indeterminate thyroid nodules. Front Endocrinol. 2019;10:438.
7. Patel KN, Angell TE, Babiarz J, Barth NM, Blevins T, Duh Q-Y, et al. Performance of a genomic sequencing classifier for the preoperative diagnosis of cytologically indeterminate thyroid nodules. JAMA Surg. 2018;153(9):817–24.
8. Krasner JR, Alyouha N, Pusztaszeri M, Forest V-I, Hier MP, Avior G, et al. Molecular mutations as a possible factor for determining extent of thyroid surgery. J Otolaryngol Head Neck Surg. 2019;48(1):51.
9. Endo M, Nabhan F, Porter K, Roll K, Shirley LA, Azaryan I, et al. Afirma gene sequencing classifier compared with gene expression classifier in indeterminate thyroid nodules. Thyroid. 2019;29(8):1115–24.
10. Haddad RI. NCCN clinical practice guidelines in oncology (NCCN guidelines): thyroid carcinoma. NCCN. 2020.
11. Ahmadi S, Herbst R, Oyekunle T, Jiang XS, Strickland K, Roman S, et al. Using the ATA and ACR TI-RADS sonographic classifications as adjunctive predictors of malignancy for indeterminate thyroid nodules. Endocr Pract. 2019;25(9):908–17.
12. Ohori NP, Landau MS, Manroa P, Schoedel KE, Seethala RR. Molecular-derived estimation of risk of malignancy for indeterminate thyroid cytology diagnoses. J Am Soc Cytopathol. 2020;9(4):213–20.
13. Angell TE, Heller HT, Cibas ES, Barletta JA, Kim MI, Krane JF, et al. Independent comparison of the Afirma genomic sequencing classifier and gene expression classifier for cytologically indeterminate thyroid nodules. Thyroid. 2019;29(5):650–6.
14. Nikiforova MN, Mercurio S, Wald AI, Barbi de Moura M, Callenberg K, Santana-Santos L, et al. Analytical performance of the ThyroSeq v3 genomic classifier for cancer diagnosis in thyroid nodules. Cancer. 2018;124(8):1682–90.
15. Cibas ES, Ali SZ. The 2017 Bethesda system for reporting thyroid cytopathology. Thyroid. 2017;27(11):1341–6.

16. Steward DL, Carty SE, Sippel RS, Yang SP, Sosa JA, Sipos JA, et al. Performance of a multi-gene genomic classifier in thyroid nodules with indeterminate cytology: a prospective blinded multicenter study. JAMA Oncol. 2019;5(2):204–12.
17. Nikiforova MN, Lepe M, Tolino LA, Miller ME, Ohori NP, Wald AI, et al. Thyroid cytology smear slides: an untapped resource for ThyroSeq testing. Cancer Cytopathol. 2021;129(1):33–42.
18. Addasi N, Fingeret A, Goldner W. Hemithyroidectomy for thyroid cancer: a review. Medicina. 2020;56(11):586.
19. Chen Y, Sadow PM, Suh H, Lee KE, Choi JY, Suh YJ, et al. BRAFV600E is correlated with recurrence of papillary thyroid microcarcinoma: a systematic review, multi-institutional primary data analysis, and meta-analysis. Thyroid. 2016;26(2):248–55.
20. Trybek T, Walczyk A, Gąsior-Perczak D, Pałyga I, Mikina E, Kowalik A, et al. Impact of BRAF V600E and TERT promoter mutations on response to therapy in papillary thyroid cancer. Endocrinology. 2019;160(10):2328–38.
21. Moon S, Song YS, Kim YA, Lim JA, Cho SW, Moon JH, et al. Effects of coexistent BRAFV600E and TERT promoter mutations on poor clinical outcomes in papillary thyroid cancer: a meta-analysis. Thyroid. 2017;27(5):651–60.
22. Chin PD, Zhu CY, Sajed DP, Fishbein GA, Yeh MW, Leung AM, et al. Correlation of ThyroSeq results with surgical histopathology in cytologically indeterminate thyroid nodules. Endocr Pathol. 2020;31(4):377–84.
23. Angell TE, Wirth LJ, Cabanillas ME, Shindo ML, Cibas ES, Babiarz JE, et al. Analytical and clinical validation of expressed variants and fusions from the whole transcriptome of thyroid FNA samples. Front Endocrinol. 2019;10:612.
24. Krane JF, Cibas ES, Endo M, Marqusee E, Hu MI, Nasr CE, et al. The Afirma Xpression atlas for thyroid nodules and thyroid cancer metastases: insights to inform clinical decision-making from a fine-needle aspiration sample. Cancer Cytopathol. 2020;128(7):452–9.
25. Nicholson KJ, Roberts MS, McCoy KL, Carty SE, Yip L. Molecular testing versus diagnostic lobectomy in Bethesda III/IV thyroid nodules: a cost-effectiveness analysis. Thyroid. 2019;29(9):1237–43.
26. Lin JF, Jonker PK, Cunich M, Sidhu SB, Delbridge LW, Glover AR, et al. Surgery alone for papillary thyroid microcarcinoma is less costly and more effective than long term active surveillance. Surgery. 2020;167(1):110–6.
27. Zhu CY, Donangelo I, Gupta D, Nguyen DT, Ochoa JE, Yeh MW, et al. Outcomes of indeterminate thyroid nodules managed nonoperatively after molecular testing. J Clin Endocrinol Metabol. 2021;106(3):e1240–e7.

Chapter 4
Active Surveillance of Low-Risk Differentiated Thyroid Cancer

Debbie W. Chen and Megan R. Haymart

Case

A 70-year-old man was incidentally found to have a solitary right thyroid nodule on a cervical spine computed tomography scan. His medical history was notable for hypertension, hyperlipidemia, and diabetes mellitus. He had no personal history of immune thyroid disorders or radiation exposure, and no family history of thyroid cancer. His current medications included hydrochlorothiazide, lisinopril, atorvastatin, and metformin.

Dedicated neck ultrasound was remarkable for a well-circumscribed solid hypoechoic right thyroid nodule that measured 0.7 cm in the largest diameter, was taller-than-wide, and without echogenic foci or extrathyroidal extension (TI-RADS 5). There appeared to be at least 2 mm of sonographically normal thyroid tissue between the nodule, which was located on the dorsal side of the right lobe, and the posterior border of the thyroid lobe. No suspicious cervical lymph nodes were seen. Fine needle aspiration of the right thyroid nodule revealed papillary thyroid cancer (Bethesda VI). Thyroid stimulating hormone level was normal (2.0 uIU/mL).

Since being diagnosed with thyroid cancer, the patient researched his treatment options on the internet. He recently read an article about active surveillance for thyroid cancer and was interested in learning more about this option. He expressed a strong preference to avoid thyroid surgery, if possible, and stated that he would be willing and able to obtain follow-up ultrasounds at your institution. Would active surveillance of thyroid cancer be feasible in this patient, and if so, what is the timing and duration of surveillance?

D. W. Chen · M. R. Haymart (✉)
Department of Medicine, University of Michigan School of Medicine, Ann Arbor, MI, USA
e-mail: chendeb@med.umich.edu; meganhay@med.umich.edu

© The Author(s), under exclusive license to Springer Nature Switzerland AG 2023
S. A. Roman et al. (eds.), *Controversies in Thyroid Nodules and Differentiated Thyroid Cancer*, https://doi.org/10.1007/978-3-031-37135-6_4

Rationale for Active Surveillance of Low-risk Thyroid Cancer

Most Thyroid Cancers Have a Favorable Prognosis

The incidence of thyroid cancer has dramatically increased over the last few decades while thyroid cancer-related mortality has remained relatively stable [1–3]. Most patients with thyroid cancer have low-risk disease with 5-year survival rates approaching 100% [3]. Studies have identified the widespread use of thyroid ultrasound as contributing to the overdiagnosis of thyroid cancer [1, 4–7]. In the United States, papillary thyroid cancer accounts for approximately 90% of all differentiated thyroid cancers, and the most common is low-risk papillary thyroid microcarcinoma (PTMC), i.e., tumors measuring up to 1 cm in the largest dimension [8, 9]. Despite risk stratification systems, including that of the American Thyroid Association (ATA) and American College of Radiology Thyroid Imaging, Reporting and Data System (ACR TI-RADS) uniformly recommending against biopsy of subcentimeter nodules, the prevalence of PTMC suggests that there continues to be inappropriate and unnecessary biopsies of subcentimeter thyroid nodules in clinical practice [10–14]. Since PTMC is associated with low risk of recurrence and low disease-specific mortality, thyroid surgery has not been proven to result in significant survival benefits [10]. As a result, the traditional course of treatment with surgery with or without radioactive iodine ablation followed by long-term thyroid-stimulating hormone (TSH) suppression therapy is no longer appropriate for most PTMC. However, marked variation still exists in the treatment of low-risk thyroid cancer, with many patients at risk for overtreatment and possible harm [15, 16]. Thyroid surgery has the potential to cause significant morbidity, including vocal fold paralysis and transient/ permanent hypoparathyroidism, with greater risk if surgery is performed by low-volume surgeons [17, 18]. Furthermore, aggressive TSH suppression can lead to patient harm with an increased risk of atrial fibrillation, osteoporosis, and cardiovascular mortality [19–23].

Data on Active Surveillance for Low-risk Thyroid Cancer from Case Series Has Been Favorable

Active surveillance was initially proposed as an alternative management strategy for patients with low-risk PTMC to minimize risk of overtreatment and patient harm. Since the early 1990s, Kuma Hospital and the Cancer Institute Hospital in Japan have been conducting prospective clinical trials of active surveillance for low-risk PTMC [24, 25]. Over the subsequent two decades, active surveillance for low-risk thyroid cancer has been studied in case series with diverse patient cohorts (N ranging from 57–1235 patients) in the United States, Korea, Colombia, and Italy with promising results [26–30]. In active surveillance, patients with low-risk thyroid cancer are closely monitored for evidence of disease progression without initial surgery. In a cohort of 1235 Japanese patients with low-risk PTMC who chose active surveillance between 1993 and 2011 at Kuma Hospital, Ito et al. showed that only 4.6% ($N = 58$) had tumor enlargement of at least 3 mm, only 1.5% ($N = 19$) had new appearance of lymph node metastasis, and none exhibited distant metastasis or died of thyroid cancer during an average observation period of 5 years (range 1.5–18.9 years) [31]. Similarly, in a different cohort of 230 Japanese patients with low-risk PTMC who chose active surveillance between 1995 and 2008 at the Cancer Institute Hospital, Sugitani et al. demonstrated that only 7.0% ($N = 22$) had increase in tumor size, 1.0% ($N = 3$) developed lymph node metastasis, and none developed extrathyroidal invasion or distant metastasis during an average observation period of 5 years (range 1–17 years) [25]. There were no life-threatening recurrences or deaths from thyroid cancer among patients who underwent surgical treatment after a period of active surveillance in both studies [25, 31].

Active surveillance for low-risk papillary thyroid microcarcinoma was adopted as a treatment option in the 2010 Japanese clinical guidelines for the treatment of thyroid nodules [32]. Five years later, the ATA guidelines recommended (1) against routine biopsy of subcentimeter thyroid nodules and (2) consideration of active surveillance as a safe and effective alternative to immediate surgery in properly selected patients, including those with cytologically confirmed very low-risk PTMC [10]. To facilitate implementation of active surveillance for patients diagnosed with low-risk thyroid cancer, the Japan Association of Endocrine Surgery (JAES) Task Force published consensus statements regarding the use of active surveillance for low-risk papillary thyroid cancer in 2021 [33].

Active Surveillance Is Standard of Care for Other Low-risk Cancers

Similar to patients with low-risk differentiated thyroid cancer, many patients with low-risk prostate and breast cancers that have 5-year survival rates approaching 100% are at risk for overtreatment. In this context, active surveillance has or is being considered as a management strategy for other low-risk cancers with an indolent course and low disease-specific mortality [34]. Studies have demonstrated that among men with localized prostate cancer, there is no significant difference in prostate cancer-specific or all-cause mortality among those who were managed with active surveillance compared to radical prostatectomy or external-beam radiotherapy [35]. In addition, men undergoing active surveillance for prostate cancer reported psychological well-being and quality of life that was comparable to their counterparts who received treatment with radical prostatectomy or radiation therapy [36–39]. Since 2010, when national guidelines began advocating for the use of active surveillance for management of low-risk prostate cancer, this conservative management strategy has become the standard of care option for very-low, low, and favorable intermediate-risk prostate cancer [40–42]. More recently, active surveillance is being examined as an alternative treatment option for women diagnosed with ductal carcinoma in situ (DCIS), or stage 0 breast cancer, which is almost always diagnosed in asymptomatic individuals and associated with a low breast cancer-specific mortality [43–45]. The use of active surveillance for other cancer types suggest that this strategy can also be considered for thyroid cancer. However, the median age of patients diagnosed with prostate cancer is 67 years, breast cancer is 63 years, and thyroid cancer is 51 years [3, 46, 47]. Thus, desire to pursue active surveillance and length of follow-up needed may differ based on age of the cancer patient cohort. Although some lessons can be learned from other cancer types, there are unique aspects of the thyroid cancer patient cohort, including younger patient age at diagnosis.

Identifying Candidates for Active Surveillance of Low-Risk Thyroid Cancer

Which Patients Are Appropriate Candidates for Active Surveillance?

Based on available studies, active surveillance as a management strategy for low-risk thyroid cancer can be considered in an adult patient who (1) has a preference for management with active surveillance over immediate surgery, (2) is able to adhere to follow-up with serial ultrasound monitoring, and (3) is treated by a multidisciplinary team experienced in managing thyroid cancer and in neck ultrasonography (Table 4.1). When determining the appropriateness of active surveillance in patients with low-risk papillary thyroid cancer, it is important to consider the following factors:

1. *Age*. Older patients with low-risk PTMC may be the most appropriate candidates for active surveillance because they are more likely to have indolent nonprogressive disease and have a shorter life expectancy compared to younger patients [25, 48]. In multivariate analysis, Ito et al. demonstrated that younger age was an independent predictor of tumor enlargement of at least 3 mm (<40 years: odds ratio 2.50 [95% confidence interval 1.36–4.61]; 40–59 years: odds ratio 2.17 [95% confidence interval 1.09–4.35]) compared to 60 years and above) [31]. In a meta-analysis, Koshkina et al. determined that the pooled risk ratio for tumor growth of 3 mm or more in patients aged 40–50 years (vs <40 years) was 0.51 when adjusted for confounders [49]. Little is known about active surveillance for thyroid cancer in patients younger than 20 years.
2. *Comorbidities*. For patients with comorbid diseases and competing risks of death, such as those with advanced cardiac disease or chronic lower respiratory disease, active surveillance of low-risk papillary thyroid cancer may be appropriate [50–52]. Life expectancy should be incorporated into treatment decisions for patients with comorbidities and low-risk thyroid cancer.

Table 4.1 Factors that influence appropriateness of active surveillance for low-risk thyroid cancer

	Appropriate for active surveillance	Not appropriate for active surveillance
Tumor characteristics		
Cytology	Classic variant papillary thyroid cancer	Aggressive subtypes of papillary thyroid cancer (i.e., tall cell variant); medullary thyroid cancer; anaplastic thyroid cancer
Tumor size	Papillary thyroid microcarcinoma measuring up to 1.0 cm	There is a limited to no data on active surveillance in patients with tumors >1 cm
Location	Tumor not invading into the trachea and is far from the course of the recurrent laryngeal nerve	Tumor invading into the trachea or recurrent laryngeal nerve
Metastasis	No evidence of lymph node or distant metastasis	Evidence of lymph node or distant metastasis at presentation
Patient characteristics		
Age	Older patients ≥60 years (caveat: While younger patients can be candidates for active surveillance, age < 40 years is associated with higher likelihood of disease progression during active surveillance)	Lack of data on active surveillance in patients <20 years
Treatment preference	For active surveillance	For surgery
Able to obtain follow-up ultrasounds?	Yes	No
Pregnancy status	Current or possible future pregnancy does not prevent patients from undergoing active surveillance	Not applicable
Multidisciplinary team characteristics		
Endocrinologist	Experience in managing thyroid cancer	Absent
Surgeon (i.e., otolaryngologist and endocrine surgeon)	Experience in managing thyroid cancer	Absent
Experience in neck ultrasonography	Yes	No

3. *Tumor size.* The initial studies on active surveillance were conducted in patients with PTMC or tumors measuring up to 1 cm in size [24, 25, 27, 28]. Given the promising results of these earlier studies, limited data on active surveillance for low-risk thyroid cancer measuring up to 1.5 cm in size has been reported in three case series [26, 29, 53]. The case series by Sakai et al. included the largest patient cohort with tumor size >1 cm followed by active surveillance for the longest time period [53]. In a cohort of 61 Japanese patients with T1bN0M0 papillary thyroid cancer (mean tumor size 1.17 cm, range 1.1–1.6 cm) who chose active

surveillance, Sakai et al. demonstrated that only 7% ($N = 4$) had tumor enlargement of at least 3 mm and only 3% ($N = 2$) had development of lymph node metastasis during a mean observation period of 7.9 years (range 1–17 years) [53]. While patients with more advanced disease may be candidates for active surveillance, evidence on its safety is lacking as all published studies have included only patients with T1N0M0 disease.

4. *Tumor location.* There are limited data on which tumor locations are optimal for an active surveillance management strategy. Patients with papillary thyroid cancers that are not invading into the trachea and are not adjacent to the posterior thyroid capsule (and presumably the underlying recurrent laryngeal nerve) can be candidates for active surveillance [33].

5. *Other factors.* Studies on active surveillance for low-risk papillary thyroid cancer have included patients with multifocal tumors and patients with family history of thyroid cancer originating from follicular cells [25, 28, 33, 54]. Less is known about the use of molecular markers to identify PTMC that will progress and spread outside of the thyroid gland.

Which Patients Should Be Considered for Transient Use of Active Surveillance?

Upon diagnosis of low-risk thyroid cancer, transient use of active surveillance prior to definitive surgical treatment may be considered in the following patient populations:

1. Patients undergoing concurrent treatments for comorbid diseases (e.g., treatment of another cancer).

2. Patients who are pregnant. In most patients, surgery for low-risk papillary thyroid cancer diagnosed during pregnancy can be delayed until the postpartum period [55, 56]. In a cohort of 50 female patients with PTMC who experienced a total of 51 pregnancies/deliveries while under active surveillance, Ito et al. found that only 8% ($N = 4$) exhibited tumor enlargement of at least 3 mm and none developed nodal metastasis during their pregnancies [57].

Which Patients Are Inappropriate Candidates for Active Surveillance?

Patients with papillary thyroid cancer with the following high-risk features at the time of diagnosis are not appropriate candidates for active surveillance:

1. *Metastasis.* Evidence of lymph node metastasis at presentation is predictive of local disease recurrence [58–60]. Although very rare in low-risk PTMC, distant

metastasis at the time of thyroid cancer diagnosis is associated with significantly increased thyroid cancer-related mortality [61].

2. *Tumor invasion* into the recurrent laryngeal nerve or trachea is associated with worse prognosis [24, 33, 58]. Furthermore, a study by Ito et al. of 1143 patients with low-risk thyroid cancer under active surveillance suggests that PTMC measuring at least 7 mm and either (1) attached to the trachea at an obtuse angle or (2) without a normal rim of thyroid tissue between the tumor and the course of the recurrent laryngeal nerve has a high risk of tumor invasion [54, 62].

3. *Aggressive subtypes* of papillary thyroid cancer (i.e., tall cell and diffuse sclerosing variants) as suggested by cytology [33].

Implementation of Active Surveillance for Low-Risk Papillary Thyroid Cancer

Importance of a Multidisciplinary Medical Team

It is important that patients with thyroid cancer who are interested in active surveillance be cared for by a multidisciplinary medical team that includes surgeons and endocrinologists (Table 4.1). While endocrinologists would typically be involved in routine follow-up during active surveillance, surgeons would be able to provide clinically relevant input to help decide when, if at all, transition from active surveillance to surgery is appropriate. In addition, it is critical that team members are experienced in performing and interpreting neck ultrasonography, which is highly operator dependent. Unfortunately, in a cross-sectional study of 320 physicians who reported involvement with differentiated thyroid cancer surveillance, Kovach et al. found that only 27% ($N = 84$) reported personally performing bedside ultrasonography [63]. Furthermore, 33% ($N = 94$) did not report high confidence in either their ability or a radiologist's ability to use ultrasonography to detect cancer recurrence [63]. Neck ultrasonography is the cornerstone of long-term surveillance for thyroid cancer and has an increasingly crucial role in active surveillance. In this context, Kovach et al.'s study highlight a major obstacle to the implementation of active surveillance protocols in the United States.

Treatment Decision-Making

The decision to pursue active surveillance for low-risk thyroid cancer is complex and multifaceted. While most low-risk papillary thyroid cancers have a good prognosis and indolent course, all the data supporting the use of active surveillance are from case series. Thus, shared decision-making between patients and their medical team that addresses the following components is critical to helping patients make informed decisions about management of their thyroid cancer (Fig. 4.1) [64–66]:

1. Treatment options (i.e., active surveillance, total thyroidectomy, and lobectomy) for thyroid cancer.
2. Patient's expectations and treatment preferences.
3. Candidacy for active surveillance and expectations for follow-up.
4. Potential risks and benefits of active surveillance.

I. What is active surveillance?

Active surveillance means that you will be closely monitored with neck ultrasounds without initial surgery. You can have thyroid surgery at a later time if you choose or if your cancer grows.

II. What are your treatment options, and how do they compare?

	Active surveillance	*Thyroid surgery*
What is usually involved?	• You will have regular checkups and tests (including neck ultrasounds) to watch for any changes in your cancer. • If your cancer grows, your doctor may recommend that you have surgery.	• You will have surgery with or without radioactive iodine therapy to remove the cancer. • Afterwards, you will have regular checkups to make sure the cancer hasn't come back.
What are the potential benefits?	• With papillary thyroid microcarcinoma, you have a very low risk of dying from thyroid cancer. Even if the cancer grows during active surveillance, existing data suggests that it can be treated. • You can decide later if you want to have surgery.	• You can treat the cancer right away.
What are the potential risks and side effects?	• The cancer may grow during active surveillance. • You may have worry or anxiety related to the thyroid cancer between checkups.	• Surgery has risks of serious side effects, including low calcium levels and vocal cord paralysis.

IV. What matters most to you?

Thinking about your thyroid cancer treatment, please choose how <u>important</u> each statement is to you …

	Not at all important	A little important	Somewhat important	Quite important	Very Important
a. I want to avoid surgery for as long as I can	❑	❑	❑	❑	❑
b. I'm willing to take the risk that the cancer will grow	❑	❑	❑	❑	❑
c. I'm worried that I might not be able to deal with the side effects of surgery	❑	❑	❑	❑	❑
d. I want to get rid of my cancer right away	❑	❑	❑	❑	❑
e. I'm worried that if I wait to have surgery, my cancer will grow	❑	❑	❑	❑	❑
f. I'm willing to deal with the potential side effects of surgery	❑	❑	❑	❑	❑

V. Which treatment option are you leaning towards?

Active surveillance VS thyroid surgery

Fig. 4.1 Content for a shared decision-making tool for physicians to discuss active surveillance with their patients who have low-risk papillary thyroid cancer

5. Potential risks and benefits of surgical treatment.
6. Limitations of existing data on active surveillance.

Monitoring with Ultrasound Exams

Patients with thyroid cancer who undergo active surveillance need to have serial neck ultrasounds that include evaluation of the thyroid and cervical lymph nodes to identify disease progression, which should prompt consideration for surgical treatment. Based on existing case series, ultrasound evaluations by experienced specialists are recommended every 6 months for the first 2 years after initiation of active surveillance, then annually thereafter if no disease progression is identified [33]. There are no data to suggest that serum thyroglobulin is helpful during active surveillance. Once active surveillance has been initiated, length of follow-up is not known as the mean duration of follow-up for existing case series is 0.5–7.9 years (range 0–17 years) [25–30, 53].

Potential Benefits of Active Surveillance

An active surveillance strategy for low-risk thyroid cancer has the potential to not only decrease over-treatment and patient harm, but also lead to improved patient-reported outcomes [67, 68]. Studies have demonstrated that patients who undergo active surveillance for thyroid cancer have a higher quality of life compared to those who undergo immediate surgery [69, 70]. In a cohort of 347 patients with low-risk PTMC, Nakamura et al. found that those who were treated with surgery had more complaints and significantly more anxiety and depression compared to those who were managed with active surveillance [71]. For older patients with low-risk PTMC, the use of active surveillance has been found to be more cost-effective than immediate surgery [72, 73].

When to Consider Transitioning to Surgical Treatment

A transition from active surveillance to surgery should be considered in patients with low-risk thyroid cancer when there is evidence of: (1) tumor enlargement, (2) new lymph nodes that are biopsy-proven thyroid cancer, (3) new evidence of extra-thyroidal extension, (4) tumor invasion into the recurrent laryngeal nerve or trachea or esophagus, or (5) new distant metastasis [24, 26, 28]. While there is controversy over the optimal definition of tumor enlargement, tumor growth of 3 mm or more in the maximal diameter has been adopted by many centers as the most practical and simple definition [33]. In addition to tumor characteristics, other factors that should influence the decision to transition to a surgical approach for treatment of thyroid cancer are patients' preference, other thyroid or parathyroid disease requiring surgery, and inability of patients to obtain follow-up ultrasounds.

Limitations of Existing Data and Challenges to Successful Uptake of Active Surveillance

Limitations of Existing Data on Active Surveillance

While the data on active surveillance for low-risk PMTC have been favorable and supportive of its use in select patient populations, there continue to be limitations in generalizing study findings to clinical practice. First, the ATA guidelines recommend against routine biopsy of subcentimeter thyroid nodules. However, the case series on active surveillance have largely focused on thyroid cancers measuring up to 1 cm in maximal diameter. Thus, more studies on low-risk papillary thyroid cancers measuring greater than 1 cm (i.e., 1.1–1.5 cm) are necessary. Second, studies with the largest patient cohorts were conducted in Japan. Thus, more studies on active surveillance in the United States are needed before there can be widespread uptake in the United States as there may be barriers to implementation of active surveillance in the United States that do not exist in Japan (e.g., loss to follow-up concerns) and enthusiasm for active surveillance may differ by region. Third, there is a lack of evidence on length of follow-up needed for low-risk papillary thyroid cancer. We only know about oncological outcomes of low-risk thyroid cancer during the follow-up period that is demonstrated by existing case series, which ranges from less than 1 year–17 years [25, 28]. In particular, the appropriate duration of active surveillance for young patients (i.e., 40 years and younger) is not known.

Challenges to Successful Uptake of Active Surveillance

Despite data on active surveillance for low-risk papillary thyroid cancer in diverse patient cohorts, there remain physician, patient, and systems factors that limit more widespread uptake of active surveillance. Physician factors include lack of awareness about active surveillance, perceptions that patients do not want active surveillance or that active surveillance will place a psychological burden on patients, and concerns about poor outcomes and malpractice lawsuits [74, 75]. Patient barriers include strong emotional reactions to the cancer label that motivate patients' preference for more aggressive treatment options, and lack of awareness about active surveillance [76–78]. Systems barriers include limitations of the current healthcare system infrastructure that would allow for long-term follow-up of patients while minimizing the potential for patients to be lost to follow-up.

To improve the acceptance and feasibility of active surveillance for low-risk papillary thyroid cancer, it is necessary to address the physician, patient, and systems barriers (Table 4.2). First, more research is necessary for larger tumors (i.e., 1.0–1.5 cm in maximal diameter) and in more diverse patient cohorts in the United States. Second, there also needs to be a greater understanding of the factors influencing physician and patient buy-in to active surveillance. Third, clinical practice guidelines and information support tools that are tailored to general endocrinologists and patients will be important in informing and addressing hesitancy about

Table 4.2 Strategies to overcome challenges to implementation of active surveillance for low-risk thyroid cancer

	Improve physician uptake	Improve patient uptake	Address systems barriers
Population-based studies of active surveillance			
To evaluate use in larger thyroid cancers (i.e., 1.0–1.5 cm)	X	X	
To determine appropriate duration of follow-up	X	X	
To evaluate use in younger patients (i.e., ≤60 years)	X	X	
To evaluate use in diverse patient cohorts in the United States	X	X	X
Mixed methods research on low-risk thyroid cancer			
On strategies to prevent patients being lost to follow-up	X	X	X
On adoption of de-implementation strategies to reduce overtreatment	X	X	X
Survey and qualitative research			
On factors influencing physician buy-in of active surveillance for low-risk thyroid cancer .	X		
On factors influencing patient buy-in (i.e., concerns about worry, anxiety, and quality of life during active surveillance)	X	X	
Development of clinical practice guidelines			
With step-by-step algorithm for physicians to implement active surveillance	X		X
To facilitate shared decision-making	X	X	X
Tailored to inform patients with thyroid cancer	X	X	X
Development of Continuing Medical Education courses			
On performing and interpreting neck ultrasounds	X		X
On use of active surveillance in thyroid cancer	X		X
Electronic health system that is easily accessible between different institutions	X	X	X
Registry for patients with thyroid cancer who are being managed with active surveillance	X	X	X

active surveillance [79]. Fourth, opportunities for physicians to develop their skills in performing and interpreting neck ultrasounds will help move active surveillance from the clinical trials arena into community practice. Finally, creation of a registry for patients with thyroid cancer who are being managed by active surveillance will assist in ensuring proper follow-up for patients.

Case Revisited

For the 70-year-old man with thyroid cancer described at the beginning of this chapter, active surveillance can be a feasible management strategy. The thyroid nodule of interest is subcentimeter in size, not posteriorly located, and without high-risk features. Additionally, the patient prefers a nonsurgical management option and reports being able to obtain follow-up ultrasounds, which are recommended to be performed every 6 months for the first 1–2 years and then annually thereafter. Given his older age, active surveillance is more cost-effective than surgery, and there is a low likelihood of disease progression during active surveillance compared to younger patients.

Conclusion

Until recently, thyroid cancer was the most rapidly increasing cancer type in the United States. In 2021, there will be an estimated 44,280 new cases of thyroid cancer [3]. For select patients with low-risk PTMC, active surveillance offers a valid and promising alternative to surgery and provides the potential benefit of decreasing overtreatment and its attendant risks. Active surveillance for PTMC was first studied in Japan in the early 1990s, and in less than three decades, its uptake by Japanese surgeons and patients has increased significantly. In 2018, a survey of member institutions of the JAES or Japanese Society of Thyroid Surgery (JSTS) to examine clinical practice patterns in the preceding 3 months showed that the majority (53.8%) of patients with PTMC underwent active surveillance [80]. With the passage of time and more research conducted outside of Japan, it is likely that the adoption of active surveillance protocols for low-risk thyroid cancer will continue to increase among both physicians and patients in the United States.

References

1. Davies L, Welch HG. Increasing incidence of thyroid cancer in the United States, 1973–2002. JAMA. 2006;295(18):2164–7.
2. Lim H, Devesa SS, Sosa JA, Check D, Kitahara CM. Trends in thyroid cancer incidence and mortality in the United States, 1974-2013. JAMA. 2017;317(13):1338–48.

3. National Cancer Institute. Cancer Stat Facts: Thyroid Cancer. https://seer.cancer.gov/statfacts/html/thyro.html. Accessed June 1, 2021.
4. Vaccarella S, Franceschi S, Bray F, Wild CP, Plummer M, Dal Maso L. Worldwide thyroid-cancer epidemic? The increasing impact of overdiagnosis. N Engl J Med. 2016;375(7):614–7.
5. Ahn HS, Kim HJ, Welch HG. Korea's thyroid-cancer "epidemic"—screening and overdiagnosis. N Engl J Med. 2014;371(19):1765–7.
6. Haymart MR, Banerjee M, Reyes-Gastelum D, Caoili E, Norton EC. Thyroid ultrasound and the increase in diagnosis of low-risk thyroid cancer. J Clin Endocrinol Metab. 2019;104(3):785–92.
7. Esfandiari NH, Hughes DT, Reyes-Gastelum D, Ward KC, Hamilton AS, Haymart MR. Factors associated with diagnosis and treatment of thyroid microcarcinomas. J Clin Endocrinol Metab. 2019;104(12):6060–8.
8. SEER Cancer Statistics Review 1975–2017: Cancer of the Thyroid (Invasive). https://seer.cancer.gov/csr/1975_2017/browse_csr.php?sectionSEL=26&pageSEL=sect_26_table.22. Accessed June 1, 2021.
9. Hughes DT, Haymart MR, Miller BS, Gauger PG, Doherty GM. The most commonly occurring papillary thyroid cancer in the United States is now a microcarcinoma in a patient older than 45 years. Thyroid. 2011;21(3):231–6.
10. Haugen BR, Alexander EK, Bible KC, Doherty GM, Mandel SJ, Nikiforov YE, Pacini F, Randolph GW, Sawka AM, Schlumberger M, Schuff KG, Sherman SI, Sosa JA, Steward DL, Tuttle RM, Wartofsky L. 2015 American Thyroid Association management guidelines for adult patients with thyroid nodules and differentiated thyroid cancer: the American Thyroid Association guidelines task force on thyroid nodules and differentiated thyroid cancer. Thyroid. 2016;26(1):1–133.
11. Tessler FN, Middleton WD, Grant EG, Hoang JK, Berland LL, Teefey SA, Cronan JJ, Beland MD, Desser TS, Frates MC, Hammers LW, Hamper UM, Langer JE, Reading CC, Scoutt LM, Stavros AT. ACR thyroid imaging, reporting and data system (TI-RADS): white paper of the ACR TI-RADS Committee. J Am Coll Radiol. 2017;14(5):587–95.
12. Lee SE, Kim EK, Moon HJ, Yoon JH, Park VY, Han K, Kwak JY. Guideline implementation on fine-needle aspiration for thyroid nodules: focusing on micronodules. Endocr Pract. 2020;26(9):1017–25.
13. Grani G, Lamartina L, Ascoli V, Bosco D, Biffoni M, Giacomelli L, Maranghi M, Falcone R, Ramundo V, Cantisani V, Filetti S, Durante C. Reducing the number of unnecessary thyroid biopsies while improving diagnostic accuracy: toward the "right" TIRADS. J Clin Endocrinol Metab. 2019;104(1):95–102.
14. Jeong C, Kim H, Lee J, Ha J, Kim MH, Kang MI, Lim DJ. Fine-needle aspiration of Subcentimeter thyroid nodules in the real-world management. Cancer Manag Res. 2020;12:7611–8.
15. Haymart MR, Esfandiari NH, Stang MT, Sosa JA. Controversies in the management of low-risk differentiated thyroid cancer. Endocr Rev. 2017;38(4):351–78.
16. Papaleontiou M, Chen DW, Banerjee M, Reyes-Gastelum D, Hamilton AS, Ward KC, Haymart MR. TSH suppression for papillary thyroid cancer: a physician survey study. Thyroid. 2021;31(9):1383–90.
17. Papaleontiou M, Hughes DT, Guo C, Banerjee M, Haymart MR. Population-based assessment of complications following surgery for thyroid cancer. J Clin Endocrinol Metab. 2017;102(7):2543–51.
18. Sosa JA, Bowman HM, Tielsch JM, Powe NR, Gordon TA, Udelsman R. The importance of surgeon experience for clinical and economic outcomes from thyroidectomy. Ann Surg. 1998;228(3):320–30.
19. Sawin CT, Geller A, Wolf PA, Belanger AJ, Baker E, Bacharach P, Wilson PW, Benjamin EJ, D'Agostino RB. Low serum thyrotropin concentrations as a risk factor for atrial fibrillation in older persons. N Engl J Med. 1994;331(19):1249–52.
20. Wang LY, Smith AW, Palmer FL, Tuttle RM, Mahrous A, Nixon IJ, Patel SG, Ganly I, Fagin JA, Boucai L. Thyrotropin suppression increases the risk of osteoporosis without decreasing

recurrence in ATA low- and intermediate-risk patients with differentiated thyroid carcinoma. Thyroid. 2015;25(3):300–7.

21. Papaleontiou M, Banerjee M, Reyes-Gastelum D, Hawley ST, Haymart MR. Risk of osteoporosis and fractures in patients with thyroid cancer: a case-control study in U.S. Veterans. Oncologist. 2019;24(9):1166–73.

22. Park J, Blackburn BE, Ganz PA, Rowe K, Snyder J, Wan Y, Deshmukh V, Newman M, Fraser A, Smith K, Herget K, Kirchhoff AC, Abraham D, Kim J, Monroe M, Hashibe M. Risk factors for cardiovascular disease among thyroid cancer survivors: findings from the Utah cancer survivors study. J Clin Endocrinol Metab. 2018;103(7):2468–77.

23. Pajamaki N, Metso S, Hakala T, Ebeling T, Huhtala H, Ryodi E, Sand J, Jukkola-Vuorinen A, Kellokumpu-Lehtinen PL, Jaatinen P. Long-term cardiovascular morbidity and mortality in patients treated for differentiated thyroid cancer. Clin Endocrinol. 2018;88(2):303–10.

24. Ito Y, Uruno T, Nakano K, Takamura Y, Miya A, Kobayashi K, Yokozawa T, Matsuzuka F, Kuma S, Kuma K, Miyauchi A. An observation trial without surgical treatment in patients with papillary microcarcinoma of the thyroid. Thyroid. 2003;13(4):381–7.

25. Sugitani I, Toda K, Yamada K, Yamamoto N, Ikenaga M, Fujimoto Y. Three distinctly different kinds of papillary thyroid microcarcinoma should be recognized: our treatment strategies and outcomes. World J Surg. 2010;34(6):1222–31.

26. Tuttle RM, Fagin JA, Minkowitz G, Wong RJ, Roman B, Patel S, Untch B, Ganly I, Shaha AR, Shah JP, Pace M, Li D, Bach A, Lin O, Whiting A, Ghossein R, Landa I, Sabra M, Boucai L, Fish S, Morris LGT. Natural history and tumor volume kinetics of papillary thyroid cancers during active surveillance. JAMA Otolaryngol Head Neck Surg. 2017;143(10):1015–20.

27. Oh HS, Ha J, Kim HI, Kim TH, Kim WG, Lim DJ, Kim TY, Kim SW, Kim WB, Shong YK, Chung JH, Baek JH. Active surveillance of low-risk papillary thyroid microcarcinoma: a multi-center cohort study in Korea. Thyroid. 2018;28(12):1587–94.

28. Moon JH, Kim JH, Lee EK, Lee KE, Kong SH, Kim YK, Jung WJ, Lee CY, Yoo RE, Hwangbo Y, Song YS, Kim MJ, Cho SW, Kim SJ, Jung EJ, Choi JY, Ryu CH, Lee YJ, Hah JH, Jung YS, Ryu J, Hwang Y, Park SK, Sung HK, Yi KH, Park DJ, Park YJ. Study protocol of multicenter prospective cohort study of active surveillance on papillary thyroid microcarcinoma (MAeSTro). Endocrinol Metab (Seoul). 2018;33(2):278–86.

29. Sanabria A. Active surveillance in thyroid microcarcinoma in a Latin-American cohort. JAMA Otolaryngol Head Neck Surg. 2018;144(10):947–8.

30. Molinaro E, Campopiano MC, Pieruzzi L, Matrone A, Agate L, Bottici V, Viola D, Cappagli V, Valerio L, Giani C, Puleo L, Lorusso L, Piaggi P, Torregrossa L, Basolo F, Vitti P, Tuttle RM, Elisei R. Active surveillance in papillary thyroid microcarcinomas is feasible and safe: experience at a Single Italian Center. J Clin Endocrinol Metab. 2020;105(3):e172–80.

31. Ito Y, Miyauchi A, Kihara M, Higashiyama T, Kobayashi K, Miya A. Patient age is significantly related to the progression of papillary microcarcinoma of the thyroid under observation. Thyroid. 2014;24(1):27–34.

32. Imai T, Kitano H, Sugitani I, Wada N. When can papillary microcarcinoma (papillary carcinoma measuring 1cm or less) be observed without immediate surgery? In: Takami H, editor. Treatment of thyroid tumor: Japanese clinical guidelines. Japan: Springer Japan; 2013. p. 119–22.

33. Sugitani I, Ito Y, Takeuchi D, Nakayama H, Masaki C, Shindo H, Teshima M, Horiguchi K, Yoshida Y, Kanai T, Hirokawa M, Hames KY, Tabei I, Miyauchi A. Indications and strategy for active surveillance of adult low-risk papillary thyroid microcarcinoma: consensus statements from the Japan Association of Endocrine Surgery Task Force on Management for Papillary Thyroid Microcarcinoma. Thyroid. 2021;31(2):183–92.

34. Haymart MR, Miller DC, Hawley ST. Active surveillance for low-risk cancers—a viable solution to overtreatment? N Engl J Med. 2017;377(3):203–6.

35. Hamdy FC, Donovan JL, Lane JA, Mason M, Metcalfe C, Holding P, Davis M, Peters TJ, Turner EL, Martin RM, Oxley J, Robinson M, Staffurth J, Walsh E, Bollina P, Catto J, Doble A, Doherty A, Gillatt D, Kockelbergh R, Kynaston H, Paul A, Powell P, Prescott S, Rosario DJ,

Rowe E, Neal DE, Protec TSG. 10-year outcomes after monitoring, surgery, or radiotherapy for localized prostate cancer. N Engl J Med. 2016;375(15):1415–24.

36. Donovan JL, Hamdy FC, Lane JA, Mason M, Metcalfe C, Walsh E, Blazeby JM, Peters TJ, Holding P, Bonnington S, Lennon T, Bradshaw L, Cooper D, Herbert P, Howson J, Jones A, Lyons N, Salter E, Thompson P, Tidball S, Blaikie J, Gray C, Bollina P, Catto J, Doble A, Doherty A, Gillatt D, Kockelbergh R, Kynaston H, Paul A, Powell P, Prescott S, Rosario DJ, Rowe E, Davis M, Turner EL, Martin RM, Neal DE, Protec TSG. Patient-reported outcomes after monitoring, surgery, or radiotherapy for prostate cancer. N Engl J Med. 2016;375(15):1425–37.

37. Carter G, Clover K, Britton B, Mitchell AJ, White M, McLeod N, Denham J, Lambert SD. Wellbeing during active surveillance for localised prostate cancer: a systematic review of psychological morbidity and quality of life. Cancer Treat Rev. 2015;41(1):46–60.

38. Jeldres C, Cullen J, Hurwitz LM, Wolff EM, Levie KE, Odem-Davis K, Johnston RB, Pham KN, Rosner IL, Brand TC, L'Esperance JO, Sterbis JR, Etzioni R, Porter CR. Prospective quality-of-life outcomes for low-risk prostate cancer: active surveillance versus radical prostatectomy. Cancer. 2015;121(14):2465–73.

39. van den Bergh RC, Essink-Bot ML, Roobol MJ, Wolters T, Schroder FH, Bangma CH, Steyerberg EW. Anxiety and distress during active surveillance for early prostate cancer. Cancer. 2009;115(17):3868–78.

40. Mahal BA, Butler S, Franco I, Spratt DE, Rebbeck TR, D'Amico AV, Nguyen PL. Use of active surveillance or watchful waiting for low-risk prostate cancer and management trends across risk groups in the United States, 2010-2015. JAMA. 2019;321(7):704–6.

41. Butler S, Muralidhar V, Chavez J, Fullerton Z, Mahal A, Nezolosky M, Vastola M, Zhao SG, D'Amico AV, Dess RT, Feng FY, King MT, Mouw KW, Spratt DE, Trinh QD, Nguyen PL, Rebbeck TR, Mahal BA. Active surveillance for low-risk prostate cancer in black patients. N Engl J Med. 2019;380(21):2070–2.

42. National Comprehensive Cancer Network. NCCN clinical practice guidelines in oncology: prostate cancer, version 2.2021. https://www.nccn.org/guidelines/guidelines-detail?category=1&id=1459. Accessed June 1, 2021.

43. Esserman L, Yau C. Rethinking the standard for ductal carcinoma in situ treatment. JAMA Oncol. 2015;1(7):881–3.

44. Ryser MD, Worni M, Turner EL, Marks JR, Durrett R, Hwang ES. Outcomes of active surveillance for ductal carcinoma in situ: a computational risk analysis. J Natl Cancer Inst. 2016;108(5):djv372.

45. Hwang ES, Hyslop T, Lynch T, Frank E, Pinto D, Basila D, Collyar D, Bennett A, Kaplan C, Rosenberg S, Thompson A, Weiss A, Partridge A. The COMET (comparison of operative versus monitoring and endocrine therapy) trial: a phase III randomised controlled clinical trial for low-risk ductal carcinoma in situ (DCIS). BMJ Open. 2019;9(3):e026797.

46. National Cancer Institute. Cancer Stat Facts: Prostate Cancer. https://seer.cancer.gov/statfacts/html/prost.html. Accessed June 1, 2021.

47. National Cancer Institute. Cancer Stat Facts: Female Breast Cancer. https://seer.cancer.gov/statfacts/html/breast.html. Accessed June 1, 2021.

48. Fukuoka O, Sugitani I, Ebina A, Toda K, Kawabata K, Yamada K. Natural history of asymptomatic papillary thyroid microcarcinoma: time-dependent changes in calcification and vascularity during active surveillance. World J Surg. 2016;40(3):529–37.

49. Koshkina A, Fazelzad R, Sugitani I, Miyauchi A, Thabane L, Goldstein DP, Ghai S, Sawka AM. Association of patient age with progression of low-risk papillary thyroid carcinoma under active surveillance: a systematic review and meta-analysis. JAMA Otolaryngol Head Neck Surg. 2020;146(6):552–60.

50. Papaleontiou M, Norton EC, Reyes-Gastelum D, Banerjee M, Haymart MR. Competing causes of death in older adults with thyroid cancer. Thyroid. 2021;31(9):1359–65.

51. Wang Z, Vyas CM, Van Benschoten O, Nehs MA, Moore FD Jr, Marqusee E, Krane JF, Kim MI, Heller HT, Gawande AA, Frates MC, Doubilet PM, Doherty GM, Cho NL, Cibas ES,

Benson CB, Barletta JA, Zavacki AM, Larsen PR, Alexander EK, Angell TE. Quantitative analysis of the benefits and risk of thyroid nodule evaluation in patients >/=70 years old. Thyroid. 2018;28(4):465–71.

52. Lohia S, Gupta P, Curry M, Morris LGT, Roman BR. Life expectancy and treatment patterns in elderly patients with low-risk papillary thyroid cancer: a population-based analysis. Endocr Pract. 2021;27(3):228–35.

53. Sakai T, Sugitani I, Ebina A, Fukuoka O, Toda K, Mitani H, Yamada K. Active surveillance for T1bN0M0 papillary thyroid carcinoma. Thyroid. 2019;29(1):59–63.

54. Ito Y, Miyauchi A, Oda H. Low-risk papillary microcarcinoma of the thyroid: a review of active surveillance trials. Eur J Surg Oncol. 2018;44(3):307–15.

55. Nam KH, Yoon JH, Chang HS, Park CS. Optimal timing of surgery in well-differentiated thyroid carcinoma detected during pregnancy. J Surg Oncol. 2005;91(3):199–203.

56. Yu SS, Bischoff LA. Thyroid cancer in pregnancy. Semin Reprod Med. 2016;34(6):351–5.

57. Ito Y, Miyauchi A, Kudo T, Ota H, Yoshioka K, Oda H, Sasai H, Nakayama A, Yabuta T, Masuoka H, Fukushima M, Higashiyama T, Kihara M, Kobayashi K, Miya A. Effects of pregnancy on papillary microcarcinomas of the thyroid re-evaluated in the entire patient series at Kuma Hospital. Thyroid. 2016;26(1):156–60.

58. Sugitani I, Fujimoto Y. Symptomatic versus asymptomatic papillary thyroid microcarcinoma: a retrospective analysis of surgical outcome and prognostic factors. Endocr J. 1999;46(1):209–16.

59. Hay ID, Hutchinson ME, Gonzalez-Losada T, McIver B, Reinalda ME, Grant CS, Thompson GB, Sebo TJ, Goellner JR. Papillary thyroid microcarcinoma: a study of 900 cases observed in a 60-year period. Surgery. 2008;144(6):980–7.

60. Pedrazzini L, Baroli A, Marzoli L, Guglielmi R, Papini E. Cancer recurrence in papillary thyroid microcarcinoma: a multivariate analysis on 231 patients with a 12-year follow-up. Minerva Endocrinol. 2013;38(3):269–79.

61. Kim H, Park SY, Jung J, Kim JH, Hahn SY, Shin JH, Oh YL, Chung MK, Kim HI, Kim SW, Chung JH, Kim TH. Improved survival after early detection of asymptomatic distant metastasis in patients with thyroid cancer. Sci Rep. 2019;9(1):18745.

62. Ito Y, Miyauchi A, Oda H, Kobayashi K, Kihara M, Miya A. Revisiting low-risk thyroid papillary microcarcinomas resected without observation: was immediate surgery necessary? World J Surg. 2016;40(3):523–8.

63. Kovatch KJ, Reyes-Gastelum D, Sipos JA, Caoili EM, Hamilton AS, Ward KC, Haymart MR. Physician confidence in neck ultrasonography for surveillance of differentiated thyroid cancer recurrence. JAMA Otolaryngol Head Neck Surg. 2020;147(2):166–72.

64. Elwyn G, Hutchings H, Edwards A, Rapport F, Wensing M, Cheung WY, Grol R. The OPTION scale: measuring the extent that clinicians involve patients in decision-making tasks. Health Expect. 2005;8(1):34–42.

65. D'Agostino TA, Shuk E, Maloney EK, Zeuren R, Tuttle RM, Bylund CL. Treatment decision making in early-stage papillary thyroid cancer. Psychooncology. 2018;27(1):61–8.

66. Thompson EG, Husney A, Romito K, Wood CG, Hoffman RM. Prostate cancer: should I choose active surveillance? https://www.upmc.com/health-library/article?hwid=abo8743&locale=en-us. Accessed June 1, 2021.

67. Smulever A, Pitoia F. High rate incidence of post-surgical adverse events in patients with low-risk papillary thyroid cancer who did not accept active surveillance. Endocrine. 2020;69(3):587–95.

68. Oda H, Miyauchi A, Ito Y, Yoshioka K, Nakayama A, Sasai H, Masuoka H, Yabuta T, Fukushima M, Higashiyama T, Kihara M, Kobayashi K, Miya A. Incidences of unfavorable events in the management of low-risk papillary microcarcinoma of the thyroid by active surveillance versus immediate surgery. Thyroid. 2016;26(1):150–5.

69. Kong SH, Ryu J, Kim MJ, Cho SW, Song YS, Yi KH, Park DJ, Hwangbo Y, Lee YJ, Lee KE, Kim SJ, Jeong WJ, Chung EJ, Hah JH, Choi JY, Ryu CH, Jung YS, Moon JH, Lee EK, Park YJ. Longitudinal assessment of quality of life according to treatment options in low-risk

papillary thyroid microcarcinoma patients: active surveillance or immediate surgery (interim analysis of MAeSTro). Thyroid. 2019;29(8):1089–96.

70. Jeon M, Lee YM, Sung TY, Han M, Shin YW, Kim WG, Kim TY, Chung KW, Shong Y, Kim WB. Quality of life in patients with papillary thyroid microcarcinoma managed by active surveillance or lobectomy : a cross-sectional study. Thyroid. 2019;29(7):956–62.

71. Nakamura T, Miyauchi A, Ito Y, Ito M, Kudo T, Tanaka M, Kohsaka K, Kasahara T, Nishihara E, Fukata S, Nishikawa M. Quality of life in patients with low-risk papillary thyroid microcarcinoma: active surveillance versus immediate surgery. Endocr Pract. 2020;26(12):1451–7.

72. White C, Weinstein MC, Fingeret AL, Randolph GW, Miyauchi A, Ito Y, Zhan T, Ali A, Gazelle GS, Lubitz CC. Is less more? A microsimulation model comparing cost-effectiveness of the revised American Thyroid Association's 2015 to 2009 guidelines for the management of patients with thyroid nodules and differentiated thyroid cancer. Ann Surg. 2020;271(4):765–73.

73. Lin JF, Jonker PKC, Cunich M, Sidhu SB, Delbridge LW, Glover AR, Learoyd DL, Aniss A, Kruijff S, Sywak MS. Surgery alone for papillary thyroid microcarcinoma is less costly and more effective than long term active surveillance. Surgery. 2020;167(1):110–6.

74. Pitt SC, Yang N, Saucke MC, Marka N, Hanlon B, Long KL, McDow AD, Brito JP, Roman BR. Adoption of active surveillance for very low-risk differentiated thyroid cancer in the United States: a National Survey. J Clin Endocrinol Metab. 2021;106(4):e1728–37.

75. Hughes DT, Reyes-Gastelum D, Ward KC, Hamilton AS, Haymart MR. Barriers to the use of active surveillance for thyroid cancer: results of a physician survey. Ann Surg. 2022;276(1):e40–7.

76. Pitt SC, Saucke MC, Wendt EM, Schneider DF, Orne J, Macdonald CL, Connor NP, Sippel RS. Patients' reaction to diagnosis with thyroid cancer or an indeterminate thyroid nodule. Thyroid. 2021;31(4):580–8.

77. Dixon PR, Tomlinson G, Pasternak JD, Mete O, Bell CM, Sawka AM, Goldstein DP, Urbach DR. The role of disease label in patient perceptions and treatment decisions in the setting of low-risk malignant neoplasms. JAMA Oncol. 2019;5(6):817–23.

78. Nickel B, Barratt A, McGeechan K, Brito JP, Moynihan R, Howard K, McCaffery K. Effect of a change in papillary thyroid cancer terminology on anxiety levels and treatment preferences: a randomized crossover trial. JAMA Otolaryngol Head Neck Surg. 2018;144(10):867–74.

79. Sawka AM, Ghai S, Yoannidis T, Rotstein L, Gullane PJ, Gilbert RW, Pasternak JD, Brown DH, Eskander A, Almeida JR, Irish JC, Higgins K, Enepekides DJ, Monteiro E, Banerjee A, Shah M, Gooden E, Zahedi A, Korman M, Ezzat S, Jones JM, Rac VE, Tomlinson G, Stanimirovic A, Gafni A, Baxter NN, Goldstein DP. A prospective mixed-methods study of decision-making on surgery or active surveillance for low-risk papillary thyroid cancer. Thyroid. 2020;30(7):999–1007.

80. Sugitani I, Ito Y, Miyauchi A, Imai T, Suzuki S. Active surveillance versus immediate surgery: questionnaire survey on the current treatment strategy for adult patients with low-risk papillary thyroid microcarcinoma in Japan. Thyroid. 2019;29(11):1563–71.

Chapter 5
Preoperative Laryngoscopy in Thyroid Surgery Patients

Arvind K. Badhey and David L. Steward

Cases

We will start by presenting three different scenarios of a patient with papillary thyroid cancer for which the question of undergoing preoperative laryngoscopy will be discussed:

Scenario 1

A 37-year-old female patient with no other risk factors was found to have a 2.1-cm left thyroid nodule that was within the mid-pole area based more anteriorly and was palpable on exam. She had no pertinent medical history, no history of prior neck surgery, no prior radiation, no family history of thyroid disease, and no preoperative complaints outside of the palpable mass. Ultrasound (US) assessment of the nodule showed a 2.1-cm nodule that appeared well circumscribed, hypoechoic with microcalcifications (Fig. 5.1). US-guided FNA of the nodule demonstrated a Bethesda 6 lesion, with features of well-differentiated papillary thyroid cancer. She had no associated lymphadenopathy, palpable or visualized on ultrasound in the central or lateral neck.

This patient appeared to have little to no risk factors for locally invasive disease that would make surgical management exceptionally challenging. The surgeon discussed the role and possibility of definitive surgical management with a thyroid lobectomy, as well as the possibility of converting to a total thyroidectomy in the event of intraoperative findings of extrathyroidal extension or nodal involvement. She had no voice complaints and did not appear to stratify into any higher-risk categories based on the ultrasound and exam findings. As a result, the surgeon discussed the role of preoperative laryngoscopy for assessment of her vocal folds.

A. K. Badhey · D. L. Steward (✉)
Department of Otolaryngology, University of Cincinnati, Cincinnati, OH, USA
e-mail: stewardd@ucmail.uc.edu

S. A. Roman et al. (eds.), *Controversies in Thyroid Nodules and Differentiated Thyroid Cancer*, https://doi.org/10.1007/978-3-031-37135-6_5

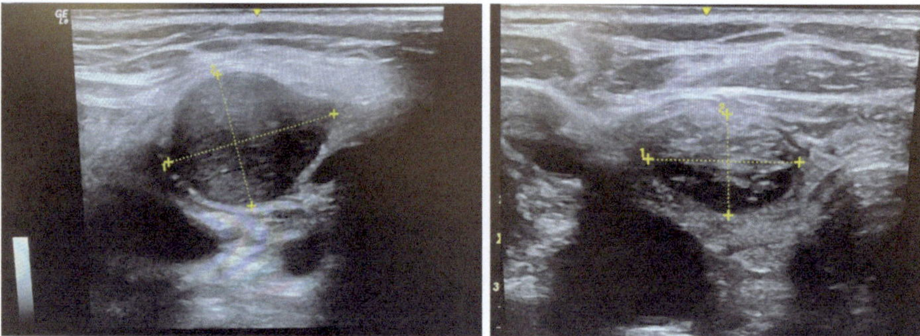

Fig. 5.1 Preoperative ultrasound of low-risk mid-pole anteriorly based nodule

Fig. 5.2 Preoperative ultrasound of a posteriorly located nodule

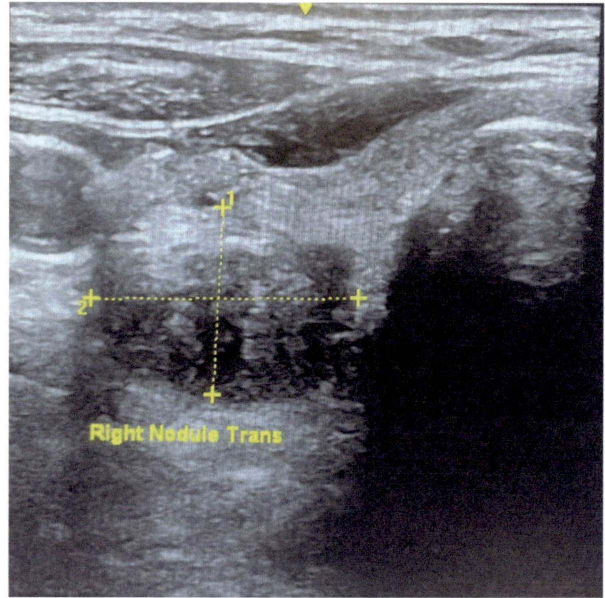

Scenario 2

In this scenario, the patient's nodule was posteriorly located on ultrasound and appeared to sit adjacent to the tracheoesophageal groove (Fig. 5.2).

Scenario 3

Finally, assume the first patient was found to have central neck lymph nodes that appeared suspicious for metastasis by ultrasound (Fig. 5.3).

Each of these scenarios begins to highlight the nuances of endocrine surgery, especially in patients that appear to be relatively low-risk surgical candidates. As surgical management of thyroid nodules has become more refined, a one-fits-all approach is no longer appropriate. The surgeon must balance oncologic outcomes with patient preferences and comfort—making patient-informed decision-making,

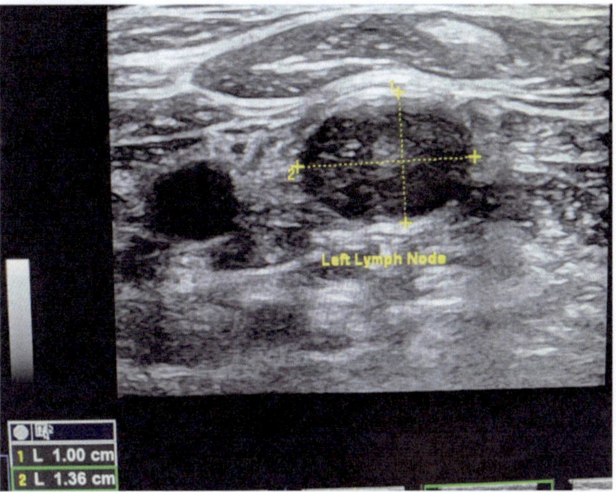

Fig. 5.3 Preoperative ultrasound demonstrating neck disease

especially important. We will review the arguments for and against the selective vs. routine approach to preoperative laryngoscopy in low-risk surgical patients using the three scenarios as examples.

Introduction

The approach to the thyroid nodule workup, pathologic diagnosis, and surgical management has gone through an evolution in the past 10 years. When approaching a patient with a thyroid nodule, along with the discussion of surgical management also comes the role of laryngoscopy for the assessment of preoperative vocal fold function.

The American Thyroid Association (ATA), the American Head and Neck Society (AHNS), the American Association of Endocrine Surgeons (AAES), and the American Academy of Otolaryngology (AAO) have published recommendations that cover multiple aspects of a surgical patient's workup; voice assessment, past surgical history, radiation therapy, pathologic diagnosis, and surgical management. They advise that all patients who are planning to have thyroid surgery should have a comprehensive voice assessment as part of their preoperative planning [1–4]. This can include the patient history, the surgeon's examination, as well as possible formal voice assessment tools [2, 5]. The examination should include an assessment of neck and chest scars, as evidence of possible prior surgery in the anatomic area of the vagus and the recurrent laryngeal nerves. This preoperative evaluation allows the surgeon and patient to properly establish surgical expectations [6, 7].

After this history is taken, the patient's overall risk should be quantified. The incidence of preoperative vocal cord paralysis or paresis can range from 0% to 8% [8–10]. Findings of vocal fold abnormalities on preoperative examination can be suggestive of local invasion. With the recent increase in surgeon-guided ultrasound, the assessment of this local invasion can be even better delineated [11, 12]. Management of possible tumor invasion is especially important during total thyroidectomy and is intimately tied to surgical planning and preoperative counseling [13]. Possible invasion can be discerned based on a combination of symptoms, physical examination findings, and imaging characteristics. Any patient who is considered high risk for vocal fold dysfunction or vocal fold pathology should be considered for preoperative laryngoscopy [3, 4]. The ATA has described patients who are considered to be high-risk surgical candidates and who should undergo routine laryngeal exam:

1. Patients with voice abnormalities or history of prior abnormalities.
2. Patients with a history of neck or chest surgery within the anatomic field of the vagus or recurrent laryngeal nerves (RLN).
3. Thyroid cancer that demonstrates posterior extrathyroidal extension (ETE) or central neck disease.

Surgeries that put patients at risk for voice issues include carotid endarterectomy, skull base resections, cervical esophagectomy, anterior cervical spine surgical approaches, prior thyroid/parathyroid surgeries, and mediastinal operations, such as coronary artery bypass with sternotomy. In addition, a history of external beam radiation can further increase surgical risk. Unfortunately, vocal fold paralysis can be asymptomatic in some patients, further complicating the role of laryngoscopy. In the patients who may have undergone the aforementioned procedures preoperative laryngoscopy is critical for both safety and surgical planning [6, 14].

The AHNS came out with a similar statement regarding laryngeal examination prior to endocrine surgery. The statement agreed on the role of laryngeal examination for patients who are at high risk for nerve injury (i.e., preoperative voice abnormalities, prior cervical or chest surgery, suspicion of posterior extension, and cervical metastasis). Furthermore, the statement concluded that flexible trans-nasal laryngoscopy is the optimal tool for vocal fold assessment. It did discuss the use of alternative techniques such as mirror examination, stroboscopy, and laryngeal ultrasound (Fig. 5.4). The statement also draws attention to the possible divergence in patient-reported vocal symptoms and objective vocal fold dysfunction seen on physical examination [3].

While guidelines offer ways to assess and treat patients who are considered high-risk, there is little discussion of the more nuanced approach of low-risk patients who are planning to undergo thyroid surgery. Franch-Arcas et al. summarizes the debate of routine versus selective preoperative laryngoscopy into four thoughtful key points for the surgeon to consider [15]:

1. The risk of detecting vocal cord paralysis in asymptomatic patients.
2. Preoperative vocal fold abnormalities can suggest an aggressive and more invasive malignancy.
3. The surgeon has a baseline for postoperative comparison.

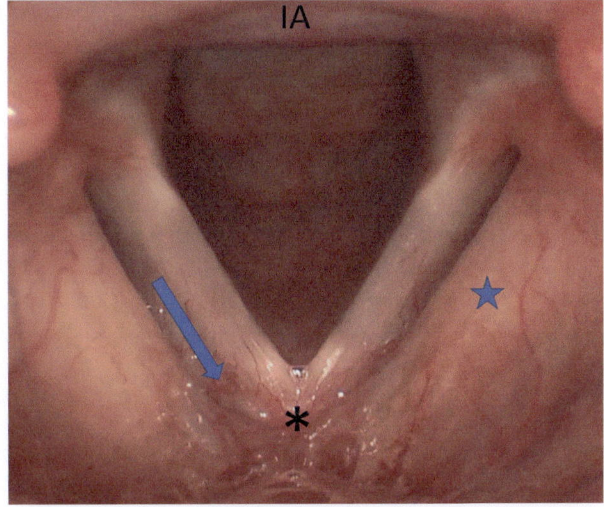

Fig. 5.4 Preoperative Fiberoptic Laryngoscopy demonstrating normal vocal cords. * Anterior commissure. Star—left false cord, Block arrow—right true vocal cord, *IA*—interarytenoid Space

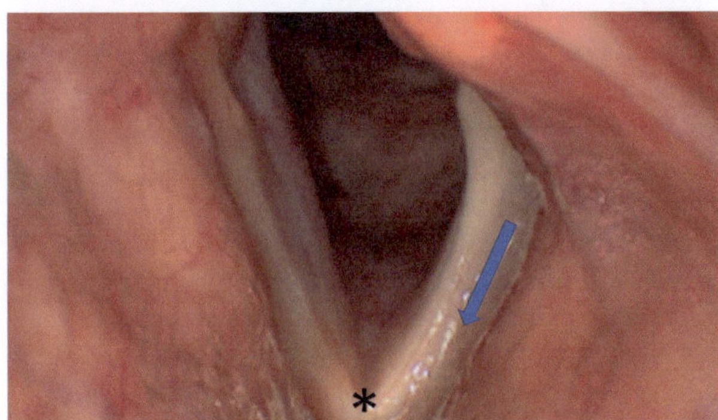

Fig. 5.5 Preoperative Fiberoptic Laryngoscopy demonstrating vocal fold paralysis. * Anterior commissure. Block arrow—left vocal cord paralyzed in the paramedian position

4. If an invaded nerve is found during surgery, knowing the preoperative function allows for informed management (Fig. 5.5).

The Routine Approach

The routine approach focuses on what can be missed based on history and physical exams, with the goal of not missing critical patient data that could be obtained with laryngoscopy. Using a patient's vocal history and symptoms as criteria for laryngoscopy is not considered reliable. Due to the lack of reliability in patient-reported outcomes the American Association of Otolaryngology and Head and Neck Surgeons recommends the use of more formal methods of measurement of voice disturbances [2]. The routine approach ultimately empowers the surgeon with knowledge that is informative during surgery and critical to vocal assessment postoperatively.

The Selective Approach

While there are multiple studies discussing the role of routine preoperative laryngoscopy, the level of evidence is relatively weak. This primarily stems from the low incidence of vocal cord palsy (VCP) in the absence of any symptoms or risk factors (as low as 0.5% of cases). A review of over 20 large studies demonstrated the incidence of VCP is between 1 and 6% [15]. Informed with these data, when thyroidectomy is performed by an experienced surgeon, it is considered a highly safe procedure with a relatively low risk of injury to the recurrent laryngeal nerve, and even more low-risk for low-risk thyroid lobectomy. While preoperative laryngeal assessment has been considered a standard of care, the data supporting its routine use are debatable [16, 17]. There are similar data in support of a selective approach, especially in patients without risk factors for preoperative VCP [18–21]. Identifying VCP preoperatively can help inform accurate interpretation of intraoperative nerve monitoring, while also serving a medico-legal purpose [7, 22]. However, in patients undergoing thyroid lobectomy with neuromonitoring, a potential loss of signal during surgery holds less risk as there is no plan to proceed to the contralateral lobe or put the contralateral nerve at risk.

When looking at the cost-effectiveness of routine laryngoscopy for patients with low-risk differentiated thyroid cancer who have no symptoms, who were planned to undergo any thyroid resection, fiberoptic laryngeal exam was generally cost-effective [23]; however, routine laryngoscopy was only cost-effective if the cost of the examination was less than $27 or the probability of asymptomatic VFP was >5% [24]. Assuming the incidence of asymptomatic vocal fold paralysis was ~3%, the number needed to "treat" (perform flexible laryngoscopy) to diagnose one patient would be 33 patients. In the workflow of a surgeon's clinic, selective laryngoscopy can be more advantageous. In the current climate of COVID-19, routine laryngoscopy of every patient would mean multiple endonasal exams and high work demand for ancillary staff. The selective approach allows the surgeon to further tailor management to the patient and his or her specific lesion. With risk stratification starting from the patient history, the surgeon can further stratify patients based on in-office ultrasound.

The use of the selective approach is contingent on a few factors that are surgeon specific. The first is that the operating surgeon is comfortable with the skills of in-office ultrasound. This allows the surgeon to have an intimate understanding of the anatomy and risk of a specific nodule. With a strong understanding of what is considered a low-risk surgical candidate, additional data from preoperative laryngoscopy may not be necessary. While routine laryngoscopy can be considered the gold standard, if the chance that a gold standard test will provide more information is low, it may not be considered a valuable test to add into the treatment algorithm. The presence of previous neck or chest scars should be noted by the endocrine surgeon, as these increase the baseline risk category of a patient. In addition, symptoms of referred otalgia should also increase risk assessment as it can be occasionally seen as a clinical sign of invasion, although coexisting inflammatory thyroid disorders may also produce otalgia. A caveat to this discussion is the nature of the surgeon's practice. A high-volume regional center where routine and complex endocrine surgery is performed regularly is likely best suited for a selective approach. This is because in such centers, clinicians can control additional variables such as reviewing outside pathology, reviewing ultrasound images, conducting in-office ultrasound, obtaining prior records and surgical history. If a high-volume, experienced endocrine surgeon is able to obtain all of this patient-specific information and feels confident in their abilities to risk stratify with in-office ultrasound, then a selective approach can be implemented.

Revisiting the Case

After review of current practice guidelines and latest literature on this subject, we can make a patient-centered and evidence-based assessment of our previous case scenarios.

Scenario 1: The patient was a low-risk surgical candidate with no risk factors for preoperative VCP.

Based on the above discussion, she would be a good candidate for "selective" laryngoscopy, and after a discussion with the patient and a surgeon's informed opinion, one could consider deferring a preoperative laryngeal exam.

Scenario 2: Based on guideline recommendations, the ultrasound findings would be considered intermediate/higher risk of VCP and nerve involvement due to the posteriorly located nodule. Surgeons should have a lower threshold to perform preoperative laryngoscopy on this patient as the RLN intraoperatively will likely be intimately associated with the posterior border of this nodule.

Scenario 3: The patient had evidence of central neck metastasis with multiple level 6 nodes running along the course of the RLN. Due to the impact that surgical dissection in this area can have on the RLN, and the close dissection of the nerve, it is recommended to assess VF mobility preoperatively. In addition, clinically detectable level 6 nodes have a higher possibility of extranodal extension, which would pose a risk for VCP.

Conclusion

The discussion of preoperative laryngoscopy in thyroidectomy patients has been debated recently due to the introduction of multiple methods to assess the larynx, including new technologies like laryngeal ultrasound. With this increased assessment has come better risk stratification of patients preoperatively, based on nodule characteristics and patient-specific factors. This has allowed for a more patient-centered and selective approach to what was previously a more routine and more weighted medical-legal approach to laryngoscopy. This chapter is not intended to dissuade the assessment of the larynx in endocrine surgical patients, but to bring up the debated topic of patients who have been preoperatively risk stratified as reasonably low risk. Selected patients with a nodule located in a favorable position, without concerning radiographic features, and without additional risk factors identified during history and physical examination, may be considered for a selective approach to laryngoscopy. The selective approach requires two key components: complete patient data for risk stratification prior to laryngoscopy and surgeon-specific abilities and experience. The surgeon must have a comprehensive history including patient-specific voice complaints, a complete surgical history with access to prior records, radiation history, and pathology review capabilities. The surgeon should be experienced in cervical endocrine operations, have an active high-volume practice at a regional center, and be comfortable performing in-office ultrasound. With the above factors in place, a selective approach to preoperative laryngoscopy can be successfully implemented in a significant number of patients planned for thyroidectomy.

References

1. Patel KN, Yip L, Lubitz CC, et al. The American Association of Endocrine Surgeons Guidelines for the definitive surgical management of thyroid disease in adults. Ann Surg. 2020;271(3):e21–93.
2. Chandrasekhar SS, Randolph GW, Seidman MD, et al. Clinical practice guideline: improving voice outcomes after thyroid surgery. Otolaryngol Head Neck Surg. 2013;148(6 Suppl):S1–37.
3. Sinclair CF, Bumpous JM, Haugen BR, et al. Laryngeal examination in thyroid and parathyroid surgery: an American Head and Neck Society consensus statement: AHNS Consensus Statement. Head Neck. 2016;38(6):811–9.
4. Haugen BR, Alexander EK, Bible KC, et al. 2015 American Thyroid Association management guidelines for adult patients with thyroid nodules and differentiated thyroid cancer: the American Thyroid Association guidelines task force on thyroid nodules and differentiated thyroid cancer. Thyroid. 2016;26(1):1–133.
5. Eadie TL, Kapsner M, Rosenzweig J, Waugh P, Hillel A, Merati A. The role of experience on judgments of dysphonia. J Voice. 2010;24(5):564–73.
6. Farrag TY, Samlan RA, Lin FR, Tufano RP. The utility of evaluating true vocal fold motion before thyroid surgery. Laryngoscope. 2006;116(2):235–8.

7. Randolph GW, Kamani D. The importance of preoperative laryngoscopy in patients undergoing thyroidectomy: voice, vocal cord function, and the preoperative detection of invasive thyroid malignancy. Surgery. 2006;139(3):357–62.
8. Shin JJ, Grillo HC, Mathisen D, et al. The surgical management of goiter: part I. Preoperative evaluation. Laryngoscope. 2011;121(1):60–7.
9. Bergenfelz A, Jansson S, Kristoffersson A, et al. Complications to thyroid surgery: results as reported in a database from a multicenter audit comprising 3,660 patients. Langenbeck's Arch Surg. 2008;393(5):667–73.
10. Green KM, de Carpentier JP. Are pre-operative vocal fold checks necessary? J Laryngol Otol. 1999;113(7):642–4.
11. Terris DJ, Snyder S, Carneiro-Pla D, et al. American Thyroid Association statement on outpatient thyroidectomy. Thyroid. 2013;23(10):1193–202.
12. Shindo ML, Caruana SM, Kandil E, et al. Management of invasive well-differentiated thyroid cancer: an American Head and Neck Society consensus statement. AHNS consensus statement. Head Neck. 2014;36(10):1379–90.
13. Falk SA, McCaffrey TV. Management of the recurrent laryngeal nerve in suspected and proven thyroid cancer. Otolaryngol Head Neck Surg. 1995;113(1):42–8.
14. Rosenthal LH, Benninger MS, Deeb RH. Vocal fold immobility: a longitudinal analysis of etiology over 20 years. Laryngoscope. 2007;117(10):1864–70.
15. Franch-Arcas G, González-Sánchez C, Aguilera-Molina YY, Rozo-Coronel O, Estévez-Alonso JS, Muñoz-Herrera Á. Is there a case for selective, rather than routine, preoperative laryngoscopy in thyroid surgery? Gland Surg. 2015;4(1):8–18.
16. Randolph GW. The importance of pre- and postoperative laryngeal examination for thyroid surgery. Thyroid. 2010;20(5):453–8.
17. Hodin R, Clark O, Doherty G, Grant C, Heller K, Weigel R. Voice issues and laryngoscopy in thyroid surgery patients. Surgery. 2013;154(1):46–7.
18. Järhult J, Lindestad PA, Nordenström J, Perbeck L. Routine examination of the vocal cords before and after thyroid and parathyroid surgery. Br J Surg. 1991;78(9):1116–7.
19. Yeung P, Erskine C, Mathews P, Crowe PJ. Voice changes and thyroid surgery: is pre-operative indirect laryngoscopy necessary? Aust N Z J Surg. 1999;69(9):632–4.
20. Schlosser K, Zeuner M, Wagner M, et al. Laryngoscopy in thyroid surgery—essential standard or unnecessary routine? Surgery. 2007;142(6):858–64. discussion 864.e851-852
21. Lang BH, Chu KK, Tsang RK, Wong KP, Wong BY. Evaluating the incidence, clinical significance and predictors for vocal cord palsy and incidental laryngopharyngeal conditions before elective thyroidectomy: is there a case for routine laryngoscopic examination? World J Surg. 2014;38(2):385–91.
22. Randolph GW, Dralle H, Abdullah H, et al. Electrophysiologic recurrent laryngeal nerve monitoring during thyroid and parathyroid surgery: international standards guideline statement. Laryngoscope. 2011;121(Suppl 1):S1-16.
23. Walgama E, Randolph GW, Lewis C, et al. Cost-effectiveness of fiberoptic laryngoscopy prior to total thyroidectomy for low-risk thyroid cancer patients. Head Neck. 2020;42(9):2593–601.
24. Zanocco K, Kaltman DJ, Wu JX, et al. Cost effectiveness of routine laryngoscopy in the surgical treatment of differentiated thyroid cancer. Ann Surg Oncol. 2018;25(4):949–56.

Chapter 6
Radiofrequency Ablation for Thyroid Nodules

Jennifer H. Kuo

Case Presentation

A 42-year-old otherwise healthy woman presented with a 43-mm right mid-thyroid nodule that she noticed several years ago as a palpable neck mass. A biopsy at that time demonstrated benign cells. The nodule had slowly grown in size, and she developed symptoms of neck pressure that bothered her constantly such that she was always thinking about the nodule. On physical examination, she had an obvious palpable goiter that was discernible without cervical extension, with the right thyroid lobe larger than the left. Ultrasound (US) revealed a 28 × 43 × 34 mm complex solid, hypoechoic mass interspersed with cystic spaces and smooth borders (Fig. 6.1). No other nodule was detected. Thyroid function tests were normal. A repeat fine needle aspiration of the nodule demonstrated a benign lesion (Bethesda II). The patient was hesitant about undergoing surgery because she did not want to take thyroid hormone replacement.

J. H. Kuo (✉)
Department of Surgery, Columbia University, New York City, NY, USA
e-mail: jhk2029@cumc.columbia.edu

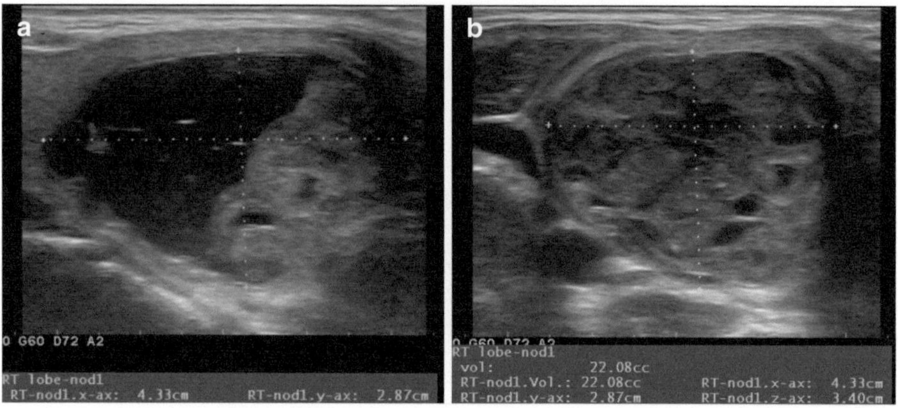

Fig. 6.1 (**a**) Pre-procedure dominant nodule located in the right mid-lower lobe measuring 43x29x34 mm, complex with isoechoic solid portion and hypoechoic cystic portion, smooth borders, with echogenic foci consistent with colloid crystals and grade 1 vascularity (TIRADS 3, ATA low suspicion) Sagittal view. (**b**) Transverse view

Background

Thyroid resection, either lobectomy or total, has traditionally been the definitive management for benign non-functioning thyroid nodules that cause compressive or cosmetic problems. In addition, thyroidectomy or radioactive iodine ablation have been the standard treatment options for benign autonomously functioning nodules [1, 2]. Although thyroidectomy is generally associated with excellent outcomes when performed by high-volume surgeons, it is still associated with complications that include recurrent or superior laryngeal nerve injury, hypoparathyroidism, hypothyroidism with need for thyroid hormone supplementation, and unsightly scarring [2, 3].

In the 2000s, thermal ablation (TA) techniques were introduced, including laser ablation (LA), radiofrequency ablation (RFA), and microwave ablation (MWA) [4, 5]. These techniques have become a popular alternative treatment option for patients who are either unsuitable or unwilling to undergo thyroid surgery. In this chapter, we will discuss the most widely adopted of these thermal techniques, RFA, and relevant considerations when this technique is used to treat benign thyroid nodules.

RFA is a minimally invasive technique using medium-frequency alternating current to generate heat in order to ablate tissue. It has gained widespread acceptance in multiple fields of medicine, ranging from treating liver tumors to treating chronic back pain [6, 7]. The first RFA of benign thyroid nodules was performed in Seoul in 2002, with the first case series published by Kim et al. in 2006, demonstrating the safety and efficacy of performing RFA on 35 benign thyroid nodules [8]. Authors in Italy published their first case series soon thereafter [9]. With reported mean nodule volume reductions of 80–85% at 12 months post-procedure, significant improvements in both cosmesis and compressive symptoms, a low complication profile, and the ability to avoid thyroid hormone dependency, thermal ablative techniques have been widely adopted for the treatment of benign thyroid nodules in Asia and Europe [10–12]. In contrast, adoption in the United States has been slower with just a single, small case series published by the Mayo Clinic in 2018 [13]. However, in the last couple of years, there have been an increasing number of institutions in the United States who have started to offer RFA for treatment of benign thyroid nodules.

Pre-procedure Considerations

In preparation for RFA, a dedicated US is performed to assess nodule characteristics and nodule volume, as well as the location of surrounding critical structures [14]. In accordance with the Korean and European Guidelines, thyroid nodules should be confirmed to be benign on at least two separate FNAs, with the exception of purely cystic lesions and spongiform nodules [15, 16]. A full evaluation of serologic tests should be performed including a complete blood count, coagulation profile, thyroid function tests, and a confirmation of a negative pregnancy test for women of childbearing age [17, 18]. Currently, only the unipolar electrode is available in the United States, which precludes those who are pregnant or who have cardiac pacemakers from undergoing the procedure. If the patient is a suitable candidate for RFA, assessment of both symptom and cosmetic impact before and after ablation should be performed; the cosmetic and symptom scoring systems described by Baek et al. have become popular systems. The symptom score is a self-measured scoring system ranging from 0 to 10. The cosmetic score ranging from 1 to 3 is graded by the provider with the following: 1 = no palpable mass, 2 = palpable mass without visible mass, 3 = visible mass on swallowing, and 4 = obviously visible mass [17, 19, 20]. All appropriate treatment options should be discussed with the patient including thyroidectomy and radioactive iodine ablation if indicated. The discussion regarding RFA should include potential complications (see below) as well as reasonably expected outcomes of the ablation. These include the incomplete disappearance of the target nodule(s), marginal regrowth, and the potential need for additional ablation sessions.

Procedure

RFA is typically performed under local anesthesia with perithyroidal lidocaine injection, ensuring adequate anesthesia at both the skin puncture site as well as the thyroid capsule [21, 22]. The electrode tip size is chosen based on the tumor size and status of the surrounding critical structures [22]. Since thyroid nodules tend to have mixed compositions and are generally intimately located next to critical structures in the neck, such as the carotid sheath, trachea, esophagus, and the recurrent laryngeal nerves, the risk for potential thermal injury to surrounding structures can be quite high even with the use of low energy settings. In order to decrease this risk, a few standard techniques have been described and widely adopted by those who

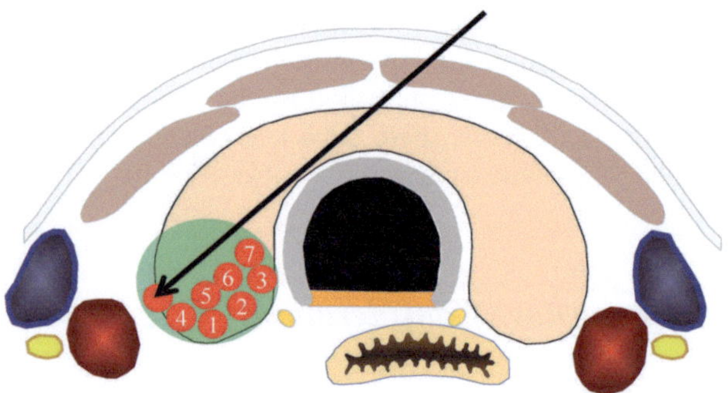

Fig. 6.2 Trans-isthmic and moving-shot techniques. The thyroid nodule (green) is compartmentalized into small units (red) and ablated systematically from deepest to most superficial (in numerical order)

perform TAs. These include the trans-isthmic approach, the moving-shot technique, and the use of hydrodissection [21–26]. The trans-isthmic approach is performed with the electrode inserted into the contralateral side of the neck first through the isthmus then into the target nodule. This approach increases the distance between the active tip and the skin to help prevent cutaneous injury, helps direct the active tip away from the "danger triangle" adjacent to the trachea that houses the recurrent laryngeal nerve, and provides greater stability of movement and access into the target nodule. The moving-shot technique involves mentally dividing the nodule into small units and ablating one unit at a time under ultrasound guidance, starting from the deepest portion to the most superficial (Fig. 6.2). The nodule is sequentially ablated, plane by plane, until post-ablation echogenic changes cover the entire volume of the nodule. Doppler flow assessment can be useful to detect under-ablated zones. By keeping the electrode in motion, this technique helps to limit the amount of energy delivered to any particular focus. Hydrodissection is the injection of fluid to increase the distance between two structures. Most commonly, lidocaine is injected along the perithyroidal capsule at the beginning of the procedure, not only to anesthetize the perithyroidal capsule, but also to increase the distance between the thyroid capsule and adjacent structures to help prevent cutaneous injury (Fig. 6.3) [27]. Hydrodissection with cold dextrose solution can be performed to create a physical margin of at least 5 mm to be achieved between the nodule and critical surrounding structures such as the recurrent laryngeal nerve [28]. The cold solution also prevents thermal propagation to the surrounding structures.

Once the ablation is completed, the electrode is gently removed and pressure held at the puncture site. It is generally recommended to observe the patient for a period of time before discharge home. Ice compresses and the use of NSAIDs can help decrease post-ablation swelling.

Post-Procedure Follow-Up

Currently, there is no consensus on the timing of follow-up after RFA. In our practice, patients are followed after the procedure with repeat thyroid function tests, repeat symptom and cosmetic scoring, and serial ultrasounds at 1, 3, 6, and 12 months, documenting the volume reduction of the thyroid nodule. The volume

Fig. 6.3 Hydrodissection of perithyroidal capsule anterior to thyroid nodule. Red arrow shows hydrodissection needle. Arrowheads delineate hydrodissection plane

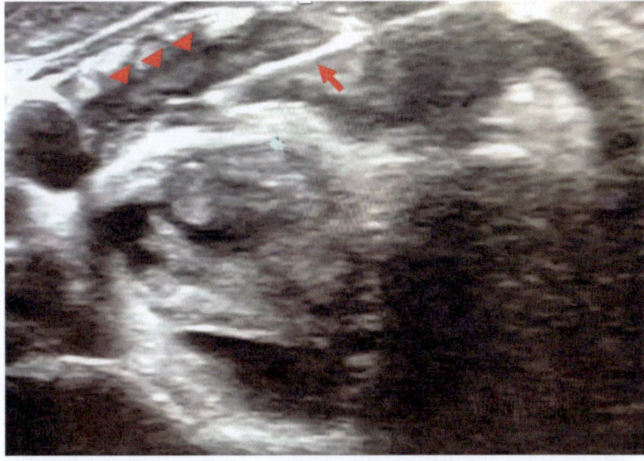

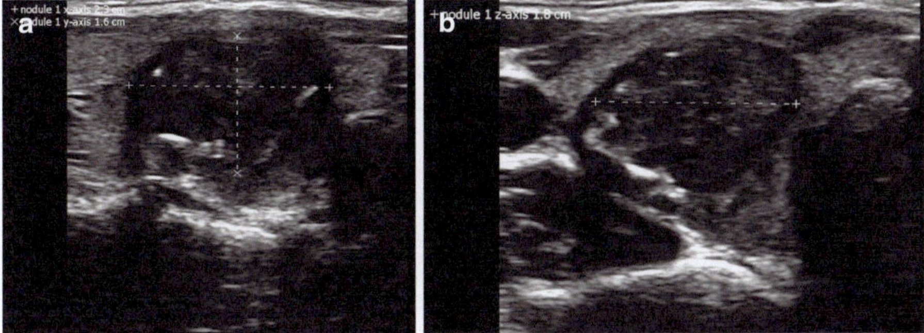

Fig. 6.4 (**a**) Right mid-lower thyroid nodule 3 months post-ablation. The nodule is solid, very hypoechoic with irregular borders and macrocalcifications; no intranodular vascularity was identified. This is a classic post-thermal ablation appearance of nodules that are often read as TIRADS 5 or ATA high suspicion and recommendation for sampling. Sagittal view. (**b**) Transverse view

reduction ratio (VRR) is calculated as ([initial volume − final volume] × 100)/initial volume [29]. It is important to note that ablated nodules often appear as very hypoechoic, solid tumors with irregular borders with occasional internal microcalcifications, which would otherwise be very suspicious characteristics (Fig. 6.4).

Discussion

With the increased use of diagnostic imaging, the incidence of benign thyroid nodules is increasing. Despite the widespread use of RFA in the treatment of benign nodules in countries such as Korea, the United States has been much slower to adopt the techniq has been much slower to adopt the technique. Factors such as cost as well as the paucity of long-term data have contributed to the reluctance. The growing evidence of the safety and efficacy of RFA have led to a surge of interest in learning and offering this minimally invasive technique in the United States. However, there remain important considerations.

Complications

Patients often misperceive these less invasive TA techniques to be "no risk" procedures. However, there have been documented associated major and minor complications with these procedures (Table 6.1). Major complications include nerve damage, nodule rupture, permanent hypothyroidism, and needle-track seeding [30]. The incidence of nerve damage with RFA range from 1.0 to 2.0% [31]. The recurrent laryngeal nerve is most commonly injured. Damage to the vagus nerve, brachial plexus, sympathetic ganglion, and other cranial nerves are also possible [32]. The Korean Society of Thyroid Radiology performed a multicenter retrospective study to delineate the complications encountered in the treatment of benign thyroid nodules with RFA [33]. Of the 1543 nodules studied, the patients with voice changes all had nodules located close to the recurrent laryngeal nerve. The voice change happened either during or immediately after the procedure with complete recovery of the voice 1–3 months post-procedure. Another patient complained of numbness and decreased sensation in the ipsilateral fourth and fifth fingers post-procedure, which gradually recovered after 2 months. If suspecting nerve damage, infusion of cold 5% dextrose in water at 0 °C around the nerve can help protect the nerve from further damage [28]. Nodule ruptures have been documented to occur between 7 and 50 days after the procedure with patients experiencing sudden onset of neck bulging and pain. US shows anterior thyroid capsule breakdown and a new anterior neck mass. Antibiotics and other supportive measures have been used in the setting of nodule ruptures. Permanent hypothyroidism has been reported secondary to RFA, for which the patient was placed on thyroid hormone supplementation. Transient hypothyroidism has also been reported, resolving by one-year post-procedure [33, 34]. Needle-track seeding is an extremely rare complication with only two reported cases after RFA of thyroid nodules [35, 36]. Minor complications include pain, hematoma, skin burn, transient thyroiditis due to an inflammatory process, fever, and post-procedure vomiting/vasovagal reaction [2, 8–11, 18, 24, 33–35, 37–52].

Marginal Regrowth

In the treatment of thyroid nodules using RFA, it is important to quantify regrowth of the nodule post-procedure. Sim et al. defined regrowth as an increase of >50% of the nodule compared to the smallest previously recorded post-procedure volume [53]. Marginal regrowth refers to the growth from insufficiently treated peripheral portions of the nodule, most commonly as a result of a larger initial nodule volume. In order to track the volume of nodule after RFA, Sim et al. divided the data into three categories: total volume, ablated volume, and viable volume [53]. Additional ablation is considered when the rate of increasing viable volume exceeds the rate of

Table 6.1 Summary of incidence, symptoms, and management principles of major and minor complications in RFA of thyroid nodules

	Complication	Incidence	Symptoms/findings	Management
Minor	**Pain/burning sensation** [9–11, 24, 35, 37–48]	1.0–100.0%	– Mild pain at site of ablation – Can radiate to head, gonial angle, ear, shoulder, jaw, teeth	– Oral analgesics (i.e., NSAIDs, acetaminophen) – Ice packs
	Hematoma/ hemorrhage [2, 33, 43, 44, 49, 50]	0.9–17.0%	– Asymptomatic to pain/swelling – Hyperechoic lesions found on US	– Usually self-resolving – Mild pressure can prevent worsening
	Vomiting/ vasovagal reactions [33, 34, 44]	0.4–2.5%	– Nausea/vomiting usually after ablation is completed – Bradycardia, defecation, sweating, dyspnea	– Antiemetics – Elevate legs – Stop ablation
	Skin burn [8, 33, 51, 52]	0.27–3.7%	– Erythematous skin – Discomfort around RFA site	– Ice packs – Oral analgesics – Surgical repair of serious skin burns
	Transient thyroiditis [18]	One case reported	– Asymptomatic – Abnormal post-procedure lab values	– Self-resolving – Serial blood tests to confirm resolution
	Fever [33, 40, 44, 45]	5.3–12.5%	– Mild-moderate fevers up to 38.5 °C	– Self-resolving – Anti-pyretic medications – Close follow-up
Major	**Nerve damage** [11, 18, 23, 32–34, 37, 53–55]	1.0–2.0%	– Voice changes, palpitations, shoulder weakness, new-onset Horner's syndrome, paresthesia	– Infuse cold solution (5% dextrose at 0 °C) – Steroids – Stop ablation
	Nodule rupture [33, 34, 53, 56]	0.2–0.5%	– Rapidly developing neck bulging – Pain at RFA site	– US/CT scan to confirm rupture – Aspirate contents if not self-resolving – Incision and drainage – Antibiotics
	Needle-seed tracking [35, 36]	Two cases reported	– Post-procedure masses around the needle track – Increased volume of nodules or lack of reduction in volume	– Surgical excision
	Permanent hypothyroidism [33]	One case reported	– Asymptomatic – Abnormal post-procedure lab values	– Thyroid hormone supplementation in patients who do not recover spontaneously

decreasing ablated volume. The potential to require multiple ablation sessions contributes to the hesitancy of performing RFA [25]. However, Huh et al. report that in nodules <20 mL, receiving an additional RFA session 1 month from the initial procedure did not show a significant difference in the 1-year follow-up results compared to undergoing only one ablation session. Additionally, there are vascular ablation techniques to limit nodule regrowth. Park et al. describe the artery-first ablation technique and the marginal venous ablation technique [22]. The artery-first technique applies to nodules with a tumor-feeding artery by first ablating the artery in order to minimize the heat-sink effect as well as to reduce the potential for nodule hemorrhage [22]. The marginal venous ablation technique not only minimizes the heat-sink effect but also allows for a complete ablation, reducing marginal regrowth [54].

Numerous studies have used VRR of solid nodules as a measure of effectiveness of RFA with 5 years as the maximum follow-up with VRR ranging between 50 and 80% [10–12]. Baek et al. conducted a randomized control trial on solid nodules, showing a VRR of 79.7 ± 14.6% at 6 months in contrast with the control group, which showed an increase in nodule volume [17]. Furthermore, a meta-analysis of studies with long-term follow-up of more than 3 years after RFA was performed showed that the pooled VRRs increased to 92% at the last follow-up, confirming the long-term efficacy of RFA as a treatment modality [55].

Potential Malignancy Risk

Controversy exists about whether RFA can induce neoplastic transformation in residual thyroid tissue. Although sonographically, post-ablated nodules behave in a benign fashion, there is a dearth of cytologic confirmation. Ha et al. performed core needle biopsies on 16 benign nodules previously treated with RFA. The biopsies were performed between 1 and 80 months following their RFA procedure with a mean interval of 37.5 months. On histopathological examination, there were no atypical cells or neoplastic changes that were detected in the undertreated peripheral portion. Additionally, the thyroid capsule was not altered nor was there evidence of perithyroidal fibrosis that could impact potential future thyroid surgery [56].

Studies have demonstrated that FNA-proven benign thyroid nodules still have malignancy potential between 2 and 6% [57, 58]. Although two separate FNAs are required prior to performing RFA on any given benign thyroid nodule, there is always a risk of sampling error causing malignancy to be missed [16]. Unfortunately, RFA does not allow for post-procedure pathological analysis of the nodule. However, the indolent nature of microcarcinoma typically behaves in a way that it may never progress to metastasis [31]. There is increasing evidence that RFA may be a safe alternative for the treatment of low-risk papillary thyroid microcarcinomas, and therefore would likely adequately treat any small incidental papillary thyroid microcarcinomas that may exist in large nodules undergoing TA. Additionally, RFA is increasingly used for treatment of recurrent thyroid cancers at the thyroidectomy bed as well as cervical lymph nodes in patients who are poor surgical candidates.

Case Conclusion

The patient underwent RFA of her right-sided nodule and was seen in a follow-up one-month post-procedure. On sonographic examination, her nodule was measured to be 21 × 32 × 20 mm, a 68% reduction in size. It was solid, hypoechoic, with macrocalcifications, indicative of a typical post-ablative appearance. Her symptom score was 3, the cosmetic score was 2. At 3 months post-procedure, the patient was seen again in follow-up appointment. This time, her thyroid nodule again demonstrated a classic post-ablative appearance and was measured to be 23 x 16 x 18 mm, an 84% reduction in size from the original nodule (Fig. 6.5). Her symptom score

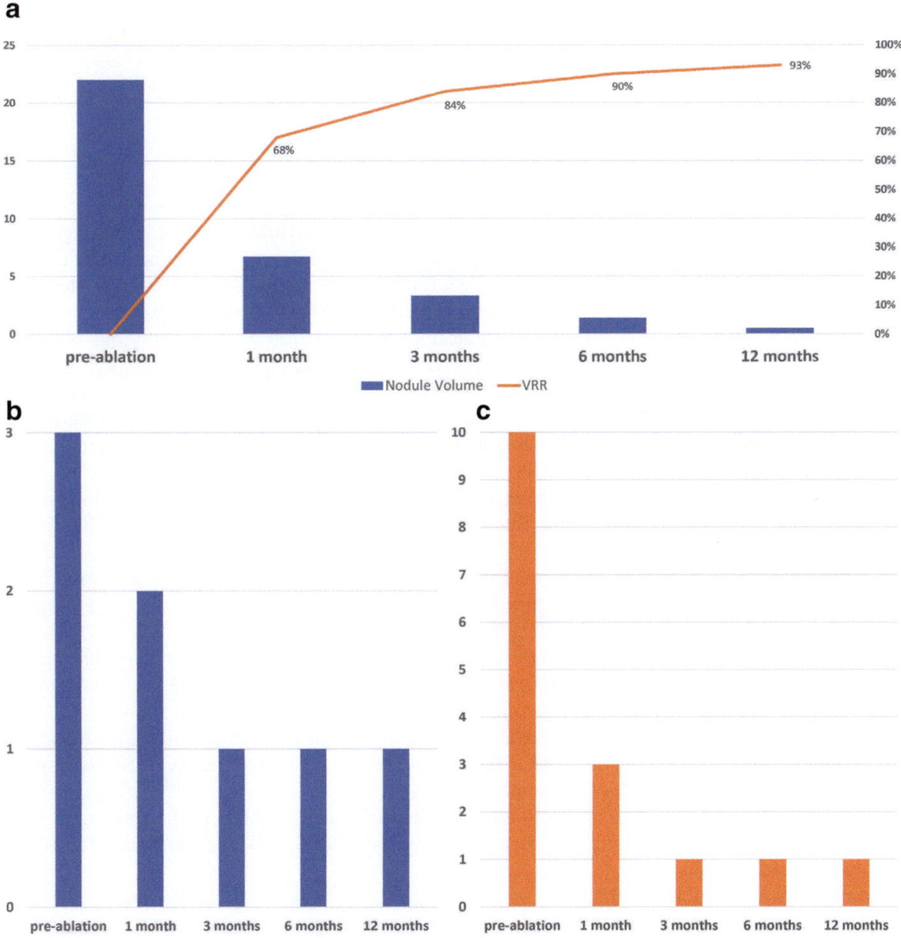

Fig. 6.5 (**a**) VRR at 1 month, 3 months, 6 months, and 12 months after RFA ablation of thyroid nodule. (**b**) Reduction in symptom score after RFA. (**c**) Reduction in cosmetic score after RFA

was 1, cosmetic score was 1. At 6 months and 12 months post-procedure, her thyroid nodule volume continued to decrease to 97% reduction in size.

Summary

- RFA is a minimally invasive, safe, and effective option in the treatment of benign thyroid nodules.
- Rare major and minor complications associated with RFA have been described; most patients recover spontaneously from complications.
- The trans-isthmic and moving-shot techniques as well as hydrodissection and vascular ablation techniques are methods to reduce RFA complications.
- Studies have used VRR to gauge the efficacy of RFA, ranging from 50 to 80% in follow-up.

References

1. Haugen BR, Alexander EK, Bible KC, et al. American Thyroid Association Management guidelines for adult patients with thyroid nodules and differentiated thyroid cancer: the American Thyroid Association guidelines task force on thyroid nodules and differentiated thyroid cancer. Thyroid. 2015;2016(1):26. https://doi.org/10.1089/thy.2015.0020.
2. Jeong WK, Baek JH, Rhim H, et al. Radiofrequency ablation of benign thyroid nodules: safety and imaging follow-up in 236 patients. Eur Radiol. 2008;18(6) https://doi.org/10.1007/s00330-008-0880-6.
3. Adam MA, Thomas S, Youngwirth L, et al. Is there a minimum number of thyroidectomies a surgeon should perform to optimize patient outcomes? Ann Surg. 2017;265(2) https://doi.org/10.1097/SLA.0000000000001688.
4. Pacella CM, Bizzarri G, Guglielmi R, et al. Thyroid tissue: US-guided percutaneous interstitial laser ablation—A feasibility study. Radiology. 2000;217(3) https://doi.org/10.1148/radiology.217.3.r00dc09673.
5. Cheng Z, Che Y, Yu S, et al. US-guided percutaneous radiofrequency versus microwave ablation for benign thyroid nodules: a prospective Multicenter study. Sci Rep. 2017;7(1) https://doi.org/10.1038/s41598-017-09930-7.
6. Leggett LE, Soril LJJ, Lorenzetti DL, et al. Radiofrequency ablation for chronic low back pain: a systematic review of randomized controlled trials. Pain Res Manag. 2014;19(5) https://doi.org/10.1155/2014/834369.
7. Rhim H, Goldberg SN, Dodd GD, et al. Essential techniques for successful radio-frequency thermal ablation of malignant hepatic tumors. Radiographics. 2001;(SPEC.ISS):21. https://doi.org/10.1148/radiographics.21.suppl_1.g01oc11s17.
8. Kim YS, Rhim H, Tae K, Park DW, Kim ST. Radiofrequency ablation of benign cold thyroid nodules: initial clinical experience. Thyroid. 2006;16(4) https://doi.org/10.1089/thy.2006.16.361.
9. Deandrea M, Limone P, Basso E, et al. US-guided percutaneous radiofrequency thermal ablation for the treatment of solid benign hyperfunctioning or compressive thyroid nodules. Ultrasound Med Biol. 2008;34(5) https://doi.org/10.1016/j.ultrasmedbio.2007.10.018.
10. Faggiano A, Ramundo V, Assanti AP, et al. Thyroid nodules treated with percutaneous radiofrequency thermal ablation: a comparative study. J Clin Endocrinol Metab. 2012;97(12) https://doi.org/10.1210/jc.2012-2251.

11. Cesareo R, Pasqualini V, Simeoni C, et al. Prospective study of effectiveness of ultrasound-guided radiofrequency ablation versus control group in patients affected by benign thyroid nodules. J Clin Endocrinol Metab. 2015;100(2) https://doi.org/10.1210/jc.2014-2186.

12. Spiezia S, Garberoglio R, Milone F, et al. Thyroid nodules and related symptoms are stably controlled two years after radiofrequency thermal ablation. Thyroid. 2009;19(3) https://doi.org/10.1089/thy.2008.0202.

13. Hamidi O, Callstrom MR, Lee RA, et al. Outcomes of radiofrequency ablation therapy for large benign thyroid nodules: a Mayo Clinic case series. Mayo Clin Proc. 2018;93(8) https://doi.org/10.1016/j.mayocp.2017.12.011.

14. Shin JH, Baek JH, Chung J, et al. Ultrasonography diagnosis and imaging-based management of thyroid nodules: revised Korean society of thyroid radiology consensus statement and recommendations. Korean J Radiol. 2016;17(3) https://doi.org/10.3348/kjr.2016.17.3.370.

15. Papini E, Monpeyssen H, Frasoldati A, Hegedüs L. European Thyroid Association clinical practice guideline for the use of image-guided ablation in benign thyroid nodules. Eur Thyroid J. 2020;2020, 9(4) https://doi.org/10.1159/000508484.

16. Kim JH, Baek JH, Lim HK, et al. Thyroid radiofrequency ablation guideline: Korean society of thyroid radiology. Korean J Radiol. 2017;2018(4):19. https://doi.org/10.3348/kjr.2018.19.4.632.

17. Baek JH, Kim YS, Lee D, Huh JY, Lee JH. Benign predominantly solid thyroid nodules: prospective study of efficacy of sonographically guided radiofrequency ablation versus control condition. Am J Roentgenol. 2010;194(4) https://doi.org/10.2214/AJR.09.3372.

18. Bernardi S, Dobrinja C, Fabris B, et al. Radiofrequency ablation compared to surgery for the treatment of benign thyroid nodules. Int J Endocrinol. 2014;2014 https://doi.org/10.1155/2014/934595.

19. Lee JH, Kim YS, Lee D, Choi H, Yoo H, Baek JH. Radiofrequency ablation (RFA) of benign thyroid nodules in patients with incompletely resolved clinical problems after ethanol ablation (EA). World J Surg. 2010;34(7) https://doi.org/10.1007/s00268-010-0565-6.

20. Jang SW, Baek JH, Kim JK, et al. How to manage the patients with unsatisfactory results after ethanol ablation for thyroid nodules: role of radiofrequency ablation. Eur J Radiol. 2012;81(5) https://doi.org/10.1016/j.ejrad.2011.02.039.

21. Baek JH, Ha EJ, Choi YJ, Sung JY, Kim JK, Shong YK. Radiofrequency versus ethanol ablation for treating predominantly cystic thyroid nodules: a randomized clinical trial. Korean J Radiol. 2015;16(6) https://doi.org/10.3348/kjr.2015.16.6.1332.

22. Park HS, Baek JH, Park AW, Chung SR, Choi YJ, Lee JH. Thyroid radiofrequency ablation: updates on innovative devices and techniques. Korean J Radiol. 2017;18(4) https://doi.org/10.3348/kjr.2017.18.4.615.

23. Lim HK, Baek JH, Lee JH, et al. Efficacy and safety of radiofrequency ablation for treating locoregional recurrence from papillary thyroid cancer. Eur Radiol. 2015;25(1) https://doi.org/10.1007/s00330-014-3405-5.

24. Ahn HS, Kim SJ, Park SH, Seo M. Radiofrequency ablation of benign thyroid nodules: evaluation of the treatment efficacy using ultrasonography. Ultrasonography. 2016;35(3) https://doi.org/10.14366/usg.15083.

25. Huh JY, Baek JH, Choi H, Kim JK, Lee JH. Symptomatic benign thyroid nodules: efficacy of additional radiofrequency ablation treatment session—prospective randomized study. Radiology. 2012;263(3) https://doi.org/10.1148/radiol.12111300.

26. Ha EJ, Baek JH, Lee JH. Moving-shot versus fixed electrode techniques for radiofrequency ablation: comparison in an ex-vivo bovine liver tissue model. Korean J Radiol. 2014;15(6) https://doi.org/10.3348/kjr.2014.15.6.836.

27. Xiaoyin T, Ping L, Dan C, et al. Risk assessment and hydrodissection technique for radiofrequency ablation of thyroid benign nodules. J Cancer. 2018;9(17) https://doi.org/10.7150/jca.26060.

28. Laeseke PF, Sampson LA, Brace CL, Winter TC, Fine JP, Lee FT. Unintended thermal injuries from radiofrequency ablation: protection with 5% dextrose in water. Am J Roentgenol. 2006;186(5 SUPPL) https://doi.org/10.2214/AJR.04.1240.

29. Tang X, Cui D, Chi J, et al. Evaluation of the safety and efficacy of radiofrequency ablation for treating benign thyroid nodules. J Cancer. 2017;8(5) https://doi.org/10.7150/jca.17655.

30. Sharma RK, Kuo JH. Complications of RFA for thyroid nodules: prevention and management. Curr Otorhinolaryngol Rep. 2021;9(1) https://doi.org/10.1007/s40136-020-00322-6.
31. Muhammad H, Santhanam P, Russell JO, Kuo JH. RFA and benign thyroid nodules: review of the current literature. Laryngoscope Investig Otolaryngol. 2021;6(1) https://doi.org/10.1002/lio2.517.
32. Chung SR, Baek JH, Choi YJ, Lee JH. Management strategy for nerve damage during radiofrequency ablation of thyroid nodules. Int J Hyperth. 2019;36(1) https://doi.org/10.1080/0265673 6.2018.1554826.
33. Baek JH, Lee JH, Sung JY, et al. Complications encountered in the treatment of benign thyroid nodules with us-guided radiofrequency ablation: a multicenter study. Radiology. 2012;262(1) https://doi.org/10.1148/radiol.11110416.
34. Kim C, Lee JH, Choi YJ, Kim WB, Sung TY, Baek JH. Complications encountered in ultrasonography-guided radiofrequency ablation of benign thyroid nodules and recurrent thyroid cancers. Eur Radiol. 2017;27(8) https://doi.org/10.1007/s00330-016-4690-y.
35. Oddo S, Spina B, Vellone VG, Giusti M. A case of thyroid cancer on the track of the radiofrequency electrode 30 months after percutaneous ablation. J Endocrinol Investig. 2017;40(1) https://doi.org/10.1007/s40618-016-0527-4.
36. Lee CU, Kim SJ, Sung JY, Park SH, Chong S, Baek JH. Needle track tumor seeding after radiofrequency ablation of a thyroid tumor. Jpn J Radiol. 2014;32(11) https://doi.org/10.1007/s11604-014-0350-9.
37. Aysan E, Idiz UO, Akbulut H, Elmas L. Single-session radiofrequency ablation on benign thyroid nodules: a prospective single center study: radiofrequency ablation on thyroid. Langenbeck's Arch Surg. 2016;401(3) https://doi.org/10.1007/s00423-016-1408-1.
38. Yoon HM, Baek JH, Lee JH, et al. Combination therapy consisting of ethanol and radiofrequency ablation for predominantly cystic thyroid nodules. Am J Neuroradiol. 2014;35(3) https://doi.org/10.3174/ajnr.A3701.
39. Ugurlu MU, Uprak K, Akpinar IN, Attaallah W, Yegen C, Gulluoglu BM. Radiofrequency ablation of benign symptomatic thyroid nodules: prospective safety and efficacy study. World J Surg. 2015;39(4) https://doi.org/10.1007/s00268-014-2896-1.
40. Spiezia S, Garberoglio R, di Somma C, et al. Efficacy and safety of radiofrequency thermal ablation in the treatment of thyroid nodules with pressure symptoms in elderly patients [5]. J Am Geriatr Soc. 2007;55(9) https://doi.org/10.1111/j.1532-5415.2007.01306.x.
41. Sung JY, Baek JH, Kim KS, et al. Single-session treatment of benign cystic thyroid nodules with ethanol versus radiofrequency ablation: a prospective randomized study. Radiology. 2013;269(1) https://doi.org/10.1148/radiol.13122134.
42. Sung JY, Baek JH, Jung SL, et al. Radiofrequency ablation for autonomously functioning thyroid nodules: a multicenter study. Thyroid. 2015;25(1) https://doi.org/10.1089/thy.2014.0100.
43. Korkusuz Y, Erbelding C, Kohlhase K, Luboldt W, Happel C, Grünwald F. Bipolar radiofrequency ablation of benign symptomatic thyroid nodules: initial experience. RoFo. 2016;188(7) https://doi.org/10.1055/s-0041-110137.
44. Valcavi R, Tsamatropoulos P. Health-related quality of life after percutaneous radiofrequency ablation of cold, solid, benign thyroid nodules: a 2-year follow-up study in 40 patients. Endocr Pract. 2015;21(8) https://doi.org/10.4158/EP15676.OR.
45. Deandrea M, Sung JY, Limone P, et al. Efficacy and safety of radiofrequency ablation versus observation for nonfunctioning benign thyroid nodules: a randomized controlled international collaborative trial. Thyroid. 2015;25(8) https://doi.org/10.1089/thy.2015.0133.
46. Kohlhase KD, Korkusuz Y, Gröner D, et al. Bipolar radiofrequency ablation of benign thyroid nodules using a multiple overlapping shot technique in a 3-month follow-up. Int J Hyperth. 2016;32(5) https://doi.org/10.3109/02656736.2016.1149234.
47. Bernardi S, Stacul F, Michelli A, et al. 12-month efficacy of a single radiofrequency ablation on autonomously functioning thyroid nodules. Endocrine. 2017;57(3) https://doi.org/10.1007/s12020-016-1174-4.

48. Yue WW, Wang SR, Lu F, et al. Radiofrequency ablation vs. microwave ablation for patients with benign thyroid nodules: a propensity score matching study. Endocrine. 2017;55(2)

49. Lim HK, Lee JH, Ha EJ, Sung JY, Kim JK, Baek JH. Radiofrequency ablation of benign non-functioning thyroid nodules: 4-year follow-up results for 111 patients. Eur Radiol. 2013;23(4) https://doi.org/10.1007/s00330-012-2671-3.

50. Zhao CK, Xu HX, Lu F, et al. Factors associated with initial incomplete ablation for benign thyroid nodules after radiofrequency ablation: first results of CEUS evaluation. Clin Hemorheol Microcirc. 2017;65(4) https://doi.org/10.3233/CH-16208.

51. Turtulici G, Orlandi D, Corazza A, et al. Percutaneous radiofrequency ablation of benign thyroid nodules assisted by a virtual needle tracking system. Ultrasound Med Biol. 2014;40(7) https://doi.org/10.1016/j.ultrasmedbio.2014.02.017.

52. Bernardi S, Lanzilotti V, Papa G, et al. Full-thickness skin burn caused by radiofrequency ablation of a benign thyroid nodule. Thyroid. 2016;26(1) https://doi.org/10.1089/thy.2015.0453.

53. Sim JS, Baek JH. Long-term outcomes following thermal ablation of benign thyroid nodules as an alternative to surgery: the importance of controlling regrowth. Endocrinol Metab. 2019;34(2) https://doi.org/10.3803/EnM.2019.34.2.117.

54. Wang B, Han ZY, Yu J, et al. Factors related to recurrence of the benign non-functioning thyroid nodules after percutaneous microwave ablation. Int J Hyperth. 2017;33(4) https://doi.org/10.1080/02656736.2016.1274058.

55. Cho SJ, Baek JH, Chung SR, Choi YJ, Lee JH. Long-term results of thermal ablation of benign thyroid nodules: a systematic review and meta-analysis. Endocrinol Metab. 2020;35(2) https://doi.org/10.3803/EnM.2020.35.2.339.

56. Ha SM, Shin JY, Baek JH, et al. Does radiofrequency ablation induce neoplastic changes in benign thyroid nodules: a preliminary study. Endocrinol Metab. 2019;34(2) https://doi.org/10.3803/EnM.2019.34.2.169.

57. Arora N, Scognamiglio T, Zhu B, Fahey TJ. Do benign thyroid nodules have malignant potential? An evidence-based review. World J Surg. 2008;32 https://doi.org/10.1007/s00268-008-9484-1.

58. Wang CCC, Friedman L, Kennedy GC, et al. A large multicenter correlation study of thyroid nodule cytopathology and histopathology. Thyroid. 2011;21(3) https://doi.org/10.1089/thy.2010.0243.

Chapter 7
Management of Low-risk Papillary Thyroid Cancer in a Patient with Familial Non-Medullary Thyroid Cancer

Wilson Alobuia and Electron Kebebew

Case Discussion

A 32-year-old woman presents to her surgeon after evaluation by her endocrinologist for management of a thyroid nodule. The patient reports a 3-month history of fatigue, intermittent neck pain, and difficulty swallowing. She denies any voice changes. She has no symptoms of hyper- or hypothyroidism. She has no significant past medical history. The patient underwent laparoscopic appendectomy 5 years ago for acute appendicitis. She takes daily multivitamins and contraceptive pills and is not allergic to any medications.

Her family history is significant for a history of differentiated thyroid cancer in multiple first- and second-degree relatives. Her 55-year-old mother underwent a total thyroidectomy at the age of 30 years for a thyroid nodule, pathology of which revealed a 3-cm papillary thyroid cancer (PTC). The patient also has two sisters, both of whom underwent total thyroidectomy in their twenties. Her older sister initially underwent a right thyroid lobectomy for a 3 cm thyroid "cyst" at the age of 26 years. She eventually required a completion total thyroidectomy and central neck lymph node dissection after she developed a recurrence. Final pathology revealed PTC with central neck lymph node metastases. Finally, her younger sister was diagnosed with a PTC at the age of 21 years (just a year prior to the patient's presentation). She underwent a total thyroidectomy and adjuvant radioactive iodine ablation. There is also a remote history of PTC in her maternal aunt, who reportedly "had some of her thyroid removed" in her late adult life. All affected family members have remained well and disease-free after their respective treatments.

Physical examination reveals a palpable thyroid nodule on the left side with no appreciable lymphadenopathy. A thyroid ultrasound showed a homogenous thyroid

W. Alobuia · E. Kebebew (✉)
Department of Surgery, Stanford University, Stanford, CA, USA
e-mail: walobuia@stanford.edu; kebebew@stanford.edu

© The Author(s), under exclusive license to Springer Nature Switzerland AG 2023
S. A. Roman et al. (eds.), *Controversies in Thyroid Nodules and Differentiated Thyroid Cancer*, https://doi.org/10.1007/978-3-031-37135-6_7

gland and an approximately 1.5 cm × 0.6 cm × 0.8 cm hypoechoic nodule in the left upper lobe, with regular margins and microcalcifications. There was no extrathyroidal extension, and no suspicious cervical lymph nodes in the central or lateral neck compartment identified on ultrasound. A fine needle aspiration biopsy was performed, and the cytologic features were consistent with PTC. Laboratory workup showed the patient was euthyroid and did not have anti-thyroglobulin or thyroid peroxidase antibodies.

Given the diagnosis of PTC and her significant family history of PTC, she was referred to an endocrine surgeon for evaluation and recommendations for surgical management. Faced with a patient with a strong family history of PTC, but an otherwise low-risk PTC, the surgeon deliberates on the extent of thyroidectomy.

Controversies in the Management of Low-risk PTC in the Setting of a Family History

The controversy underlying the surgical management of patients with low-risk PTC has been longstanding and requires complex decision-making [1–4]. Low-risk PTCs are defined as tumors measuring between 1 and 4 cm in maximum diameter, without extrathyroidal extension and no clinical (by physical examination) or radiographic (by ultrasonography) suspicion of lymph node metastases [5]. Controversy regarding the optimal surgical management of low-risk PTC has been enduring; partly because studies investigating the non-inferiority of thyroid lobectomy versus total thyroidectomy have not been performed in any prospective randomized controlled trials due to the large sample size and long-term follow-up that would be required of such a study [6–8]. As a result, recommendations for management and clinical practice guiding the management of patients with low-risk PTC have been based on retrospective data, almost all of which have inherent flaws related to methodology, data collection, and analytical and retrospective bias [8–10]. Based on retrospective studies that showed higher rates of overall survival and reduced rates of disease recurrence among patients with PTC who underwent total thyroidectomy [11–14], previous guidelines from the American Thyroid Association (ATA) recommended total thyroidectomy as the initial choice of surgical management for all patients with PTC greater than 1 cm in maximum diameter [15, 16]. However, more recent studies using institutional data, AND the National Cancer Database (NCDB) and the National Cancer Institute Surveillance, Epidemiology, and End Results (SEER) database, found no significant differences in the overall survival and rates of disease recurrence between thyroid lobectomy versus total thyroidectomy in patients with low-risk PTC [17–21]. A recent meta-analysis (including 16 studies and 175,430 patients) evaluating the impact of the extent of surgery on long-term outcomes of patients with low-risk differentiated thyroid cancer showed no statistically significant differences in the rates of recurrence, disease-free survival and disease-specific survival over a median follow-up period of seven to 10 years [22].

In a study that evaluated cost-effectiveness, thyroid lobectomy was found to be more cost-effective than total thyroidectomy for low-risk PTC [23]. Given these findings, the most recent guidelines from both the ATA in 2015 [5] and the National Comprehensive Cancer Network in 2018 [24] now recommend both thyroid lobectomy and total thyroidectomy as reasonable options for the management of low-risk PTC after careful evaluation by the patient's management team and based on patient preferences. While some subsequent studies have reported a higher trend in the use of thyroid lobectomy for thyroid cancer without the need for completion thyroidectomies [25, 26], others have reported that up to 58% of patients who undergo thyroid lobectomy may require completion thyroidectomies based on final histopathologic findings [27–29]. In general, the advantages of thyroid lobectomy include shorter operative time, lower rates of peri-operative complications, as well as the potential to avoid iatrogenic hypothyroidism. Conversely, total thyroidectomy may be preferred due to its lower risk of residual disease and disease recurrence by removing all multifocal and/or microscopic tumors [30, 31].

Family history plays an important role in the diagnosis and management of patients with PTC. There are two forms of inherited PTC: syndromic and nonsyndromic (Table 7.1). The majority of familial PTC are nonsyndromic (90%). Syndromic familial PTC includes Cowden's, DICER1, Werner's, and familial adenomatous polyposis syndromes, for which the susceptibility genes are known, and most patients are diagnosed by screening ultrasound because of positive germline mutation results. The natural history and outcome of patients with syndromic familial PTC appear to be similar to sporadic PTC, but there is scant literature to make any robust surgical management recommendations. Those for sporadic PTC are reasonable to use, except for the risk of the remaining thyroid gland to develop thyroid cancer due to the presence of a germline mutation. Nonsyndromic familial PTC has been defined based on two first-degree relatives who are affected with PTC, which is based on population-based studies that have depicted increased risk among patients with a family history of thyroid cancer [32]. However, we believe it should only be diagnosed in kindred with three or more first-degree relatives affected with PTC, based on prospective screening and surveillance studies we conducted that demonstrated that the rate of thyroid cancer is similar to the general population (4.6%) for those with only two affected first-degree relatives [33]. This is extremely important when interpreting the literature, as the susceptibility gene(s) for nonsyndromic familial PTC is not yet known and its classification is based on clinical criteria. Moreover, statistical simulation based on the incidence of thyroid cancer has shown that having two first-degree relatives affected with thyroid cancer can be a chance occurrence in 62–69% of such cases [34].

It is controversial whether familial PTC is more aggressive than sporadic PTC. In a meta-analysis performed by Wang and colleagues that included 12 studies with 12,741 patients, it was reported that patients with familial non-medullary thyroid cancer (mostly cases of classic and follicular variants of PTC) had a higher risk of disease recurrence and lower disease-free survival compared to those with sporadic disease [35]. They also found that patients with familial disease presented at a younger age, and had higher rates of multifocal and bilateral disease, extrathyroidal

Table 7.1 Nonsyndromic and syndromic familial thyroid cancers of follicular cell origin

Nonsyndromic	Susceptibility gene	Type of thyroid cancer	Clinical features
Isolated cases of thyroid cancer in first-degree relatives	Not known	PTC most common	Isolated family history of thyroid cancer. Early age of onset. Higher rate of multifocal and bilateral tumors, extrathyroidal extension, and lymph node metastasis. Possible higher rate of recurrence. Disease may be more aggressive in index case
Syndrome	**Susceptibility gene(s)**	**Type of thyroid cancer**	**Clinical features**
Cowden syndrome	*PTEN*	PTC, FTC	Hamartomas and epithelial tumors of the breast, kidney, colon, endometrium, and brain; mucocutaneous lesions; macrocephaly
Werner syndrome	*WRN*	PTC, FTC, ATC	Premature aging; scleroderma-like skin changes; cataracts; premature graying and/ or thinning of scalp hair; short stature
Carney complex	*PRKAR1*	PTC, FTC	Myxomas of soft tissues; skin and mucosal pigmentation (blue nevi); schwannomas; tumors of the adrenals, pituitary gland, and testicles
Familial adenomatous polyposis	*APC*	PTC	Multiple adenomatous polyps with malignant potential lining mucosa of GI tract, particularly colon
Pendred syndrome	*SLC26A4, FOXI1, KCNJ10*	PTC, FTC, ATC	Hearing impairment and benign multinodular goiter
Ataxia-telangiectasia	*ATM*	PTC	Impaired coordination of voluntary movements (cerebral ataxia); apraxia of eye movements; oculocutaneous telangiectasia; the absence or rudimentary appearance of a thymus; immunodeficiency; lymphoid tumors; insulin-resistant diabetes; and radiosensitivity
Bannayan-Riley-Ruvalcaba syndrome	*PTEN*	PTC, FTC	Macrocephaly; intestinal hamartomatous polyps; lipomas; pigmented maculae of the glans penis; developmental delay and mental retardation
DICER1 syndrome	*DICER1*	DTC	Familial pleuropulmonary blastoma; cystic nephroma; ovarian Sertoli-Leydig cell tumors
Peutz-Jeghers syndrome	*STK11*	PTC, DTC	Hamartomatous polyps in the gastrointestinal tract; epithelial malignancies, such as pancreas, breast, uterus, ovaries, and testes

Table 7.1 (continued)

PTEN hamartoma tumor syndrome	*PTEN, SDH, PIK3CA, C16ORF72, PTPN2, SEC23B, KLLN*	FTC	Cowden syndrome; Bannayan-Riley-Ruvalcaba syndrome; Proteus syndrome; and Proteus-like syndrome

PTC papillary thyroid cancer, *FTC* follicular thyroid cancer, *ATC* anaplastic thyroid cancer, *DTC* differentiated thyroid cancer

extension, and cervical lymph node metastases [35]. Specifically, in most, but not all studies, familial PTC has been associated with more aggressive features and higher rates of disease recurrence, as well as lower overall survival [36–40]. While family history is not routinely utilized in the assessment of low- versus high-risk PTC, it is of importance and should be considered when faced with a patient with PTC and a family history of PTC in three or more first-degree relatives.

Studies evaluating the influence of family history on patient outcomes after thyroid lobectomy versus total thyroidectomy are limited. Several reports have shown that patients with familial PTC have more biologically aggressive diseases [37, 40, 41]. Capezzone et al., in their study comparing the long-term clinical outcomes in patients with familial versus sporadic PTC, found that while patients with familial PTC were more likely to have bilateral tumors and had more aggressive clinico-pathological features, the long-term outcomes were not different between the two groups [41]. It is noteworthy, however, that patients with familial PTC had higher rates of persistent disease at short-term follow-up (1–2 years after initial treatment) [41]. Similarly, family history has not significantly been associated with poor prognosis in patients with PTC in a retrospective, individual risk factor-matched cohort study [42], as well as in a single institutional study of 42 patients [43]. Another recent study evaluating the risk of requiring completion thyroidectomy among patients with low-risk PTC found that family history was not an independent predictor of the final surgical management [44]. Family history, however, was associated with a higher likelihood of disease recurrence in other studies [40, 45, 46]. As a result, patients with family history tend to undergo higher rates of total thyroidectomy, compared to those without family history.

It is clear that the extent of surgery in the management of patients with low-risk PTC is controversial. However, the overall low risk of disease recurrence and comparable rates of overall survival seen in numerous recent studies suggests that thyroid lobectomy may indeed be a safe option for patients with low-risk PTC. However, in the presence of a significant family history (three or more affected first-degree relatives), total thyroidectomy may be a better operative choice, given the higher risk of harboring microscopic disease (multifocal tumors and bilateral disease) and the risk for disease recurrence. It is important, however, that all relative risks and benefits of the proposed surgery are fully discussed with the patient in detail (especially in a patient with significant family history), as they may have a significant influence on patient decision-making. In patients diagnosed with low-risk PTC in a prospective screening protocol with a family history of nonsyndromic differentiated thyroid cancer, we presented both surgical treatment options (thyroid lobectomy or total thyroidectomy) and 23.5% of patients elected to undergo thyroid lobectomy [33]. In comparison, 17.6% of patients underwent therapeutic lymph node dissection due to central neck lymph node metastases detected at the time of thyroidectomy that was not seen on preoperative ultrasound [33]. The final decision regarding the extent of surgery should, therefore, depend heavily on a discussion involving all members of the multidisciplinary care team: the patient, endocrinologist, and endocrine surgeon.

Case Summary and Evidence-Based Recommendations for Management

The case at the beginning of this chapter involves a 32-year-old woman without a significant past medical or surgical history with a newly diagnosed 1.5 cm PTC without clinical or radiographic evidence of lymphadenopathy. She has a significant family history of PTC in three first-degree relatives, all of whom required total thyroidectomy. One relative required a completion thyroidectomy for a "benign" neck mass after pathology revealed PTC.

Table 7.2 Important factors to consider when determining the appropriate extent of thyroidectomy in a patient with low-risk PTC and a family history of differentiated thyroid cancer

Factors to consider	Thyroid lobectomy	Total thyroidectomy
Patient factors	• Prefers to avoid iatrogenic hypothyroidism. • Diagnosed on screening with small tumor. • Male sex.	• Prefers to have definitive evidence of cure. • Clinically presents with symptoms. • On thyroid hormone replacement. • Female sex[a].
Type of family history	• Two first-degree relatives affected.	• Three or more first-degree relatives affected including the patient being evaluated. • Family members with a history of advanced disease.
Preoperative diagnosis and laboratory findings	• Biopsy conclusive for classic papillary thyroid cancer. • TSH < 2.0 μIU/mL[a].	• Biopsy cannot exclude aggressive features and show lymphocytic infiltration. • TSH ≥ 2.0 μIU/mL[a]. • Positive for serum anti-thyroglobulin and or thyroid peroxidase antibodies[a].
Preoperative ultrasound imaging findings	• Solitary thyroid nodule.	• Multiple nodules even if smaller than 1 cm and no suspicious ultrasound features.

[a]Factors reported to be associated with a higher risk of postsurgical (hemithyroidectomy) hypothyroidism include female sex, TSH ≥ 2.0 μIU/mL, and autoimmune thyroid disease (anti-thyroglobulin and or thyroid peroxidase antibodies, lymphocytic thyroiditis) [48]

The important factors to deliberate when considering the appropriate extent of thyroidectomy in a patient with low-risk PTC and familial nonsyndromic PTC are summarized in Table 7.2. According to the 2015 ATA consensus guideline on the management of low-to-intermediate-risk thyroid cancers (Recommendation 35): *"thyroid lobectomy alone is sufficient treatment for small, unifocal, intrathyroidal carcinomas in the absence of prior head and neck radiation, familial thyroid carcinoma, or clinically detectable cervical nodal metastases."* Considering this patient's significant history of familial PTC, thyroid lobectomy may not be appropriate, and it is therefore necessary to proceed with total thyroidectomy with the possibility of therapeutic central/lateral neck dissection, should there be any evidence of lymph node involvement at the time of surgery. While the data from currently available research show no significant differences in the outcomes between patients treated with thyroid lobectomy and total thyroidectomy, a history of PTC among first-degree relatives (three or more) theoretically places patients at a higher risk for multifocal and bilateral tumors, recurrence and more aggressive disease. As a result, these patients are more likely to benefit from total thyroidectomy. However, patients with familial PTC diagnosed by screening have been shown to have a lower extent of disease and can undergo less extensive treatment, depending on patient preference and commitment to close follow-up [33].

Given the controversy that exists related to the extent of surgical management of these patients, a multidisciplinary approach and inclusion of the patient in all decisions are essential in providing the best care for patients with familial PTC. In the discussion of all relative risks and benefits of thyroid lobectomy versus total thyroidectomy, it is also important to remind patients who are faced with this dilemma that total thyroidectomy (especially when performed by a high-volume thyroid surgeon) is safe, overall, and associated with a lower risk of/need for reoperation [47].

References

1. Haymart MR, Esfandiari NH, Stang MT, Sosa JA. Controversies in the management of low-risk differentiated thyroid cancer. Endocr Rev. 2017;38(4):351.
2. McDow AD, Pitt SC. Extent of surgery for low-risk differentiated thyroid cancer. Surg Clin North Am. 2019;99(4):599.
3. Liu WYX, Cheng R. Continuing controversy regarding individualized surgical decision-making for patients with 1-4 cm low-risk differentiated thyroid carcinoma: a systematic review. Eur J Surg Oncol. 2020;46:12.
4. McLeod DS, Sawka AM, Cooper DS. Controversies in primary treatment of low-risk papillary thyroid cancer. Lancet (London, England). 2013;381(9871):1046.
5. Haugen BR, Alexander EK, Bible KC, Doherty GM, Mandel SJ, Nikiforov YE, Pacini F, Randolph GW, Sawka AM, Schlumberger M, Schuff KG, Sherman SI, Sosa JA, Steward DL, Tuttle RM, Wartofsky L. 2015 American Thyroid Association management guidelines for adult patients with thyroid nodules and differentiated thyroid cancer: the American Thyroid Association guidelines task force on thyroid nodules and differentiated thyroid cancer. Thyroid. 2016;26:1.

6. Mazzaferri EL, Jhiang SM. Long-term impact of initial surgical and medical therapy on papillary and follicular thyroid cancer. Am J Med. 1994;97(5):418.
7. Udelsman R, Lakatos E, Ladenson P. Optimal surgery for papillary thyroid carcinoma. World J Surg. 1996;20(1):88.
8. Gibelli B, Dionisio R, Ansarin M. Role of hemithyroidectomy in differentiated thyroid cancer. Curr Opin Otolaryngol Head Neck Surg. 2015;23(2):99.
9. Sedgwick P. Retrospective cohort studies: advantages and disadvantages. BMJ (onlinw). 2014;348(nov08 1)
10. Sica GT. Bias in research studies. Radiology. 2006;238(3):780. https://doi.org/10.1148/radiol2383041109.
11. Hay ID, Grant CS, Bergstralh EJ, Thompson GB, van Heerden JA, Goellner JR. Unilateral total lobectomy: is it sufficient surgical treatment for patients with AMES low-risk papillary thyroid carcinoma? Surgery. 1998;124(6):958.
12. Bilimoria KY, Bentrem DJ, Ko CY, Steward AK, Winchester DP, Talamonti MS, et al. Extent of surgery affects survival for papillary thyroid cancer. Ann Surg. 2007;246(3):375.
13. Ito Y, Masuoka H, Fukushima M, Inoue H, Kihara M, Tomoda C, Higashiyama T, Takamura Y, Kobayashi K, Miya A, Miyauchi A. Excellent prognosis of patients with solitary T1N0M0 papillary thyroid carcinoma who underwent thyroidectomy and elective lymph node dissection without radioiodine therapy. World J Surg. 2010;34(6):1285.
14. Ebina A, Sugitani I, Fujimoto Y, Yamada K. Risk-adapted management of papillary thyroid carcinoma according to our own risk group classification system: is thyroid lobectomy the treatment of choice for low-risk patients? Surgery. 2014;156(6):1579.
15. Cooper DS, Doherty GM, Haugen BR, Kloos RT, Lee SL, Mandel SJ, Mazzaferri EL, McIver B, Pacini F, Schlumberger M, Sherman SI, Steward DL, Tuttle RM. Revised American Thyroid Association management guidelines for patients with thyroid nodules and differentiated thyroid cancer. Thyroid. 2009;19(11):1167.
16. Cooper DS, Doherty GM, Haugen BR, Kloos RT, Lee SL, Mandel SJ, Mazzaferri EL, McIver B, Sherman SI, Tuttle RM. Management guidelines for patients with thyroid nodules and differentiated thyroid cancer. Thyroid. 2006;16(2):109.
17. Díez JJ, Alcázar V, Iglesias P, Romero-Lluch A, Sastre J, Corral BP, Zafón C, Galofré JC, Pamplona MJ. Thyroid lobectomy in patients with differentiated thyroid cancer: an analysis of the clinical outcomes in a nationwide multicenter study. Gland Surg. 2021;10(2):678.
18. Barney BM, Hitchcock YJ, Sharma P, Shrieve DC, Tward JD. Overall and cause-specific survival for patients undergoing lobectomy, near-total, or total thyroidectomy for differentiated thyroid cancer. Head Neck. 2011;33(5):645.
19. Adam MA, Pura J, Gu L, Dinan MA, Tyler DS, Reed SD, Scheri R, Roman SA, Sosa JA. Extent of surgery for papillary thyroid cancer is not associated with survival: an analysis of 61,775 patients. Ann Surg. 2014;260(4):601.
20. Haigh PI, Urbach DR, Rotstein LE. Extent of thyroidectomy is not a major determinant of survival in low- or high-risk papillary thyroid cancer. Ann Surg Oncol. 2005;12(1):81.
21. Nixon IJ, Ganly I, Patel SG, Palmer FL, Whitcher MM, Tuttle RM, Shaha A, Shah JP. Thyroid lobectomy for treatment of well differentiated intrathyroid malignancy. Surgery. 2012;151(4):571.
22. Bojoga A, Koot A, Bonenkamp J, de Wilt J, IntHout J, Stalmeier P, Hermens R, Smit J, Ottevanger P, Netea-Maier R. The impact of the extent of surgery on the long-term outcomes of patients with low-risk differentiated non-medullary thyroid cancer: a systematic meta-analysis. J Clin Med. 2020;9(7):2316.
23. Lang BH, Wong CKH. Lobectomy is a more cost-effective option than Total thyroidectomy for 1 to 4 cm papillary thyroid carcinoma that do not possess clinically recognizable high-risk features. Ann Surg Oncol. 2016;23(11):3641.
24. Haddad RI, Nasr C, Bischoff L, Busaidy NL, Byrd D, Callender G, Dickson P, Duh QY, Ehya H, Goldner W, Haymart M, Hoh C, Hunt JP, Iagaru A, Kandeel F, Kopp P, Lamonica DM, McIver B, Raeburn CDRJA, Ringel MD, Scheri RP, Shah JP, Sippel R, Smallridge

RC, Sturgeon C, Wang TN, Wirth LJ, Wong RJ, Johnson-Chilla A, Hoffmann KG, Gurski LA. NCCN guidelines insights: thyroid carcinoma, version 2.2018. J Natl Compr Cancer Netw. 2018;16(12):1429.

25. Ullmann TM, Gray KD, Stefanova D, Limberg J, Buicko JL, Finnerty B, Zarnegar R, Fahey TJ, Beninato T. The 2015 American Thyroid Association guidelines are associated with an increasing rate of hemithyroidectomy for thyroid cancer. Surgery. 2019;166(3):349.

26. Toumi A, DiGennaro C, Vahdat V, Jalali MS, Gazelle GS, Chhatwal J, Kelz RR, Lubitz CC. Trends in thyroid surgery and guideline-concordant Care in the United States, 2007–2018. Thyroid. 2021;31(6):941.

27. Kluijfhout WP, Pasternak JD, Lim J, Kwon JS, Vriens MR, Clark OH, Shen WT, Gosnell JE, Suh I, Duh QY. Frequency of high-risk characteristics requiring Total thyroidectomy for 1-4 cm well-differentiated thyroid cancer. Thyroid. 2016;26(6):820.

28. Kluijfhout WP, Pasternak JD, Drake FT, Beninato T, Shen WT, Gosnell JE, Suh I, Liu C, Duh QY. Application of the new American Thyroid Association guidelines leads to a substantial rate of completion total thyroidectomy to enable adjuvant radioactive iodine. Surgery. 2017;161(1):127.

29. Anda Apiñániz E, Zafon C, Ruiz Rey I, Perdomo C, Pineda J, Alcalde J, García Goñi M, Galofré JC. The extent of surgery for low-risk 1-4 cm papillary thyroid carcinoma: a catch-22 situation. A retrospective analysis of 497 patients based on the 2015 ATA guidelines recommendation 35. Endocrine. 2020;70(3):538.

30. Kluijfhout WP, Rotstein LE, Pasternak JD. Well-differentiated thyroid cancer: thyroidectomy or lobectomy? Can Med Assoc J. 2016;188(17–18):E517.

31. Welch HG, Doherty GM. Saving thyroids—overtreatment of small papillary cancers. N Engl J Med. 2018;379(4):310.

32. Frank C, Fallah M, Sundquist J, Hemminki A, Hemminki K. Population landscape of familial cancer. Sci Rep. 2015;5:12891.

33. Klubo-Gwiezdzinska J, Yang L, Merkel R, Patel D, Nilubol N, Merino MJ, et al. Results of screening in familial non-medullary thyroid cancer. Thyroid. 2017;27(8):1017.

34. Charkes ND. On the prevalence of familial nonmedullary thyroid cancer in multiply affected kindreds. Thyroid. 2006;16(2):181.

35. Wang X, Cheng W, Li J, Su A, Wei T, Liu F, et al. Endocrine tumours: familial nonmedullary thyroid carcinoma is a more aggressive disease: a systematic review and meta-analysis. Eur J Endocrinol. 2015;172(6):R253.

36. Muallem Kalmovich L, Jabarin B, Koren S, Or K, Marcus E, Tkacheva I, Benbassat C, Steinschneider M. Is familial nonmedullary thyroid cancer a more aggressive type of thyroid cancer? Laryngoscope. 2021;131(2):E677.

37. El Lakis M, Giannakou A, Nockel PJ, Wiseman D, Gara SK, Patel D, Sater ZA, Kushchayeva YY, Klubo-Gwiezdzinska J, Nilubol N, Merino MJ, Kebebew E. Do patients with familial nonmedullary thyroid cancer present with more aggressive disease? Implications for initial surgical treatment. Surgery. 2019;165(1):50.

38. Kebebew E. Hereditary non-medullary thyroid cancer. World J Surg. 2008;32:5.

39. Klubo-Gwiezdzinska J, Yang L, Merkel R, Patel D, Nilubol N, Merino M, Skarulis M, Sadowski SM, Kebebew E. Results of screening in familial non-medullary thyroid cancer. Thyroid. 2017;27(8):1017.

40. Cao J, Can C, Chen C, Wang QL, Ge MH. Clinicopathological features and prognosis of familial papillary thyroid carcinoma—a large-scale, matched, case-control study. Clin Endocrinol. 2016;84(4):598.

41. Capezzone M, Fralassi N, Secchi C, Cantara S, Brilli L, Pilli T, Maino F, Forleo R, Pacini F, Cevenini G, Cartocci A, Castagna MG. Long-term clinical outcome in familial and sporadic papillary thyroid carcinoma. Eur Thyroid J. 2020;9(4):213.

42. Lee YM, Jeon MJ, Kim WW, Chung KW, Baek JH, Shong YK, Sung TY, Hong SJ. Comparison between familial and sporadic non-medullary thyroid carcinoma: a retrospective individual risk factor-matched cohort study. Ann Surg Oncol. 2021;28(3):1722.

43. Rosario PW, Calsolari MR. Should a family history of papillary thyroid carcinoma indicate more aggressive therapy in patients with this tumor? Arq Bras Endocrinol Metabol. 2014;58(8):812.
44. DiMarco AN, Wong MS, Jayasekara J, Cole-Clark D, Aniss A, Glover AR, Delbridge LW, Sywak MS, Sidhu SB. Risk of needing completion thyroidectomy for low-risk papillary thyroid cancers treated by lobectomy. BJS Open. 2019;3(3):299.
45. Jauculan MC, Buenaluz-Sedurante M, Jimeno CA. Risk factors associated with disease recurrence among patients with low-risk papillary thyroid cancer treated at the University of The Philippines-Philippine general hospital. Endocrinol Metab (Seoul, Korea). 2016;31(1):113.
46. Lee YM, Yoon JH, Yi O, Sung TY, Chung KW, Kim WB, Hong SJ. Familial history of non-medullary thyroid cancer is an independent prognostic factor for tumor recurrence in younger patients with conventional papillary thyroid carcinoma. J Surg Oncol. 2014;109(2):168.
47. Hauch A, Al-Qurayshi Z, Randolph G, Kandil E. Total thyroidectomy is associated with increased risk of complications for low- and high-volume surgeons. Ann Surg Oncol. 2014;21(12):3844.
48. Li Z, Qiu Y, Fei Y, Xing Z, Zhu J, Su A. Prevalence of and risk factors for hypothyroidism after hemithyroidectomy: a systematic review and meta-analysis. Endocrine. 2020;70(2):243.

Chapter 8
Intraoperative Nerve Monitoring in Thyroid Operations

Martin Almquist

Case

A 37-year-old woman, internationally renowned opera singer, is referred for a 1.5 × 1.7 cm large nodule in her left thyroid lobe. The ultrasonographic report describes an intrathyroidal, irregularly demarcated, calcified, hypoechoic nodule, classified as TiRADS 5. A fine-needle biopsy shows sparse cellularity, with some features suggestive of papillary thyroid cancer; it has been classified as Bethesda V. Serum calcitonin is below the detection limit, and serum thyroid function tests are normal. There is no clinical or ultrasonographical evidence of lymph node metastasis. The right thyroid lobe appears sonographically to be normal size, without any suspicious nodules. Family history is non-remarkable, and she has no radiation exposure.

The patient is otherwise healthy. She is worried about her nodule. She has considered several options but has decided that she wishes to have it removed. She is reluctant to undergo total thyroidectomy but would consent to lobectomy. She is dependent on her voice and wants to know how you as a thyroid surgeon will make sure her voice is not impaired by the surgery. She wants to know whether you use intraoperative neuromonitoring, if it lowers the risk of voice impairment after surgery, which type of neuromonitoring you use, and what your strategy is to preserve your patients' voice during surgery.

M. Almquist (✉)
Department of Surgery, Lund University, Lund, Sweden
e-mail: martin.almquist@med.lu.se

Importance of Recurrent and Superior Laryngeal Nerves for Voice

Voice impairment is common after thyroid surgery [1]. The most serious cause of voice impairment is damage to the recurrent laryngeal nerve (RLN). The importance of the RLN, and the peculiar, recurrent aspect of its anatomy was known already to Galen, who in the second century demonstrated that a piglet's squeal could be silenced by sectioning this nerve [2]. Loss of function of the RLN leads to immobility of the ipsilateral vocal cord, due to lack of neuromuscular activation of the vocal cord muscles, the thyroarytenoid, and the vocalis, which some authors also consider to be part of the thyroarytenoid. Vocal immobility can also cause impaired breathing, since the immobilized vocal cord obstructs airflow in the upper airway, or chronic cough as compensatory muscles can spasm. Bilateral vocal fold paralysis can cause complete obstruction of the upper airway and may require tracheostomy. The RLN also innervates muscles involved in swallowing, which is why dysphagia and aspiration often accompany voice impairment after RLN damage. Thus, minimizing the risk of damage to the RLN is of paramount importance in thyroid surgery, and especially so in patients depending on their voice for their livelihood, such as singers [1].

Throughout the history of thyroid surgery, most focus was placed on the RLN. The importance of the exterior branch of the superior laryngeal nerve (EBSLN) for voice modulation was not recognized until much later [3]. The case of the loss of the magic voice of the opera singer Amelita Galli Curci illustrates the dramatic consequences of loss of function of the EBSLN [4]. The EBSLN, referred to as the "neglected nerve" [5], has often been overlooked in thyroid surgery [6]. This nerve innervates the cricothyroid muscle (CTM), which is involved in producing sounds of higher pitch, in projecting the voice, and hence important for shouting, calling, and singing high-pitched notes. The EBSLN is a small nerve, and it runs along the superior thyroid vessels, after which it penetrates between the two heads of the cricothyroid muscle. The EBSLN is therefore at risk when dissecting the upper pole. Several anatomic variations of its relation to the upper pole of the thyroid and to the superior thyroid vessels have been observed. Well-recognized anatomical classifications of the relation between the EBSLN and the upper pole of the thyroid include Cernea's [7] and Friedman's [8]. Diagnosis of pre- and postoperative CTM function is difficult to ascertain, since it cannot be evaluated reliably with laryngoscopy. Instead, registration of CTM movement depends on electromyography, which requires needles to be placed in the CTM [9]. This is technically difficult and invasive, and not without risk and pain to the patient [9]. Evaluation of CTM function using acoustic analysis has been investigated but is too unreliable to be used in clinical practice [10].

Other potential causes of voice impairment after thyroid surgery, such as scarring, endotracheal intubation damage to the upper airway, and injury to the strap muscles, will not be covered in this chapter.

Intraoperative RLN and EBSLN Management

As late as 1933, Prioleau stated that "a nerve seen is a nerve injured." However, early thyroid surgeons, such as Lahey [11] realized the need for visual identification of the RLN to preserve its integrity. Due to its anatomy, with the distal part of the RLN running in the ligament of Berry, which attaches the thyroid gland to the trachea, the RLN is at risk of damage during thyroid surgery [12]. As noted, the EBSLN is also at risk, due to its small size, and its intimate relation with the superior pole and vessels of the thyroid. Nerve damage can be caused by transection, clamping, heat, and stretch. If a nerve is transected or otherwise permanently damaged, Wallerian degeneration [13] with axonal loss distal to the point of damage will occur. This causes permanent immobility of the muscles innervated by the nerve, i.e. the thyroarytenoid and vocalis muscles, and the cricothyroid muscle. Not surprisingly, damage to the RLN causes less morbidity if the ipsilateral EBSLN is preserved [14].

Electrical stimulation of the vagus proximal to the RLN branching, or stimulation of the RLN itself causes activation of the vocal cord muscles. This leads to a depolarization–repolarization sequence which can be recorded as an electromyogram (EMG). Electrodes on the endotracheal tube register this electrical activity in the vocal cord muscles and transmit a signal to a recording instrument, which displays a typical EMG curve on the screen [15]. One of the first reports on intraoperative neuromonitoring of the RLN in human thyroid surgery was published in 1970 [16]. Several groups in Germany developed and refined the technique. Today, a number of commercially and practically usable applications of IONM exist. IONM can be used intermittently (iIONM), or continuously (cIONM) [17]. In cIONM, a soft silicone electrode is attached to the vagus nerve [18], and the vagus nerve is continuously stimulated with a regular frequency.

Both the amplitude (the voltage elicited from the vocal cord muscles in the EMG) and the latency (the time in milliseconds from stimulation to activation) are registered in IONM. In cIONM, baseline values of amplitude and latency are established, and a reduction in amplitude or an increase in latency, signaling damage to the RLN, informs the surgeon of the risk of imminent damage to the RLN.

There have been no randomized trials comparing the risk of RLN damage with or without IONM; neither with intermittent nor continuous IONM. However, several large observational studies [19–21] strongly suggest that the risk of vocal cord paresis is lower if IONM is used during surgery. Hence, uptake of intermittent IONM has been strong. Surveys in Italy [22] and the US [23, 24] show that a majority of thyroid surgeons now use IONM. Continuous IONM has in single-center studies been reported to yield even better results, with a near total absence of RLN damage and vocal cord immobilization after thyroid surgery [25]. Inadvertent effects of cIONM seem to be rare; however, cardiac arrest has been reported [26].

The identification of the EBSLN is much facilitated by the use of IONM. The EBSLN is thin, often covered by the pharyngeal muscles, or intertwined with the vessels of the upper pole of the thyroid lobe. The interest in the EBSLN has increased in recent years, and some [6, 27] thyroid surgeons [23] but not all try to identify and preserve this nerve. Intraoperative electrical stimulation of the EBSLN results in contraction of the CTM, which can be observed as a "twitch" in this muscle, located on the anterior of the laryngeal cartilage. Recent developments in endotracheal tubes for neuromonitoring make it possible to also record the EMG of the CTM, making it visible on the neuromonitor [28]. Sometimes, a connection between the EBSLN and the RLN is present (Galens anastomosis). This is important—damage to both the EBSLN and the RLN is related to worse outcomes than damage to the RLN alone [14]. Several randomized trials have been performed, showing improved identification and less damage to the EBSLN, when IONM is used. This was summarized in a recent meta-analysis suggesting that by using IONM, the EBSLN can be identified and preserved in almost all thyroid operations [29]. Despite this strong evidence for the benefit of IONM in preserving EBSLN function, only a minority of surgeons attempt to identify and preserve this nerve during thyroid surgery [23].

Evidence Based Case Management

Every effort should be made to preserve the voice of this patient. Preoperative laryngoscopy is important, since it informs the surgeon about silent, non-clinical vocal cord immobility and any other potential abnormalities of the larynx. It also carries some potential legal implications.

Generally, an atraumatic technique should be used; dissection kept to a minimum; utmost care should be taken when intubating the patient.

A wealth of pre-clinical, clinical observational, and experimental data strongly suggests that intermittent intraoperative neuromonitoring, IONM, is related to a lower risk of damage to the recurrent and superior laryngeal nerves in thyroid surgery and that this translates to improved voice outcomes. Results from single-center studies regarding continuous intraoperative neuromonitoring (cIONM) show impressively low rates of RLN palsy; the benefits of cIONM remain to be proven in multicenter trials. Familiarity with the technique of IONM, pitfalls, and problem-solving algorithms, together with expert knowledge of thyroid, recurrent and superior laryngeal nerve anatomy, and experience in thyroid surgery, will yield the best outcomes for the individual patient.

References

1. Chandrasekhar SS, Randolph GW, Seidman MD, Rosenfeld RM, Angelos P, Barkmeier-Kraemer J, et al. Clinical practice guideline: improving voice outcomes after thyroid surgery. Otolaryngol Head Neck Surg (United States). 2013;148(6 SUPPL)
2. Gross CG. Galen and the squealing pig. Neuroscientist. 1998;4(3):216–21.

3. Kochilas X, Bibas A, Xenellis J, Anagnostopoulou S. Surgical anatomy of the external branch of the superior laryngeal nerve and its clinical significance in head and neck surgery. Clin Anat. 2008;21(2):99–105.

4. Marchese-Ragona R, Restivo DA, Mylonakis I, Ottaviano G, Martini A, Sataloff RT, et al. The superior laryngeal nerve injury of a famous soprano, Amelita Galli-Curci. Acta Otorhinolaryngol Ital [Internet]. 2013;33(1):67–71. Available from: http://www.ncbi.nlm.nih.gov/pubmed/23620644%0A; http://www.pubmedcentral.nih.gov/articlerender.fcgi?artid=PMC3631811

5. Delbridge L. The 'neglected' nerve in thyroid surgery: the case for routine identification of the external laryngeal nerve. ANZ J Surg. 2001;71(4):199. https://doi.org/10.1046/j.1440-1622.2001.02120.x.

6. Almquist M, Nordenström E. Management of the exterior branch of the superior laryngeal nerve among thyroid surgeons—results from a nationwide survey. Int J Surg. 2015;20:46.

7. Cernea CR, Ferraz AR, Nishio S, Dutra A, Hojaij FC, Dos Santos LRM. Surgical anatomy of the external branch of the superior laryngeal nerve. Head Neck [Internet]. 1992;14(5):380–3. https://doi.org/10.1002/hed.2880140507.

8. Friedman M, Wilson MN, Ibrahim H. Superior laryngeal nerve identification and preservation in thyroidectomy. Oper Tech Otolaryngol Head Neck Surg. 2009;20(2):145–51.

9. Sung ES, Chang JH, Kim J, Cha W. Is cricothyroid muscle twitch predictive of the integrity of the EBSLN in thyroid surgery? Laryngoscope. 2018;128(11):2654–61.

10. Aluffi P, Policarpo M, Cherovac C, Olina M, Dosdegani R, Pia F. Post-thyroidectomy superior laryngeal nerve injury. Eur Arch Oto-Rhino-Laryngol [Internet]. 2001;258(9):451–4. https://doi.org/10.1007/s004050100382.

11. Lahey F. Routine dissection and demonstration of the laryngeal nerve in subtotal thyroidectomy. Surg Obstet Gynecol. 1938;66:775–7.

12. Delbridge L. Total thyroidectomy: the evolution of surgical technique. ANZ J Surg. 2003;73(9):761–8.

13. Gordon T. Peripheral nerve regeneration and muscle reinnervation. Int J Mol Sci. 2020;21(22):1–24.

14. Pei YC, Lu YA, Wong AMK, Chuang HF, Li HY, Fang TJ. Two trajectories of functional recovery in thyroid surgery related unilateral vocal cord paralysis. Surg (United States). 2020;168(4):578–85.

15. Randolph GW, Dralle H. Electrophysiologic recurrent laryngeal nerve monitoring during thyroid and parathyroid surgery: international standards guideline statement. Laryngoscope. 2011;121(SUPPL. 1)

16. Flisberg K, Lindholm T. Electrical stimulation of the human recurrent laryngeal nerve during thyroid operation. Acta Otolaryngol. 1970;69(S263):63–7.

17. Schneider R, Machens A, Randolph GW, Kamani D, Lorenz K, Dralle H. Opportunities and challenges of intermittent and continuous intraoperative neural monitoring in thyroid surgery. Gland Surg. 2017;6(5):537–45.

18. Schneider R, Przybyl J, Hermann M, Hauss J, Jonas S, Leinung S. A new anchor electrode design for continuous neuromonitoring of the recurrent laryngeal nerve by vagal nerve stimulations. Langenbeck's Arch Surg. 2009;394(5):903–10.

19. Bergenfelz A, Salem AF, Jacobsson H, Nordenström E, Almquist M, Wallin GW, et al. Risk of recurrent laryngeal nerve palsy in patients undergoing thyroidectomy with and without intraoperative nerve monitoring. Br J Surg. 2016;103:13.

20. Abdelhamid A, Aspinall S. Intraoperative nerve monitoring in thyroid surgery: analysis of United Kingdom registry of endocrine and thyroid surgery database. Br J Surg. 2021;108(2):182–7.

21. Staubitz JI, Watzka F, Poplawski A, Riss P, Clerici T, Bergenfelz A, et al. Effect of intraoperative nerve monitoring on postoperative vocal cord palsy rates after thyroidectomy: European multicentre registry-based study. BJS Open. 2020;4(5):821–9.

22. Dionigi G, Lombardi D, Lombardi CP, Carcoforo P, Boniardi M, Innaro N, et al. Intraoperative neuromonitoring in thyroid surgery: a point prevalence survey on utilization, management, and documentation in Italy. Updat Surg. 2014;66(4):269–76.
23. Ritter A, Ganly I, Wong RJ, Randolph GW, Shpitzer T, Bachar G, et al. Intraoperative nerve monitoring is used routinely by a significant majority of head and neck surgeons in thyroid surgery and impacts on extent of surgery—Survey of the American Head and Neck society. Head Neck. 2020;42(8):1757–64.
24. Horne SK, Gal TJ, Brennan JA. Prevalence and patterns of intraoperative nerve monitoring for thyroidectomy. Otolaryngol Head Neck Surg. 2007;136(6):952–6.
25. Schneider R, Machens A, Sekulla C, Lorenz K, Elwerr M, Dralle H. Superiority of continuous over intermittent intraoperative nerve monitoring in preventing vocal cord palsy. Br J Surg. 2020:566–73.
26. Almquist M, Thier M, Salem F, Terris D. Cardiac arrest with vagal stimulation during intraoperative nerve monitoring. Head Neck. 2016;38
27. Barczyński M, Randolph GW, Cernea C. International survey on the identification and neural monitoring of the EBSLN during thyroidectomy. Laryngoscope. 2016;126(1):285–91.
28. Barczyński M, Randolph GW, Cernea CR, Dralle H, Dionigi G, Alesina PF, et al. External branch of the superior laryngeal nerve monitoring during thyroid and parathyroid surgery: international neural monitoring study group standards guideline statement. Laryngoscope. 2013;123(SUPPL. 4)
29. Naytah M, Ibrahim I, da Silva S. Importance of incorporating intraoperative neuromonitoring of the external branch of the superior laryngeal nerve in thyroidectomy: a review and meta-analysis study. Head Neck. 2019;41(6):2034–41.

Chapter 9
Extent of Surgery for Low-Risk Papillary Thyroid Cancer

Jessica Dahle and Hadiza S. Kazaure

Case

A 34-year-old woman with a history of anxiety presented to the office to discuss treatment options for a left-sided 1.5 cm thyroid nodule with cytology diagnostic of papillary thyroid cancer. On physical examination augmented by surgeon-directed ultrasound, the nodule was noted to be in the mid-left thyroid pole and measured 1.5 cm in greatest dimension. The nodule was hypoechoic, smooth, and did not appear to involve the thyroid capsule or trachea. No abnormal cervical lymph nodes were seen on sonography.

Introduction

Papillary thyroid cancer (PTC) is the most common subtype of thyroid carcinoma and the incidence has increased over the last several decades. This is in large part due to increased diagnosis of microcarcinomas [1, 2]. PTC is approximately three times more common in females than males. Studies have postulated that thyroid cancer may soon become the third or fourth most common cancer diagnosis among women; disease-specific mortality remains low [2–4].

J. Dahle
Department of Surgery, Section of Endocrine Surgery, Duke University Medical Center, Durham, NC, USA

Endocrine and General Surgery, Ochsner Health, New Orleans, LA, USA
e-mail: jessica.dahle@ochsner.org

H. S. Kazaure (✉)
Department of Surgery, Section of Endocrine Surgery, Duke University Medical Center, Durham, NC, USA
hadiza.kazaure@duke.edu

© The Author(s), under exclusive license to Springer-Nature Switzerland AG 2023
S. A. Roman et al. (eds.), *Controversies in Thyroid Nodules and Differentiated Thyroid Cancer*, https://doi.org/10.1007/978-3-031-37135-6_9

In recognition of the relatively indolent behavior and overall favorable prognosis of PTC, evidence-based support for the reclassification of one low-risk variant of PTC to a noninvasive thyroid neoplasm, revision of the well-differentiated thyroid cancer staging system, and adoption of more conservative treatment strategies for the management of PTC have followed [4, 5]. The current 2015 American Thyroid Association (ATA) guidelines allow flexibility between total thyroidectomy and lobectomy for low-risk PTC—tumors that are less than 4 cm in size and are without evidence of extra-thyroidal extension or nodal disease (in patients without a family history of thyroid cancer or personal history of radiation to the head and neck) [5]. In addition, there has been growing evidence in support of nonoperative management—*active surveillance*—for select low-risk PTCs [6–11]. At present, the management of low-risk PTC espouses individualization of oncologic therapy, and this is heavily dependent on fine-tuned risk stratification and patient preference.

Risk Stratification

Once a diagnosis of PTC is made, risk stratification dictates appropriate management. In conjunction with a thorough physical examination assessing for mobility of the thyroid gland, voice quality, and lymphadenopathy, ultrasonographic assessment of the neck assessing for extracapsular extension, involvement of surrounding structures such as strap muscles, as well as presence of abnormal central and lateral neck lymph nodes constitute the first steps toward risk stratification (Fig. 9.1). It is useful to review the fine-needle biopsy slides with an experienced pathologist. Although final diagnosis is made on final pathologic specimens, some aggressive variants, such as tall cell variant of PTC may have identifiable cytologic features on fine needle aspiration biopsy, and such features can influence management considerations [12, 13].

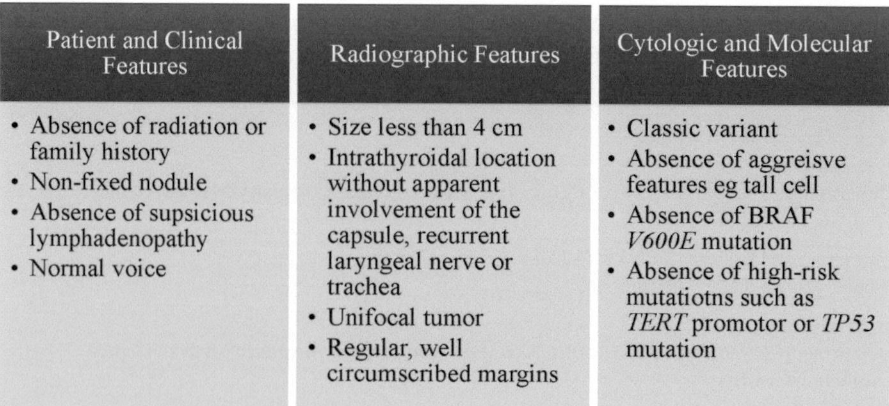

Patient and Clinical Features	Radiographic Features	Cytologic and Molecular Features
• Absence of radiation or family history • Non-fixed nodule • Absence of supsicious lymphadenopathy • Normal voice	• Size less than 4 cm • Intrathyroidal location without apparent involvement of the capsule, recurrent laryngeal nerve or trachea • Unifocal tumor • Regular, well circumscribed margins	• Classic variant • Absence of aggreisve features eg tall cell • Absence of BRAF *V600E* mutation • Absence of high-risk mutatiotns such as *TERT* promotor or *TP53* mutation

Fig. 9.1 General features of low-risk papillary thyroid cancers

Risk stratification of tumors based on molecular features could assist in determining appropriate treatment plans. The presence of BRAF *V600E* mutation compared to the wild-type allele is associated with extra-thyroidal extension, capsular invasion, and lymph node metastasis with increased risk of persistent or recurrent disease [14]. Additionally, the presence of *TERT* promoter and *TP53* mutations, which have been associated with a more aggressive papillary thyroid cancer and less favorable outcome when coexisting with BRAF *V600E* mutations, could sway management decisions [15, 16]. At present, there are no guidelines recommending the use of molecular testing to risk stratify PTC in order to determine *initial* treatment approach, however, as the molecular profiling of thyroid cancer becomes more refined, molecular testing could be useful in aiding the decision about the extent of initial surgery for PTC [16].

Management Strategies for Low-Risk PTC

Evolving understanding of the natural history and molecular basis of PTC has prompted a trend toward less aggressive management and individualized therapy. Historically treated with total thyroidectomy with/without neck dissection, along with adjuvant radioiodine therapy, current evidence-based practice for managing a 1.5-cm low-risk PTC as presented in this case, allows for consideration of thyroid lobectomy and potentially active surveillance. Nonetheless, the debate on appropriate management of low-risk PTC is ongoing.

Surgical Treatment

Operative management of PTC measuring <4 cm can involve either a lobectomy or total thyroidectomy (Fig. 9.2). For low-risk PTC, lobectomy has a survival rate similar to total thyroidectomy, even when stratified by tumor size [2, 17, 18]. Locoregional recurrence rate following thyroid lobectomy is estimated at less than 6% [18, 19]. Although the presence of the remaining thyroid lobe may obviate the need for lifelong exogenous thyroid hormone, up to 66% of patients may require thyroid replacement to maintain a euthyroid state [5, 20, 21].

Compared to total thyroidectomy, thyroid lobectomy is associated with fewer surgical complications (20.4% vs.10.8%, $p < 0.001$) including a lower risk of temporary hypocalcemia (relative risk [RR]: 3.17, 95% confidence interval [CI]:1.72–5.83), permanent hypocalcemia (RR: 1.69, 95% CI: 1.30–2.20), temporary recurrent laryngeal nerve injury (RR:1.69, 95% CI: 1.30–2.20), permanent recurrent laryngeal nerve injury (RR: 1.85, 95% CI 1.28–2.69), and hemorrhage (RR: 2.58, 95% CI: 1.69–3.93) [22–24]. Additionally, procedure charges are lower ($15,602 vs $19,365, $p < 0.0001$) and length of stay is shorter (1.29 vs 1.63 days, $p < 0.0001$) for thyroid lobectomy compared to total thyroidectomy [24].

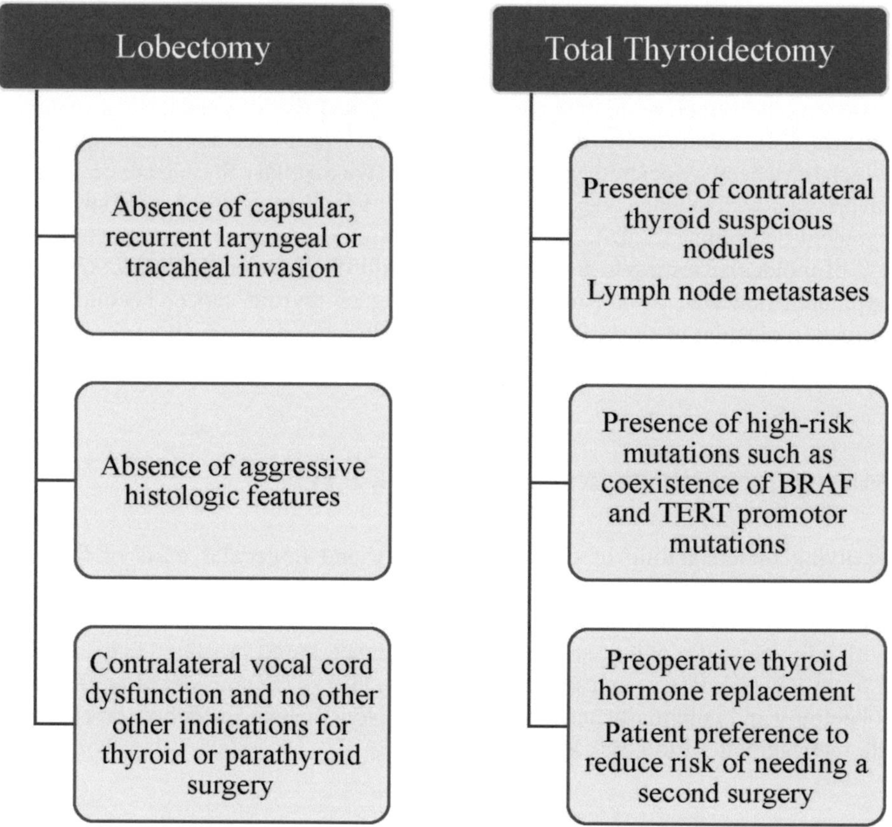

Fig. 9.2 Determination of extent of initial surgery for PTC measuring <4 cm

Nonetheless, depending on the final pathology, a completion thyroidectomy following lobectomy for low-risk PTC may be necessary. High-risk features such as aggressive histology, capsular and/or vascular invasion, microscopic extra-thyroidal extension, and multi-focality warrant consideration of completion thyroidectomy. A recent systemic review showed that the proportion of patients meeting the 2015 ATA guidelines criteria for thyroid lobectomy who subsequently needed completion thyroidectomy was variable but averaged approximately 34% [18].

Surgeon experience and familiarity with guidelines can influence surgical management options provided to patients. McDow et al.'s nationwide survey of 320 surgeons found that low-volume surgeons who performed less than 25 thyroidectomies annually were less likely than high-volume surgeons to be aware that thyroid lobectomy is supported by guidelines as a treatment option for patients with low-risk thyroid cancer (72.5% vs. 92.0%, respectively, $p < 0.001$); low-volume surgeons were also less likely to report using clinical practice guidelines (84.0% vs. 94.7%, $p = 0.004$) [25]. Tumor size influenced treatment recommendations: when respondents (surgeons) were asked which management option they would choose for themselves if diagnosed with a 1.5-cm low-risk PTC, only 38.4% of low-volume and 43.8% of high-volume surgeons would choose a thyroid lobectomy [25].

Active Surveillance

As a management option that enables monitoring disease progression while allowing for rescue surgery, active surveillance is a potential management strategy for low-risk PTC. Active surveillance is recommended in the 2015 ATA guidelines for low-risk tumors that are without evidence of metastatic disease or local invasion and those tumors without aggressive cytology [5]. Active surveillance is also acceptable in patients with prohibitive surgical risk or considerable comorbidities as well as patients with short life expectancy [5]. The American Association of Endocrine Surgeons' executive summary guidelines cite active surveillance as a possible management strategy for small PTC which requires an informed surgical discussion, patient motivation, potentially more cost, an experienced multidisciplinary team, and high-quality neck ultrasounds [26].

Data supporting active surveillance for low-risk PTC is largely based on international studies; these have consistently demonstrated the feasibility and safety of active surveillance [7–9, 27–29]. Initial studies were focused on papillary microcarcinomas (tumor size ≤ 1 cm) but have gradually incorporated PTCs measuring >1 cm. The vast majority of studies have shown that more than 90% of surveilled papillary microcarcinomas do not progress significantly in size [8, 9]. Most patients showed stable tumor size with follow-up averaging 60 months (range 18–227 months with 5% showing tumor enlargement of greater than 3 mm at 5 years and 8% at 10 years) [30]. Small growth of 3 mm or more has been seen in 11 of 291 (3.8%) patients in a US cohort undergoing active surveillance, with a cumulative incidence of 2.5% noted at 2 years and 12.1% at 5 years [9]. Lymph node metastases were seen in 1.7% at 5 years and 3.8% at 10 years [31]. In a review of 18,445 cases of papillary microcarcinoma, disease-specific survival at 10 and 15 years was 99.5% and 99.3% respectively [6].

The size criterion for active surveillance was extended to 1.5 cm in a cohort study conducted at a high-volume center in the United States [9]. Further, a recent meta-analysis of nine studies comprising patients from the United States, Japan, South Korea, and Columbia concluded that active surveillance is a reasonable treatment option and there were equivalent outcomes with a broader size criterion of tumors measuring up to 1.5 cm [9, 30]. In the meta-analysis, 4.4% demonstrated tumor growth with only 1.0% and 0.04% developing cervical lymph node and metastatic disease, respectively, with a pooled thyroid-specific mortality of 0.03% [32].

Several active surveillance protocols for low-risk PTC have been described; key elements are summarized in Fig. 9.3 [32–36]. Informed consent and multidisciplinary coordination of patient care are essential. Currently, potential candidates for active surveillance are those at least age 18 years with low-risk PTC measuring ≤ 1.5 cm who are not at high risk of loss to follow-up. More data are needed to

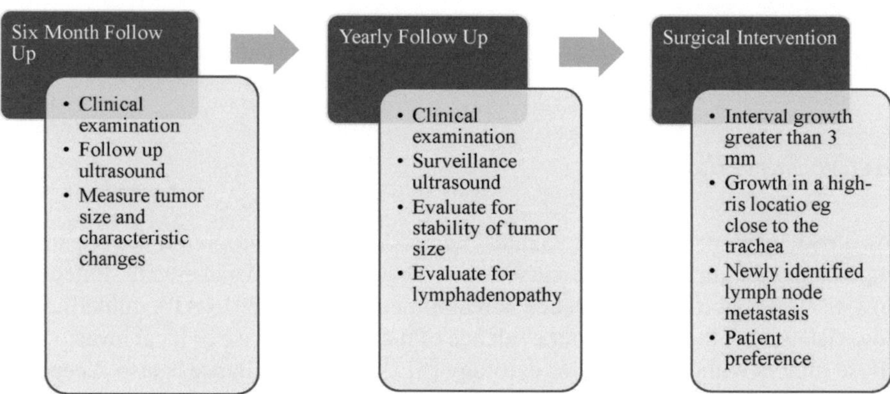

Fig. 9.3 Active surveillance protocol for low-risk PTC

investigate the potential influence of patient age, molecular tumor features, and comorbid thyroid diseases such as thyroiditis or multinodular goiters on the safety and feasibility of active surveillance for low-risk PTC.

Emerging Data on Patient Perspectives for the Management of Low-Risk PTC

Once classified as a low-risk PTC, the shared decision-making process for management should focus on a comprehensive explanation of risks and potential outcomes of active surveillance vs. surgical intervention. For patients leaning toward surgical intervention, a thorough discussion of the pros and cons of lobectomy vs. total thyroidectomy is paramount in determining the appropriate intervention for that particular patient.

A number of studies utilizing discrete choice experiments have evaluated patient selections of two or more hypothetical treatment options for thyroid cancer, and investigated trade-offs between positive and negative patient perspectives of the interventions. In Ahmadi et al.'s study, 150 patients with low-risk thyroid cancer or thyroid nodules necessitating surgery (lobectomy or thyroidectomy) were administered a survey to identify acceptable trade-offs patients would be willing to make to balance risks and benefits of thyroid lobectomy versus total thyroidectomy [37]. The authors found that patient treatment preferences were influenced most strongly by perceptions of thyroid cancer recurrence risk, followed by risk of requiring a second surgery, risk of recurrent laryngeal nerve damage, and risk of hypocalcemia and need for thyroid hormone supplementation [37]. When accounting for differences in postoperative risks, the average patient favored lobectomy over total thyroidectomy as long as the chance of needing a second (i.e., completion) surgery after initial lobectomy remained below 30%. Participants would also accept a 4.1%

risk of cancer recurrence if the risk of a second surgery could be reduced from 40% to 10% [37].

Another discrete choice experiment evaluated preferences of 2054 participants in treating PTC via lobectomy, total thyroidectomy, or active surveillance [38]. The study found that in general, participants preferred management strategies that required less frequent follow-up, lower out-of-pocket costs, lower likelihood of having voice changes or hypocalcemia and a lower risk of developing invasive thyroid cancer or dying of thyroid cancer. Lower health literacy was also found to have an association with significantly lower preference for a less invasive treatment option. Moreover, the study provided insight into how terminologies used by providers could influence patient treatment preferences; if the term "lesion" was used to describe the tumor instead of the term "cancer," participants judged the need for lifelong thyroid replacement medication, higher costs, and a higher risk of developing invasive thyroid cancer more negatively compared to when the term "cancer" was used. Further, when the tumor was described as a "cancer," there was a lower preference for active surveillance, and when the condition was described as a "lesion," there was a higher preference for lobectomy. Overall, patients were more willing to accept potential treatment harms when the condition was described using the term "cancer" [38]. In contrast, a single-center Canadian study assessing the treatment preferences of 100 patients for managing low-risk PTC <2 cm found that approximately 71% of patients who were offered the choice of active surveillance or surgery (thyroidectomy or lobectomy), chose active surveillance [39]. Factors reported by patients as influencing their treatment decision included perceived risk of thyroidectomy or cancer, family considerations, treatment timing in the context of life circumstances, and trust in health care providers [39]. A major limitation of the study is that lobectomy was not analyzed as a distinct treatment option.

Case Conclusion

Our patient presented with a low-risk classic PTC measuring 1.5 cm. She had no family history of thyroid cancer or cranio-cervical radiation exposure. Clinical exam revealed a mobile thyroid gland with a palpable nodule. There was no palpable lymphadenopathy. Voice was normal. High-resolution ultrasound revealed a completely intra-thyroidal tumor without evidence of extra-thyroidal extension or invasion. Lymph node mapping was negative for any lymphadenopathy. After confirming the low-risk nature of this PTC, the patient was offered active surveillance or thyroid lobectomy with possibility of total thyroidectomy. The pros and cons of each intervention were discussed. Considering that she was an anxious patient, discussions were held over multiple visits to allow ample opportunity for the patient to fully consider all options. After extensive discussions, the patient elected to undergo a thyroid lobectomy with possibility of total thyroidectomy depending on intraoperative findings. There was no intraoperative evidence of extra-thyroidal extension, involvement of strap muscles, or abnormal lymph nodes. Final pathology showed a classical, unifocal PTC without capsular, lymphatic or vascular invasion, and with negative resection margins. Thyroid function tests were normal at 6 weeks after surgery, obviating thyroid hormone therapy. She was referred to an endocrinologist for cancer surveillance.

Summary

The goals of surgical intervention for thyroid cancer include improvement of overall and disease-specific survival, reduction of persistent or recurrent disease risk and associated morbidity, as well as reduction of treatment-related morbidity and unnecessary therapy [2]. Since publication of the 2015 ATA guidelines which supported lobectomy as a treatment option for low-risk PTC, emerging evidence has also shown that select low-risk PTC could be safely managed with active surveillance with a low risk of disease progression. Overall, the management of low-risk PTC remains an area of active research and ongoing controversy. If active surveillance is considered, a clear surveillance plan should be delineated with the patient, and the patient should be unlikely to be lost to follow-up. If surgical intervention is preferred, thyroid lobectomy can be considered while maintaining overall low risk of recurrent disease or disease-specific mortality. Ultimately, fastidious evaluation of the clinical, radiographic, cytologic, and molecular features of cancer, as well as involving the patient in a comprehensive discussion about risks and benefits of treatment options are important in determining an appropriate management plan for low-risk PTC.DisclosuresThe authors have no disclosures.

References

1. Roman BR, Morris LG, Davies L. The thyroid cancer epidemic, 2017 perspective. Curr Opin Endocrinol Diabetes Obes. 2017;24:332–6.
2. SEER Cancer Stat Facts. Thyroid cancer. Bethesda, MD: National Cancer Institute. https://seer.cancer.gov/statfacts/html/thyro.html
3. Rahib L, Smith BD, Aizenberg R, et al. Projecting cancer incidence and deaths to 2030: the unexpected burden of thyroid, liver, and pancreas cancers in the United States. Cancer Res. 2014;74:2913–21.
4. Nikiforov YE, Seethala RR, Tallini G, et al. Nomenclature revision for encapsulated follicular variant of papillary thyroid carcinoma: a paradigm shift to reduce overtreatment of indolent Tumors. JAMA Oncol. 2016;2(8):1023–9. https://doi.org/10.1001/jamaoncol.2016.0386.
5. Haugen BR, Alexander EK, Bible KC, et al. 2015 American Thyroid Association management guidelines for adult patients with thyroid nodules and differentiated thyroid cancer: the American Thyroid Association guidelines task force on thyroid nodules and differentiated thyroid cancer. Thyroid. 2016;26:1–133.
6. Yu XM, Wan Y, Sippel RS, et al. Should all papillary thyroid microcarcinomas be aggressively treated? An analysis of 18,445 cases. Ann Surg. 2011;254:653–60.
7. Ito Y, Uruno T, Nakano K, et al. An observation trial without surgical treatment in patients with papillary microcarcinoma of the thyroid. Thyroid. 2003;13:381–7.

8. Ito Y, Miyauchi A, Inoue H, et al. An observational trial for papillary thyroid microcarcinoma in Japanese patients. World J Surg. 2010;34:28–35.
9. Tuttle RM, Fagin JA, Minkowitz G, et al. Natural history and tumor volume kinetics of papillary thyroid cancers during active surveillance. JAMA Otolaryngol Head Neck Surg. 2017;143:1015–20.
10. Macedo FI, Mittal VK. Total thyroidectomy versus lobectomy as initial operation for small unilateral papillary thyroid carcinoma: a meta-analysis. Surg Oncol. 2015;24:117–22.
11. Mazzaferri EL. Management of low-risk differentiated thyroid cancer. Endocr Pract. 2007;13:498–512.
12. Guan H, Vandenbussche CJ, Erozan YS, et al. Can the tall cell variant of papillary thyroid carcinoma be distinguished from the conventional type in fine needle aspirates? A cytomorphologic study with assessment of diagnostic accuracy. Acta Cytol. 2013;57:534–42.
13. Das DK, Mallik MK, Sharma P, et al. Papillary thyroid carcinoma and its variants in fine needle aspiration smears. A cytomorphologic study with special reference to tall cell variant. Acta Cytol. 2004;48:325–36.
14. Xing M, Clark D, Guan H, et al. BRAF mutation testing of thyroid fine-needle aspiration biopsy specimens for preoperative risk stratification in papillary thyroid cancer. J Clin Oncol. 2009;27:2977–82.
15. Xing M, Liu R, Liu X, et al. BRAF V600E and TERT promoter mutations cooperatively identify the most aggressive papillary thyroid cancer with highest recurrence. J Clin Oncol. 2014;32:2718–26.
16. Yip L, Gooding WE, Nikitski A, Wald AI, Carty SE, Karslioglu-French E, Seethala RR, Zandberg DP, Ferris RL, Nikiforova MN, Nikiforov YE. Risk assessment for distant metastasis in differentiated thyroid cancer using molecular profiling: a matched case-control study. Cancer. 2021;127(11):1779–87. https://doi.org/10.1002/cncr.33421. Epub 2021 Feb 4. PMID: 33539547; PMCID: PMC8113082
17. Adam MA, Pura J, Gu L, et al. Extent of surgery for papillary thyroid cancer is not associated with survival: an analysis of 61,775 patients. Ann Surg. 2014;260:601–5.; discussion 605-7.
18. Vargas-Pinto S, Romero Arenas MA. Lobectomy compared to total thyroidectomy for low-risk papillary thyroid cancer: a systematic review. J Surg Res. 2019;242:244–51. https://doi.org/10.1016/j.jss.2019.04.036. Epub 2019 May 16. PMID: 31103828
19. Vaisman F, Shaha A, Fish A, Tuttle AS. Initial therapy with either thyroid lobectomy or total thyroidectomy without radioactive iodine remnant ablation is associated with very low rates of structural disease recurrence in properly selected patients with differentiated thyroid cancer. Clin Endocrinol. 2011;75:112–9.
20. Matsuzu K, Sugino K, Masudo K, et al. Thyroid lobectomy for papillary thyroid cancer: long-term follow-up study of 1,088 cases. World J Surg. 2014;38:68–79.
21. Kim SY, Kim HJ, Kim SM, et al. Thyroid hormone supplementation therapy for differentiated thyroid cancer after lobectomy: 5 years of follow-up. Front Endocrinol (Lausanne). 2020;11:520.
22. Park JO, Bae JS, Lee SH, et al. The Long-term prognosis of voice pitch change in female patients after thyroid surgery. World J Surg. 2016;40:2382–90.
23. Kandil E, Krishnan B, Noureldine SI, et al. Hemithyroidectomy: a meta-analysis of postoperative need for hormone replacement and complications. ORL J Otorhinolaryngol Relat Spec. 2013;75:6–17.
24. Hauch A, Al-Qurayshi Z, Randolph G, et al. Total thyroidectomy is associated with increased risk of complications for low- and high-volume surgeons. Ann Surg Oncol. 2014;21:3844–52.
25. McDow AD, Saucke MC, Marka NA, Long KL, Pitt SC. Thyroid lobectomy for low-risk papillary thyroid cancer: a National Survey of low- and high-volume surgeons. Ann Surg Oncol. 2021;28(7):3568–75. https://doi.org/10.1245/s10434-021-09898-9. Epub 2021 May 3
26. Patel KN, Yip L, Lubitz CC, et al. Executive summary of the American Association of Endocrine Surgeons Guidelines for the definitive surgical management of thyroid disease in adults. Ann Surg. 2020;271:399–410.

27. Cho SJ, Suh CH, Baek JH, Chung SR, Choi YJ, Chung KW, Shong YK, Lee JH. Active surveillance for small papillary thyroid cancer: a systematic review and meta-analysis. Thyroid. 2019;29(10):1399–408. https://doi.org/10.1089/thy.2019.0159.
28. Sawka AM, Thabane L. Active surveillance of low-risk papillary thyroid cancer: a meta-analysis-methodologic critiques and tips for addressing them [published online ahead of print, 2020 Apr 9]. Surgery. 2020;168(5):975.
29. Miyauchi A. Clinical trials of active surveillance of papillary microcarcinoma of the thyroid. World J Surg. 2016;40(3):516–22. https://doi.org/10.1007/s00268-015-3392-y.
30. Saravana-Bawan B, Bajwa A, Paterson J, et al. Active surveillance of low-risk papillary thyroid cancer: a meta-analysis. Surgery. 2020;167:46–55.
31. Ito Y, Miyauchi A, Kihara M, et al. Patient age is significantly related to the progression of papillary microcarcinoma of the thyroid under observation. Thyroid. 2014;24:27–34.
32. Brito JP, Ito Y, Miyauchi A, et al. A clinical framework to facilitate risk stratification when considering an active surveillance alternative to immediate biopsy and surgery in papillary microcarcinoma. Thyroid. 2016;26:144–9.
33. Sawka AM, Ghai S, Tomlinson G, et al. A protocol for a Canadian prospective observational study of decision-making on active surveillance or surgery for low-risk papillary thyroid cancer. BMJ Open. 2018;8(4):e020298. https://doi.org/10.1136/bmjopen-2017-020298.
34. Davies L, Chang CH, Sirovich B, Tuttle RM, Fukushima M, Ito Y, Miyauchi A. Thyroid cancer active surveillance program retention and adherence in Japan. JAMA Otolaryngol Head Neck Surg. 2021;147(1):77–84. https://doi.org/10.1001/jamaoto.2020.4200.
35. McCaffery KJ, Nickel B. Clinician be my guide in active surveillance of papillary thyroid microcarcinoma. JAMA Otolaryngol Head Neck Surg. 2021;147(1):7–8. https://doi.org/10.1001/jamaoto.2020.4237.
36. Sugitani I, Ito Y, Takeuchi D, Nakayama H, Masaki C, Shindo H, Teshima M, Horiguchi K, Yoshida Y, Kanai T, Hirokawa M, Hames KY, Tabei I, Miyauchi A. Indications and Strategy for Active Surveillance of Adult Low-Risk Papillary Thyroid Microcarcinoma: Consensus Statements from the Japan Association of Endocrine Surgery Task Force on Management for Papillary Thyroid Microcarcinoma. Thyroid. 2021;31(2):183–92. https://doi.org/10.1089/thy.2020.0330. Epub 2020 Nov 2. PMID: 33023426; PMCID: PMC7891203.
37. Ahmadi S, Gonzalez JM, Talbott M, et al. Patient preferences around extent of surgery in low-risk thyroid cancer: a discrete choice experiment. Thyroid. 2020;30:1044–52.
38. Nickel B, Howard K, Brito JP, et al. Association of preferences for papillary thyroid cancer treatment with disease terminology: a discrete choice experiment. JAMA Otolaryngol Head Neck Surg. 2018;144:887–96.
39. Sawka AM, Ghai S, Yoannidis T, Rotstein L, Gullane PJ, et al. A prospective mixed-methods study of decision-making on surgery or active surveillance for low-risk papillary thyroid cancer. Thyroid. 2020;30(7):999–1007. https://doi.org/10.1089/thy.2019.0592.

Chapter 10
Surgical Management of Locally Advanced Thyroid Cancer with Tracheal Invasion

Christopher M. K. L. Yao, Maureen V. Hill, and John A. (Drew) Ridge

Case

A 62-year-old woman presented after a "health fair screening" neck ultrasound demonstrated multiple bilateral thyroid nodules. She was free of symptoms and had no family history of thyroid cancer or external beam radiation treatment. She had a normal-appearing gland, with a dominant right central solid nodule measuring 13x11x12 mm that was internally hypoechoic with ill-defined margins (TIRADS 5) (Fig. 10.1). In the left lobe there was a second circumscribed hypoechoic nodule measuring $7 \times 6 \times 8$ mm (TIRADS 4). Office physical examination was notable for a normal head and neck examination. The dominant right thyroid nodule was not palpable and her cords moved bilaterally on mirror examination. Fine needle aspiration was performed of both lesions which demonstrated bilateral papillary thyroid carcinoma. A repeat neck ultrasound showed no lymphadenopathy and she was assigned clinical Stage I (cT1bN0M0) papillary thyroid cancer.

She was taken to the operating room, planning a total thyroidectomy. Upon dissection of the right side of the gland, at the location of cancer there were dense adhesions to the trachea, medial to the suspensory ligament.

In the absence of clinical tracheal invasion with the surface area of the tumor adherent to the tracheal rings <1 cm^2, the thyroid was sharply dissected from the trachea without clinical tumor transection (tracheal shave). Removal of the left side of the gland was uneventful. No suspicious lymph nodes were encountered. Postoperative vocal cords and parathyroid function were normal.

Surgical pathology revealed multifocal papillary carcinoma with a 1.2-cm classic variant of the isthmus with posterior extra-thyroidal extension (ETE), an involved tracheal margin, and a 0.7-cm tall cell variant of the left lobe with clear margins and

Christopher M. K. L. Yao (✉) · M. V. Hill · J. A. (Drew) Ridge
Department of Surgical Oncology, Fox Chase Cancer Center, Philadelphia, PA, USA
e-mail: john.ridge@fccc.edu

Fig. 10.1 Pre-operative ultrasound. White arrow: Right lobe/isthmus cancer

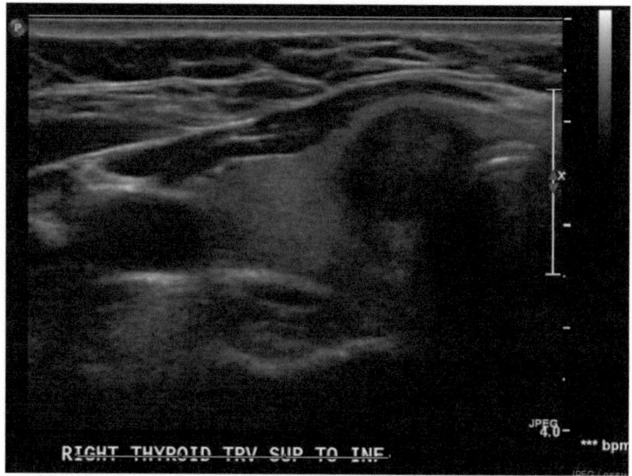

no ETE. Lymphovascular invasion was not identified in either tumor. A third 0.3 cm papillary microcarcinoma was incidentally found in the left lower pole. In view of this, her pathologic stage III pT4a(m)N0M0 papillary thyroid cancer, radioactive iodine (RAI), and thyroid suppression were recommended. More than 2 years have passed since completion of her RAI treatment, and her thyroglobulin remains undetectable.

Discussion

Locally advanced thyroid cancer, defined by the presence of ETE of the tumor through the thyroid capsule into surrounding anatomic structures occurs in 10–15% of patients [1]. While minimal invasion into structures such as the strap muscles can be readily treated with en bloc removal of the muscle with excellent outcomes and essentially no morbidity [2], invasion of the trachea, larynx, esophagus, or superior and recurrent laryngeal nerves poses more challenging problems because incomplete surgical excision is associated with higher mortality [3, 4]. ETE is recognized by the American Joint Committee on Cancer (AJCC) as an important prognostic factor and is incorporated into the "T Category" of the primary tumor. Any ETE beyond the strap muscles, regardless of primary tumor size, is categorized as T4, with extension into the subcutaneous soft tissues, larynx, trachea, esophagus, or recurrent laryngeal nerve designated categorized as T4a. Invasion of great vessels or prevertebral fascia is considered "very locally advanced" and termed T4b [5, 6].

ETE occurs more frequently in older patients (over 55 years old) and with large tumors (larger than 3.7–4 cm) [7, 8]. The percent of ETE into various structures has been estimated in two case series of locally advanced thyroid cancers (of 153 and 262 patients, respectively), with invasion of the recurrent laryngeal nerve being most common (47–51%), followed by the trachea (37–46%), the esophagus

(21–39%), and the larynx (12%) [9, 10]. The true incidence of extrathyroidal invasion into the trachea varies depending upon the chosen definitions of invasion, ranging from adherence to gross tumor penetration. However, in a comprehensive review of 10,251 thyroid cancer patients, Honings et al. estimated a rate of 5.8% [11].

Extra-Thyroidal Extension to the Airway

The anatomic relationship between thyroid cancer and tracheal invasion was classically described by Shin et al. [12] (Fig. 10.2). According to their histologic studies, the collagen fibers abutting the thyroid gland run parallel to the outer wall of the trachea, but the more posterior fibers course in curves into the intercartilaginous space, running perpendicular to the tracheal lumen, along with nerves, blood vessels, and lymphatics that course within the intercartilaginous plates. It is along these perpendicular vessels that extra-thyroidal cancer cells can invade the trachea, typically by the following progression: Stage 1—carcinoma extends through the capsule of the gland and abuts the external perichondrium. Stage 2—carcinoma invades between the rings of cartilage or destroys the cartilage. Stage 3—carcinoma extends through the cartilage or between cartilaginous rings to the lamina propria of the tracheal mucosa without elevating or invading the tracheal epithelium. Stage

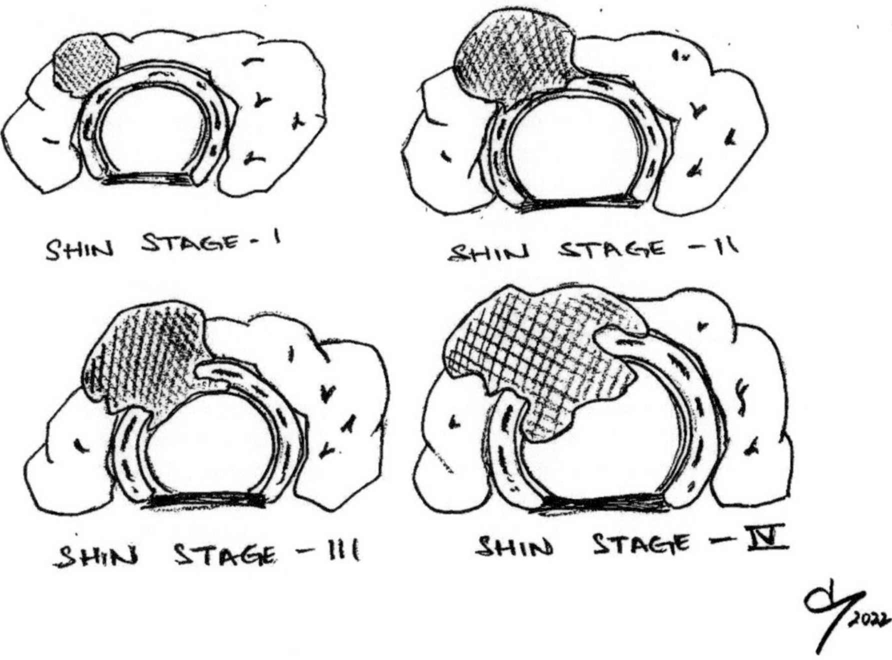

Fig. 10.2 Shin classification of tracheal invasion

4—carcinoma extends through the thickness of the tracheal mucosa and is visible bronchoscopically as a nodule or ulcerated mass [12].

With locally advanced differentiated thyroid cancer, one of the challenges in management is the frequent absence of pre-operative symptoms of tracheal involvement, leading to identification of ETE only in the operating room. Even among patients with thyroid cancer invading into the lumen of the trachea, only 22% report hoarseness, 11% hemoptysis, or dyspnea in 5% [13]. While other studies have suggested a higher prevalence of some form of dyspnea at presentation [13–15], a high degree of suspicion is necessary. Even in the setting of vocal cord paralysis from nerve invasion, frequency of voice change ranges from 33 to 68% [16, 17]. Thus, the American Head and Neck Society recommends laryngeal evaluation for all patients with thyroid cancer [1].

If tracheal invasion is suspected pre-operatively, cross-sectional imaging in the form of a fine-cut computed tomography (CT) of the larynx and an ultrasound are recommended means for assessment of the trachea [1]. While the accuracy of CT has been estimated to range from 83 to 99%, with a specificity of 90–99% [18]; it only has a sensitivity of 59% [19]. The main signs of tracheal invasion with either CT or magnetic resonance imaging (MRI) is contact of tumor with the trachea of 180° or more of the circumference, deformity of the lumen, focal mucosal irregularity, or an intraluminal mass [18, 20]. While ultrasound accuracy, sensitivity, and specificity are operator dependent, in experienced hands invasion was correctly identified before surgery in 83–85% of cases [21, 22], and found to have higher sensitivity for minimal ETE than MRI [23].

In addition to pre-operative imaging, bronchoscopic examination should be performed either before or at the time of the initial tumor resection in the setting of symptoms or radiographic evidence of tracheal invasion. Bronchoscopy may identify frank mucosal invasion, luminal compression (Shin Stage 4), or subtler mucosal changes such as erythema and edema (Shin Stage 3). Koike and co-workers described using the bronchoscopic findings as the basis for a tracheal shave vs. resection [24].

Prognosis of Locally Advanced Thyroid Cancer

Well-differentiated thyroid cancers have excellent prognosis, with some 97% of patients surviving 10 years, and 90% at 20 years [25], those with tracheal invasion have lower long-term survival [26, 27]. While the nature of resection typically varies with the extent of disease, with circumferential resection more likely with more extensive tracheal involvement, a recent meta-analysis showed a local-regional recurrence rate of 15% following circumferential resection (19 pooled studies) and 25.6% following window resection (7 pooled studies) [28]. In another recent study of patients with locally advanced thyroid cancer, where disease-free survival was measured against completeness of resection, patients were found to have 5-year disease-specific survivals of 94%, 88%, and 68%, with higher survival in patients with a R0 resection, compared to R1 and R2, respectively [9]. This series was not limited to patients with tracheal invasion (46% of the cohort), and site of invasion was not correlated with margin status. In view of the morbidity associated en bloc laryngeal or esophageal resections, margin positivity and therefore local recurrence could be strongly informed by site of invasion.

There is no argument that primary treatment of locally invasive thyroid cancer is surgical, however, one must carefully balance the oncologic benefits of a complete resection with the potential morbidity, which has been reported between 14 and 39% after a tracheal resection [28, 29]. This has led many surgeons to pursue more limited techniques (such as "shaving" disease from the trachea in the absence of its invasion). While such approaches may be followed by the delivery of adjuvant post-operative radioactive iodine (RAI) with or without external beam radiotherapy (EBRT), there has been concern that the tumor biology of the invading front of thyroid cancer may become dedifferentiated; tumors in these patients may not be RAI-avid [14].

Surgical Techniques

Surgical techniques addressing tracheal invasion include sharp "shaved" resection, windowed tracheal resection, and complete circumferential tracheal ring resection with primary anastomosis. The use of a knife to separate the tumor or gland from the trachea sharply has been shown to have similar survival and local control rates to more radical resection in appropriately selected patients [8, 10]. The extent and definition of the "shave" vary by practitioner, including sharp dissection of the investing adventitia from the trachea, as well as superficial tangential cartilaginous resection. However, the challenges with shave procedures include difficulty confirming tumor-free margins intraoperatively due to the lack of a continuous plane between the external perichondrium of a tracheal ring and the dense fibrous inter-cartilaginous tissue, as well as the potential for tumor spread via intercartilaginous space [1]. Such approaches are not typically technically demanding and add little, if any, additional morbidity to the usual thyroidectomy.

McCarty and co-workers found that of 35 shave procedures performed, all resulted in residual microscopic disease on the tracheal margin [13]. Some series have shown higher recurrence rates and worse survival for patients submitted to less aggressive approaches to dense tracheal invasion; they should be anticipated when performing another shave procedure to treat tracheal recurrence after a prior shave procedure [30–32]. Nevertheless, there have been reports of local control as high as 95% if the tumor does not penetrate the perichondrium [33]. Patient selection is thus important and may prove challenging.

While the presence of gross positive margins and extrathyroidal extension indicate higher risk of disease, the impact of a microscopic positive margin noted only on final pathology is less clear. In a large case series including 3664 patients, Ganley and co-workers demonstrated that microscopic positive margins did not predict local failure, with a 5-year local-regional failure-free survival rate of 99% [34]. Indeed, in a selected group of patients with small tumors and positive margins without gross ETE; adjuvant RAI was not administered, and no recurrences were reported. Though this review did not differentiate between microscopically involved anterior or posterior thyroid margins, other high-risk features including T and N category or gross ETE, rather than the margin status alone, should inform adjuvant treatment decisions making.

Our approach is to employ tracheal shaving in settings where the tumor factors are favorable: small surface area of suspected invasion (Shin Stage 1); pre-operatively unheralded superficial tumor adherence to the trachea, with no signs or symptoms of tracheal invasion; or when patient factors preclude more aggressive operative intervention (e.g., poor performance status or prohibitive comorbidities). In all other cases, when tracheal invasion is encountered resection with a window or sleeve resection is undertaken (Fig. 10.3).

For patients with known intraluminal cancer, or destroyed tracheal cartilage, an en bloc tracheal cartilage resection is indicated. A window resection can be safely performed when tumor invasion is limited to an anterior or lateral location; the defect can be closed with either strap muscles or periosteum [35]. Where more than a single ring is excised, circumferential resection with primary re-anastomosis is often indicated. While many series have demonstrated low mortality and moderate morbidity with segmental resections, complications can be life threatening, with mortality rates as high as 5–9%. Serious complications include anastomotic dehiscence, laryngeal stenosis, and stricture [28, 29, 33, 36, 37]. To minimize complications, surgeons engaging in airway surgery should be familiar with the tracheal blood supply and techniques to mobilize both the trachea and the larynx to produce minimal tension along the anastomosis [38].

In view of the difficulty in predicting ETE and tracheal resection pre-operatively, the surgeon may be faced with the need to perform a tracheal resection without pre-operative consent. In this setting, shave resection might be undertaken and tracheal resection delayed until appropriate discussion and consent can be obtained. However, while tracheal resection can be performed in a staged procedure after a shave procedure with known residual disease, complication rates are higher when

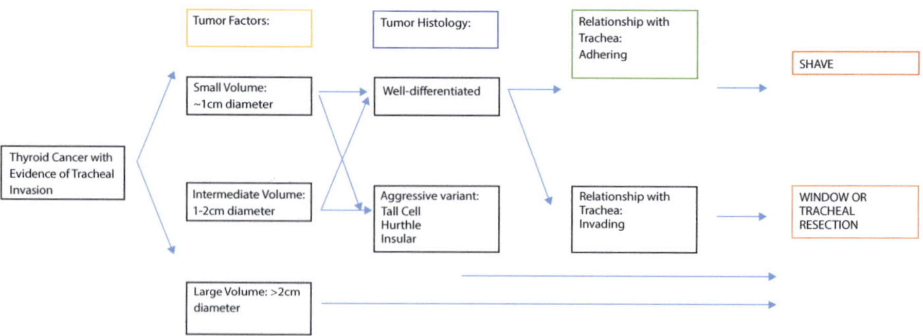

Fig. 10.3 Decision tree

secondary surgery is performed and this warrants consideration when entertaining such an approach [39, 40]. Surgeons should endeavor to perform thorough resections to decrease the incidence of recurrence and reoperation.

Adjuvant therapy including postoperative RAI and thyroid-stimulating hormone suppression remain the mainstay. In the setting of residual disease external beam radiotherapy may warrant consideration in patients of suitable age [34, 41, 42].

Case Discussion

While the right lobe/isthmus thyroid cancer was not believed pre-operatively to have invaded the trachea, the pre-operative ultrasound reveals that the cancer was situated in the posterior aspect of the gland without a clear margin between the trachea and tumor (which is not uncommon for isthmus lesions). Shadowing due to the tracheal rings makes detailed evaluation of this area challenging on static images.

Shave resection of the adventitia only was performed with the small primary tumor in view of the absence of aggressive features on pre-operative biopsy, and a relatively small area of contact between the tumor and the trachea. While the final surgical margin was microscopically involved (R1), as the pathology demonstrated classical papillary thyroid carcinoma without any other concerning pathology features (beyond ETE) no additional resection was undertaken. RAI and thyroid suppression have thus far proven effective, however, the risk of local recurrence cannot be ignored, and continued surveillance is appropriate.

Conclusion

Locally advanced thyroid cancer with invasion of the trachea remains rare, but it is helpful for the surgeon to identify these patients pre-operatively. While the problem may be unheralded a high degree of suspicion is appropriate for older patients, those with large tumors, and the presence of suggestive symptomatology including hoarseness, hemoptysis, or dyspnea. Ultrasound and bronchoscopic evaluation are important for evaluation of suspected tracheal invasion. Tracheal invasion may reflect dedifferentiation of thyroid cancer, which might be less RAI and radiation sensitive. Complete surgical resection provides accurate pathologic assessment, and lower recurrence rates, however, more aggressive resection must be balanced against increased surgical morbidity. For selected patients, formal tracheal resection can be performed with acceptable morbidity and mortality, and should be offered pre-operatively to patients suspected of tracheal invasion.

References

1. Shindo ML, Caruana SM, Kandil E, et al. Management of invasive well-differentiated thyroid cancer: an American Head and Neck Society consensus statement. AHNS consensus statement. Head Neck. 2014;36:1379–90.
2. Nixon IJ, Ganly I, Patel S, et al. The impact of microscopic extrathyroid extension on outcome in patients with clinical T1 and T2 well-differentiated thyroid cancer. Surgery. 2011;150:1242–9.
3. Shaha AR. Implications of prognostic factors and risk groups in the management of differentiated thyroid cancer. Laryngoscope. 2004;114:393–402.
4. Kowalski LP, Filho JG. Results of the treatment of locally invasive thyroid carcinoma. Head Neck. 2002;24:340–4.
5. Kim H, Choi N, Baek CH, Son YI, Jeong HS, Chung MK. Comparison of prognostic implications between the 7th and 8th edition of AJCC TNM staging system for head and neck soft-tissue sarcoma in adult patients. Eur Arch Otorhinolaryngol. 2019;276:3195–202.
6. NCCN Guidelines Version 3.2020 Thyroid Carcinoma. 2020. (Accessed 3.2.2021, at https://www.nccn.org/professionals/physician_gls/pdf/thyroid.pdf.)
7. Ortiz S, Rodríguez JM, Soria T, et al. Extrathyroid spread in papillary carcinoma of the thyroid: clinicopathological and prognostic study. Otolaryngol Head Neck Surg. 2001;124:261–5.
8. Segal K, Shpitzer T, Hazan A, Bachar G, Marshak G, Popovtzer A. Invasive well-differentiated thyroid carcinoma: effect of treatment modalities on outcome. Otolaryngol Head Neck Surg. 2006;134:819–22.
9. Wang LY, Nixon IJ, Patel SG, et al. Operative management of locally advanced, differentiated thyroid cancer. Surgery. 2016;160:738–46.
10. McCaffrey TV, Bergstralh EJ, Hay ID. Locally invasive papillary thyroid carcinoma: 1940-1990. Head Neck. 1994;16:165–72.
11. Honings J, Stephen AE, Marres HA, Gaissert HA. The management of thyroid carcinoma invading the larynx or trachea. Laryngoscope. 2010;120:682–9.
12. Shin DH, Mark EJ, Suen HC, Grillo HC. Pathologic staging of papillary carcinoma of the thyroid with airway invasion based on the anatomic manner of extension to the trachea: a clinicopathologic study based on 22 patients who underwent thyroidectomy and airway resection. Hum Pathol. 1993;24:866–70.
13. McCarty TM, Kuhn JA, Williams WL Jr, et al. Surgical management of thyroid cancer invading the airway. Ann Surg Oncol. 1997;4:403–8.
14. Tsumori T, Nakao K, Miyata M, et al. Clinicopathologic study of thyroid carcinoma infiltrating the trachea. Cancer. 1985;56:2843–8.
15. Ishihara T, Yamazaki S, Kobayashi K, et al. Resection of the trachea infiltrated by thyroid carcinoma. Ann Surg. 1982;195:496–500.
16. Randolph GW, Kamani D. The importance of preoperative laryngoscopy in patients undergoing thyroidectomy: voice, vocal cord function, and the preoperative detection of invasive thyroid malignancy. Surgery. 2006;139:357–62.
17. Farrag TY, Samlan RA, Lin FR, Tufano RP. The utility of evaluating true vocal fold motion before thyroid surgery. Laryngoscope. 2006;116:235–8.
18. Seo YL, Yoon DY, Lim KJ, et al. Locally advanced thyroid cancer: can CT help in prediction of extrathyroidal invasion to adjacent structures? AJR Am J Roentgenol. 2010;195:W240-4.
19. Hoang JK, Branstetter BFT, Gafton AR, Lee WK, Glastonbury CM. Imaging of thyroid carcinoma with CT and MRI: approaches to common scenarios. Cancer Imaging. 2013;13:128–39.
20. Wang JC, Takashima S, Takayama F, et al. Tracheal invasion by thyroid carcinoma: prediction using MR imaging. AJR Am J Roentgenol. 2001;177:929–36.
21. Yamamura N, Fukushima S, Nakao K, et al. Relation between ultrasonographic and histologic findings of tracheal invasion by differentiated thyroid cancer. World J Surg. 2002;26:1071–3.
22. Tomoda C, Uruno T, Takamura Y, et al. Ultrasonography as a method of screening for tracheal invasion by papillary thyroid cancer. Surg Today. 2005;35:819–22.

23. Kim H, Kim JA, Son EJ, et al. Preoperative prediction of the extrathyroidal extension of papillary thyroid carcinoma with ultrasonography versus MRI: a retrospective cohort study. Int J Surg. 2014;12:544–8.
24. Koike E, Yamashita H, Noguchi S, et al. Bronchoscopic diagnosis of thyroid cancer with laryngotracheal invasion. Arch Surg. 2001;136:1185–9.
25. Ito Y, Miyauchi A, Kihara M, Fukushima M, Higashiyama T, Miya A. Overall survival of papillary thyroid carcinoma patients: a single-institution long-term follow-up of 5897 patients. World J Surg. 2018;42:615–22.
26. Ito Y, Tomoda C, Uruno T, et al. Prognostic significance of extrathyroid extension of papillary thyroid carcinoma: massive but not minimal extension affects the relapse-free survival. World J Surg. 2006;30:780–6.
27. McCaffrey JC. Aerodigestive tract invasion by well-differentiated thyroid carcinoma: diagnosis, management, prognosis, and biology. Laryngoscope. 2006;116:1–11.
28. Allen M, Spillinger A, Arianpour K, et al. Tracheal resection in the management of thyroid cancer: an evidence-based approach. Laryngoscope. 2020;
29. Rotolo N, Cattoni M, Imperatori A. Complications from tracheal resection for thyroid carcinoma. Gland Surg. 2017;6:574–8.
30. Gaissert HA, Honings J, Grillo HC, et al. Segmental laryngotracheal and tracheal resection for invasive thyroid carcinoma. Ann Thorac Surg. 2007;83:1952–9.
31. Friedman M, Danielzadeh JA, Caldarelli DD. Treatment of patients with carcinoma of the thyroid invading the airway. Arch Otolaryngol Head Neck Surg. 1994;120:1377–81.
32. Park CS, Suh KW, Min JS. Cartilage-shaving procedure for the control of tracheal cartilage invasion by thyroid carcinoma. Head Neck. 1993;15:289–91.
33. Tsukahara K, Sugitani I, Kawabata K. Surgical management of tracheal shaving for papillary thyroid carcinoma with tracheal invasion. Acta Otolaryngol. 2009;129:1498–502.
34. Wang LY, Ghossein R, Palmer FL, et al. Microscopic positive margins in differentiated thyroid cancer is not an independent predictor of local failure. Thyroid. 2015;25(9):993–8.
35. Czaja JM, McCaffrey TV. The surgical management of laryngotracheal invasion by well-differentiated papillary thyroid carcinoma. Arch Otolaryngol Head Neck Surg. 1997;123:484–90.
36. Machens A, Hinze R, Dralle H. Surgery on the cervicovisceral axis for invasive thyroid cancer. Langenbeck's Arch Surg. 2001;386:318–23.
37. Gillenwater AM, Goepfert H. Surgical management of laryngotracheal and esophageal involvement by locally advanced thyroid cancer. Semin Surg Oncol. 1999;16:19–29.
38. Price DL, Wong RJ, Randolph GW. Invasive thyroid cancer: management of the trachea and esophagus. Otolaryngol Clin N Am. 2008;41(1155–68):ix–x.
39. Grillo HC, Suen HC, Mathisen DJ, Wain JC. Resectional management of thyroid carcinoma invading the airway. Ann Thorac Surg. 1992;54:3–9. discussion -10
40. Brauckhoff M, Meinicke A, Bilkenroth U, et al. Long-term results and functional outcome after cervical evisceration in patients with thyroid cancer. Surgery. 2006;140:953–9.
41. Lee N, Tuttle M. The role of external beam radiotherapy in the treatment of papillary thyroid cancer. Endocr Relat Cancer. 2006;13(4):971–7.
42. Kiess AP, Agrawal N, Brierley JD, et al. External-beam radiotherapy for differentiated thyroid cancer locoregional control: a statement of the American Head and Neck Society. Head Neck. 2016;38:493–8.

Chapter 11
Management of Central Neck Nodes in Papillary Thyroid Cancer

Iuliana Bobanga and Christopher R. McHenry

Case Presentation

A 48-year-old woman was found to have a 3-cm thyroid nodule on a routine physical examination. She had no compressive symptoms, no prior history of head or neck irradiation, and had no family history of thyroid cancer or other endocrinopathies.

On physical examination, she had a 3-cm firm nodule palpable in the right lobe of the thyroid gland. She had no palpable nodules in the isthmus or the left lobe of the thyroid gland. Her trachea was midline. She had no palpable cervical or supraclavicular lymphadenopathy.

Her serum TSH level was 2.107 uIU/ml (0.450–5.330 uIU/ml). A comprehensive ultrasound examination of the neck revealed a $3.0 \times 1.6 \times 2.9$ cm solid, hypoechoic nodule with irregular margins and punctate calcifications in the right lobe of the thyroid gland, classified as TI-RADS 5 (highly suspicious for cancer). There was a $1.3 \times 0.8 \times 1.2$ cm solid, isoechoic nodule in the posterior, superior aspect of left lobe of the thyroid gland, classified as TI-RADS 3. There were no enlarged or abnormal lymph nodes in the central or lateral compartments of the neck.

A fine needle aspiration biopsy (FNAB) of the 3.0-cm nodule in the right lobe of the thyroid gland revealed papillary cancer. After extensive discussion with the

I. Bobanga
MatSu Surgical Associates, MatSu Regional Medical Center, Palmer, AK, USA

C. R. McHenry (✉)
Case Western Reserve University School of Medicine, Cleveland, OH, USA

Department of Surgery, MetroHealth Medical Center, Cleveland, OH, USA

Division of General Surgery, MetroHealth Medical Center, Cleveland, OH, USA
e-mail: cmchenry@metrohealth.org

S. A. Roman et al. (eds.), *Controversies in Thyroid Nodules and Differentiated Thyroid Cancer*, https://doi.org/10.1007/978-3-031-37135-6_11

115

patient, she elected for total thyroidectomy. The patient and her endocrinologist ask whether a central neck dissection will be performed during the total thyroidectomy.

Background

Lymph node (LN) metastases are common in patients with papillary thyroid cancer (PTC). LN metastases from PTC most commonly occur in the central compartment of the neck and spread sequentially via the lymphatics to the lateral neck and the superior mediastinum. Risk factors for LN metastases and recurrence include increased tumor size, extrathyroidal extension (ETE), multifocal disease, and extremes of age. In contrast to other malignancies, clinically apparent LN metastases in patients with PTC have no effect on survival in younger patients and likely have only a small effect on disease-specific survival in patients 45 years or older [1, 2]. LN metastases, however, are associated with increased rates of recurrence [3].

Clinically apparent macroscopic LN metastases (cN1) occur in 20–31% of patients with PTC [4] and are associated with increased regional recurrence. LN metastases have been associated with reduced survival in older patients [1, 2]. Total thyroidectomy and therapeutic central compartment neck dissection (CND) are the recommended surgical treatment for cN1 disease in order to reduce recurrence and improve survival [5, 6].

The role of prophylactic central neck dissection (pCND) for patients with no evidence of LN metastases on physical examination, preoperative imaging, or intra-operative evaluation remains controversial. This is due to the significant limitations of retrospective studies and the fact that only two small randomized controlled trials (RCTs) have been published to date [7, 8]. Studies differ in their definitions of recurrence, extent of thyroidectomy (hemithyroidectomy versus total thyroidectomy), extent of pCND (unilateral or bilateral), administration and dosing of radioiodine, and length of follow-up. Most of the published studies have significant selection bias.

Approximately 40–50% of patients with PTC have occult micrometastases in central neck LNs [4, 9]. Micrometastases are defined by sizes less than <2 mm [6]. Despite the high incidence of occult micrometastases, the rate of recurrence in the central neck has been reported to be only 2% whether or not a pCND is performed [10]. This relatively low recurrence rate, combined with the overall excellent prognosis for patients with PTC and central neck micrometastases suggests that micrometastases rarely progress to clinically significant disease. As a result, the benefit of pCND for clinically node-negative disease (cN0) is questionable.

The anatomic boundaries of the central compartment of the neck (Fig. 11.1) are the hyoid bone superiorly, the innominate artery inferiorly, the common carotid arteries laterally, the prevertebral fascia posteriorly, and the superficial layer of the deep cervical fascia anteriorly [11]. The LNs in the central compartment of the neck are categorized as level VI and level VII LNs. Level VI LNs include the

Fig. 11.1 Anatomic boundaries for the central compartment of the neck and the lymph nodes that are removed in a central compartment neck dissection. (*C* common carotid artery, *H* hyoid bone, *I* innominate artery, *LIV* left innominate vein, *RLN* recurrent laryngeal nerve)

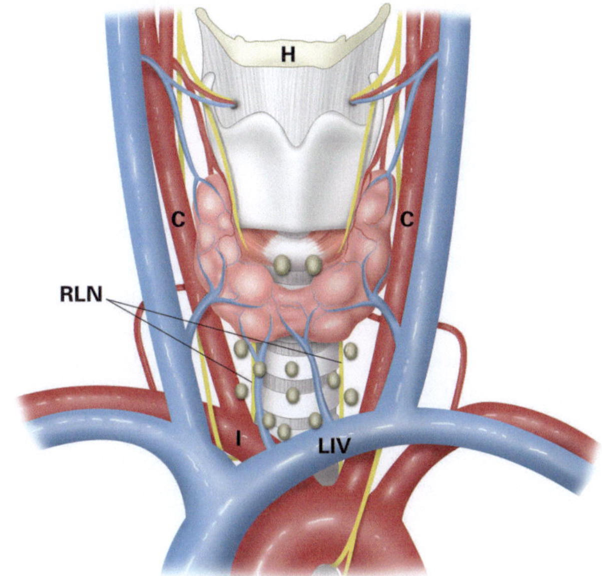

prelaryngeal (Delphian) LNs, which are superior to the isthmus in the midline of the neck; the pretracheal LNs, which are inferior to the isthmus along the anterior surface of the trachea; and the right and left paratracheal lymph nodes, which are present along the course of the RLNs between the common carotid arteries and the trachea. Level VII lymph nodes are the superior mediastinal LNs associated with the innominate artery and veins.

A CND involves removal of all lymph nodes and fibrofatty tissue from the central compartment of the neck. A unilateral CND includes removal of the prelaryngeal, pretracheal, superior mediastinal, and paratracheal LNs on the side of cancer. A bilateral CND includes removal of the prelaryngeal, pretracheal, superior mediastinal, and the right and left paratracheal LNs. A CND is classified as therapeutic when performed for the treatment of cN1 disease and as prophylactic when performed in patients with cN0 disease.

Prophylactic CND has been advocated by some surgeons because of its potential benefits, which include improved accuracy of staging and better selection of patients for I-131 administration, reduced postoperative thyroglobulin levels, reduced recurrence rates, and reduced need for reoperation in the central neck with its potential morbidity. However, pCND has been associated with higher risk of complications compared to thyroidectomy alone [7, 9, 12, 13]. Because of the potentially higher risk of complications following pCND, a unilateral CND has been recommended as an alternative for patients with cN0 disease to reduce potential injury to contralateral RLN and parathyroid glands. Alternatively, some surgeons have recommended that pCND not be performed at all because of lack of significant effect on locoregional recurrence, higher postoperative complication rates, and the potential for overuse of RAI without significant benefit. In our opinion, deciding whether to perform a pCND comes down to weighing the risks of permanent hypoparathyroidism and RLN injury versus the benefit of preventing recurrence and reoperation in the central compartment of the neck.

It has been estimated that a prospective RCT to study the effectiveness of pCND would require 5840 patients at a cost exceeding 15 million dollars [14]. This would be impractical and logistically challenging. As a result, review of data from high-quality observational studies and small prospective randomized controlled studies is required to determine the value, if any, of pCND in patients with cN0 PTC.

In this chapter, we will make recommendations and summarize the best available evidence regarding optimal pre- and intraoperative evaluation and management of central neck nodes for a patient with low risk, cN0 PTC. To determine whether or not pCND is of value in a patient with low risk, cN0 PTC, three questions will need to be addressed: (1) Is the rate of recurrence in the central compartment of the neck lower following pCND? (2) Is the rate of complications higher with pCND? and (3) Does the balance of potential risks and benefits justify performing pCND?

Preoperative Evaluation

Physical exam and comprehensive ultrasound (US) of the central and lateral neck are essential components of the preoperative evaluation of patients with PTC. Physical examination should include palpation of the thyroid gland, with attention to tumor size, location, consistency, mobility, additional nodules, tracheal deviation, and substernal extension. Palpation of the neck to evaluate for clinically apparent LN metastases should include the anterior and posterior cervical, supraclavicular, prelaryngeal, pretracheal, and paratracheal lymph node basins. Palpable cervical lymphadenopathy in a patient with PTC is suggestive of metastatic disease and requires further evaluation with ultrasound and fine needle aspiration biopsy (FNAB) of any abnormal nodes.

The positive predictive value of physical exam in detecting metastatic lateral neck disease in patients with PTC approaches 100%. However, the sensitivity of physical examination in detecting low-volume metastatic lymphadenopathy is only 19% [15]. High-resolution US is a much more sensitive method for detecting metastatic lateral neck disease [15, 16]. Preoperative neck US to evaluate for central and lateral neck compartment LNs is recommended in all patients with biopsy-proven PTC [5, 6].

In patients with a normal physical exam and known PTC, the US was able to identify metastatic disease in LNs of the lateral neck in 14–34% of patients and in the central compartment of the neck in 2–6% of patients [15, 17, 18]. Preoperative US identified suspicious cervical adenopathy in 20–31% of cases, altering the surgical approach in approximately 20% of patients [6, 15, 19]. Additional cross-sectional imaging, most commonly computed tomography with intravenous contrast, may augment ultrasound assessment in patients with a bulky primary, extensive nodal disease, nodes that extend inferiorly that cannot be fully evaluated by ultrasound, or if significant central neck nodal disease is suspected [20].

Preoperative neck ultrasound should be performed or interpreted by a clinician trained in thyroid pathology, using a high-resolution ultrasound scanner with a 7–14 mHz linear array transducer with real-time grayscale and color Doppler imaging [15, 18]. The central compartment (level VI) and the lateral compartments (levels II–V) of the neck should be examined. Sonographic features suggestive of a metastatic LN include size ≥10 mm, loss of a normal fatty hilum, rounded shape, hypoechogenicity, cystic change, microcalcifications, and peripheral vascularity [6, 15, 17, 18]. Confirmation of malignancy in LNs with suspicious US characteristics or enlarged physical exam is achieved by FNAB or intraoperative frozen section exam.

Preoperative FNAB of suspicious lymph nodes should be performed if it will change surgical management [5, 6]. If abnormal nodes are present in the lateral neck compartment, FNAB is performed to confirm metastatic disease to the lateral neck prior to performing a lateral neck dissection. Measurement of thyroglobulin from the needle washout of a FNAB may be helpful to diagnose metastasis in LNs that are cystic or specimens with inadequate cellularity for cytological evaluation [21, 22].

In the central neck, US evaluation of abnormal LNs is limited by the presence of the thyroid gland, and only half of abnormal central neck lymph nodes are detected preoperatively [23]. In addition, patients who have a history of Hashimoto thyroiditis commonly have benign reactive LNs in the central neck that may mimic metastatic disease. FNAB of suspicious central neck LNs can be avoided if intraoperative evaluation with a frozen section is planned or if therapeutic CND is planned based on US findings.

Intraoperative Evaluation

A systematic search and evaluation for abnormal LNs in the central compartment of the neck are routinely performed in patients with nodular thyroid disease and a FNAB that is malignant (Bethesda VI), indeterminate (Bethesda III, IV, and V), or nondiagnostic (Bethesda I). Abnormal LNs are enlarged, firm or rubbery, darker in color, or more rounded in shape.

A preliminary evaluation of the prelaryngeal and pretracheal regions for abnormal LNs occurs during the separation of the sternohyoid muscles in the midline of the neck to expose the thyroid gland. The search for abnormal prelaryngeal LNs is completed during the evaluation for a pyramidal lobe of the thyroid gland and exposure and resection of the pyramidal lobe. The area from the thyroid isthmus inferiorly to the hyoid bone superiorly is carefully examined.

The paratracheal areas, from the common carotid artery laterally to the trachea medially, are examined during the exposure and dissection of the RLNs. Special attention should be paid to the area dorsal to the RLN where abnormal LNs may be present, especially inferiorly on the right. Exposure of the paratracheal areas is optimized by retraction of the trachea medially.

The pretracheal area is further examined during the ligation of the inferior pole vessels and mobilization of the thyroid lobe and isthmus to the contralateral side of the trachea. The area from the inferior margin of the isthmus to the innominate artery is inspected. Inspection of the inferior aspect of the pretracheal area may be best accomplished after the exploration of the right paratracheal area and exposure of the innominate artery. Final evaluation of the pretracheal area is completed during the division of the ligament of Berry and removal of the contralateral lobe of the thyroid gland.

Discovery of an Abnormal LN

When abnormal LNs are discovered intraoperatively in the central neck of patients with PTC, there should be high suspicion of metastatic disease. In patients with concomitant Hashimoto thyroiditis and PTC, intraoperative nodal assessment is more challenging due to the frequent presence of inflammatory lymphadenopathy [20, 24]. A frozen section may be useful for evaluation of suspicious nodes. If positive for metastatic disease, therapeutic CND should be performed.

In patients with cN1 disease, a therapeutic bilateral CND is indicated. The operative report should specify that this is a therapeutic node dissection, and should specify the extent of dissection [11]. The goals of resection of clinically evident nodal metastasis are to decrease recurrence and improve survival [20].

If enlarged nodes are seen on both sides, bilateral CND should be performed [24]. In contrast, if only enlarged ipsilateral nodes are present, the surgeon has the option to perform a unilateral therapeutic node dissection alone, in order to minimize the risk of injury to the contralateral recurrent laryngeal nerve and parathyroid glands [20].

Several studies have shown that bilateral CND may be associated with higher morbidity, primarily RLN injury, and transient hypoparathyroidism, with no reduction in recurrence [12, 20, 25–27]. Extent of therapeutic CND should be adjusted based on surgeon judgement, but "berry picking" or removing only the obviously enlarged lymph nodes should be avoided [5, 6, 11, 20]. The number of nodes in the paratracheal regions ranges from 3 to 30 [20]. Nodal yield from a CND has an average of 8 nodes on pathologic exams [12].

Management of Patients with cN0 Disease

For patients with a 1–4 cm low-risk PTC, without evidence of LN metastasis on preoperative and intraoperative evaluation, surgical options include thyroid lobectomy (TL) or total thyroidectomy (TT) with or without pCND. The decision to perform a TL or TT for unilateral PTC must take into account patient and tumor characteristics, risk of loco-regional recurrence, and rate of operative complications. Previous guidelines have recommended TT for all differentiated thyroid cancers >1 cm based on data showing improved survival and decreased recurrence rates [6, 28]. Additional benefits of TT include optimization of the use of serum thyroglobulin for detection of recurrent disease and the use of RAI for imaging and treatment of metastatic disease.

More recent data has demonstrated, that in select patients with unilateral differentiated thyroid cancer <4 cm in size, without ETE, LN metastasis, history of neck radiation exposure or familial thyroid cancer, survival outcomes are similar in patients undergoing TL or TT [29–31]. Although some studies have demonstrated a lower risk of locoregional recurrence following TT compared to TL, the overall risk of recurrence after TL in low-risk cN0 PTC is between 1 and 4% [32–34]. With proper long-term follow-up, recurrence can be readily detected and treated without impact on overall survival [33–35].

Multiple studies comparing TT alone to TT with pCND for cN0 PTC have reported variable rates of recurrence and complications with different conclusions (Table 11.1). The majority of studies are single-institution retrospective cohort studies [4, 9, 13, 36–44]. There has been one multicenter retrospective study [45], two prospective RCTs [7, 8] and one prospective non-randomized study [46]. Most studies have not found a significant difference in the overall rate of recurrence and the rate of recurrence in the central neck for patients who underwent TT alone versus patients who underwent TT with pCND.

The first published RCT by Viola et al. included 93 patients randomized to TT with pCND and 88 patients treated with TT alone [7]. The primary endpoints of the study were successful radioiodine ablation with a stimulated thyroglobulin level < 1 ng/ml and recurrence; both were similar in the two groups after 5 years of follow-up. Ninety-nine percent of patients in the study received RAI ablation, however, a higher percentage of the TT group were treated with more than one dose of RAI to achieve successful ablation. Permanent hypoparathyroidism was higher with TT and pCND than with TT alone (19% vs. 8%, $p = 0.2$). The authors concluded that there was no significant benefit to pCND, with an increased risk of permanent hypoparathyroidism for patients with cN0 PTC.

A recent RCT by Sippel et al. also showed no clear benefit to pCND in patients with cN0 PTC [8]. This trial randomized 30 patients to TT with pCND and 30 patients to TT alone. There was no difference in recurrence and postoperative complication rates were similar between the two groups. However, the duration of follow-up was only 1 year.

Table 11.1 Publications comparing recurrence and complications rates for TT with pCND versus TT alone for treatment of cN0 papillary thyroid cancer

Author	Publication year	Study type	Sample size		Country	Follow-up duration (years)	Unilateral or bilateral pCND	Criteria for recurrent PTC	Total recurrence rate (%)	Central neck recurrence n (%)	RLN dysfunction (%) TT + pCND vs. TT		Hypoparathyroidism (%) TT + pCND vs. TT	
			TT + pCND	TT					TT + pCND vs. TT	TT + pCND vs. TT)	Transient	Permanent	Transient	Permanent
Barczynski	2013	Retrospective	358	282	Poland	10	B	FNA or path	* 4 vs. 13	* 1 vs 8	NS 3.6 vs 3.2	NS 1 vs 1	* 30 vs. 13	NS 2 vs. 0.7
Calo	2014	Retrospective	65	220	Italy	8.3	NR	US, Tg	NS 3 vs. 2	NS 0 vs. 0.5	NS 3 vs. 1	NS 0 vs 0	* 38 vs. 25	NS 11 vs. 5
Conzo	2014	Retrospective	362	390	Italy	9.5	B	FNA	NS 3.3 vs. 3.8	NS 1.4 vs 1.5	* 3.5 vs 1	NS 1.6 vs 0.7	* 15 vs 7	* 3.5 vs 1
Dobrinja	2017	Retrospective	74	112	Italy	3–6.3	NR	US, Tg	NS 5 vs. 4	–	* 10 vs 3	NS 4 vs 1	NS 15 vs. 8	* 8 vs. 1
Hughes	2010	Retrospective	78	65	USA	1.6–2	B	US, CT	NS 5 vs. 5	–	–	NS 0 vs. 3	* 27 vs. 8	NS 2.6 vs. 0
Kim	2016	Retrospective	8735	2834	S. Korea	5.2	U & B	FNA cytology	2 vs 3	0.3 vs 0.5	* 6 vs 3	NS 0.2 vs 0	* 32 vs 16	* 4 vs 2
Lang	2012	Retrospective	82	103	China	2	U	sTg @ 6mo postop	NS 4 vs. 3	–	NS 2 vs 0	NS 0.6 vs 0.5	* 18 vs. 9	NS 2.4 vs 1
Perrino	2009	Retrospective	82	159	Italy	5.7	U & B	Tg levels	* 5 vs. 37	–	NS 3 vs 3	Ns 2 vs 2	NS 9 vs 7	NS 2 vs 4
Popadich	2011	Retrospective	259	347	Australia, US & England	2.7–4	U & B	Reoperation	NS 5 vs. 8	* 1.5 vs. 6	NS 0.4 vs. 2	NS 0.4 vs. 2	* 10 vs. 4	NS 0.4 vs. 2
Raffaelli	2012	Prospective, nonrandom	124 62 ipsi 62 bi	62	Italy	2	U & B	US, FNA	NS 0.5 vs 0	–	NS 1 vs. 0	NS 1 vs. 0	* 43 vs. 18	NS 1 vs. 0

			TT + pCND	TT					TT + pCND vs. TT	TT + pCND vs. TT)	Transient	Permanent	Transient	Permanent
Sadowski	2009	Retrospective	180	130	USA	3.2	U & B	Reoperation	* 0 vs. 8	* 0 vs. 3	NS 9 vs. 5	NS 2 vs. 3	–	–
Sippel	2020	RCT	30	30	USA	1	U	US, Tg	–	–	NS 13 vs. 10	NS -	NS 33 vs. 24	NS -
Sywak	2006	Retrospective	56	391	Australia	2–5.8	U	NR	NS 3.5 vs. 5	–	NS 1.8 vs. 1	NS 0 vs. 1	NS 18 vs. 8	NS 1.8 vs. 0.5
Viola	2015	RCT	93	88	Italy	5	B	US, Tg	NS 7.5 vs 8	–	–	NS 4 vs 8	–	* 19 vs 8
Yazici	2020	Retrospective	258	100	Turkey	6.5	NR	Reoperation	* 3 vs. 19	–	NS 6 vs. 5	NS 0.4 vs. 1	* 27 vs. 10	NS 1 vs. 2
Ywata de Carvalho	2015	Retrosepctive	102	478	Brazil	6	NR	US	NS 4 vs 1.5	NS 0 vs 0.4	* 12 vs. 6	* 6 vs 1.5	* 46 vs 32%	* 12 vs 2
Total significant (of 16 studies)									4	3	4	1	10	5

U unilateral, *B* bilateral, *NR* not reported, *NS* not significant, *RCT* randomized controlled trial
*Statistically significant

A prospective study by Raffaelli et al. evaluated TT alone vs. TT with ipsilateral pCND vs. TT with bilateral pCND in patients with cN0 PTC [46]. A total of 186 patients were assigned to one of the three groups based on surgeon preference and the need to have three equal groups with similar baseline characteristics. With a short follow-up duration of 2 years, there were no significant differences in recurrence between groups, and complication rates were similar except for higher rate of transient hypocalcemia in the patients who underwent TT with bilateral pCND.

Kim et al. retrospectively evaluated the role of pCND in 11,569 cases from a single institution in South Korea [9]. The study included: 1259 patients with TL, 1575 patients with TT, 2107 patients with TL and ipsilateral pCND, 3377 patients with TT and ipsilateral pCND, and 3251 patients with TT and bilateral pCND. The mean tumor size for the thyroidectomy groups vs. pCND groups was 0.8 and 0.9 cm, respectively. There were significant differences in age, T stage, multifocality, ETE, and BRAF positivity between the thyroidectomy groups and the thyroidectomy with pCND groups, which may have affected results. The study showed no benefit to pCND in preventing recurrence and significantly higher rates of temporary RLN palsy and permanent hypoparathyroidism with pCND.

Four of the 16 studies outlined in Table 11.1 found a significantly lower rate of overall recurrence with TT and pCND compared to TT alone, while three studies found a significantly lower rate of central neck recurrence. One of the studies by Barczynski et al. had the longest duration of follow-up of two cohorts that were historically consecutive to each other: a TT group treated between 1993 and 1997 and a TT with pCND group treated between 1998 and 2002 [36]. Overall recurrence and central neck recurrence were significantly lower in the pCND group. The rate of recurrence for the TT group was 13%, higher than the average recurrence rate of 3–5% observed in most other studies. At 10 years, disease-specific survival was higher in the pCND group (98% vs. 92.5%).

A study by Perrino et al. also demonstrated a reduction in recurrence with TT and pCND compared to TT alone [41]. One limitation of this study, however, was that persistent or recurrent disease was defined based on Tg levels. Of those patients who were considered to have persistent or recurrent disease, 72% had an elevated Tg level without evidence of metastatic disease in US [41]. The definition of persistent and recurrent disease varies among the studies detailed in Table 11.1, resulting in varying rates of recurrence.

Popadich et al. performed a multicenter retrospective cohort study with pooled data from 3 Endocrine Surgery units, one each from Australia, the United States, and England [45]. This study showed a significantly lower rate of stimulated Tg level in the pCND group before initial I^{131} ablation. The total recurrence rate between the group with and without pCND was not significantly different; however, the rate of reoperation in the central neck compartment was lower in the pCND group (1.5% vs. 6%, $p = 0.004$). The number needed to treat (NNT) with a pCND to prevent 1 recurrence was 20. Effectiveness of pCND was greater for T3 and T4 tumors, with NNT with a pCND to prevent 1 recurrence being 16 and 5, respectively.

The rates of temporary RLN dysfunction were significantly higher with pCND in four studies, while permanent RLN dysfunction was not significantly different in all but one study (Table 11.1) [44]. The rates of temporary hypoparathyroidism were significantly higher with pCND in ten studies, while permanent hypoparathyroidism was significantly higher with pCND in five studies (Table 11.1).

Many of the retrospective studies summarized in Table 11.1 have similar limitations. For the non-randomized studies, the decision for TT vs. TT with pCND was most commonly based on surgeon preference, which created a significant selection bias. In several studies, tumor size, ETE, or the appearance of LNs at operation were used to decide whether or not to perform pCND. The TT group included patients who did not have a preoperative diagnosis of PTC but were found to have PTC on final pathology, another example of selection bias [4]. Both ipsilateral and bilateral pCND were included, however, some studies did not specify the extent of pCND. This resulted in a large variability in the extent of neck dissection, with varying numbers of LNs removed. Although the goal of pCND is to prevent recurrence and need for reoperation in the central neck, many studies did not specify rates of central neck recurrence.

Six meta-analyses have combined data from a variable number of the studies outlined in Table 11.1 [10, 47–51]. Five of them also included studies that only evaluated a pCND cohort without a comparison TT group [47–51]. Four of the 6 meta-analyses found a significantly lower rate of overall locoregional recurrence with pCND compared to the TT alone. Of the three studies that analyzed the rate of central neck recurrence, two meta-analyses noted this to be significantly lower with pCND [47, 49]. Of the three meta-analyses that analyzed complications, two noted significantly higher rates or permanent hypoparathyroidism with TT and pCND compared to TT alone [48, 49].

The five most recent meta-analyses included the study by Barczynski et al. that has an unusually large difference in recurrence rates between the TT with pCND and TT alone, much higher than reported in most other studies (4% vs. 13% for overall recurrence, 1% vs. 8% for central neck recurrence, Table 11.1). The meta-analysis by Lang et al., which included 14 studies, found that the study by Barczynski et al. had a profound impact on the overall incidence rate ratio of locoregional recurrence rate in the two groups. Because the study by Barczynski et al. was close to but within the margin of the funnel plot, it was not excluded from the meta-analysis. This study may have had a significant effect on the final rates of recurrence in several of the meta-analyses outlined in Table 11.2.

A sub-analysis was performed by Liu et al. to evaluate the difference between ipsilateral pCND and bilateral pCND. When comparing TT with ipsilateral CND vs TT alone, there was no difference in recurrence rates; however, TT with bilateral CND had a significantly lower rate of recurrence than TT alone [47]. In the meta-analysis by Chen et al., when the subgroups were compared, there was no difference in local-regional recurrence or complication rates between ipsilateral and bilateral pCND [48].

In several meta-analyses, patients who underwent pCND received higher doses of RAI, which was another confounding factor that may have had a significant impact on recurrence [48–50]. Zhao et al. reported a higher rate of recurrence in the lateral neck versus the central neck (3.3% vs. 1.1%) with TT and pCND, whereas

Table 11.2 Meta-analysis of recurrence and complication rates for TT with pCND versus TT alone for treatment of cN0 papillary thyroid cancer

Author, year	Number of studies included	TT + pCND (*n*)	TT (*n*)	Total recurrence rate		Central neck recurrence		Permanent RLN dysfunction		Permanent hypoPTH	
				TT + pCND	TT	TT + pCND	TT	TT + pCND	TT	TT + pCND	TT
Liu 2019	25	3413	3639	3.9%*	6%*	0.8%*	2.6%*	–	–	–	–
Chen 2018	23	11,098	5583	2.5%*	4.6%*	–	–	0.9%	0.75%	4.1%*	1.95%*
Zhao 2017	17	1969	2468	4.6%*	6.9%*	1.1%*	3.4%*	–	–	4.1%*	2.3%*
Lang 2013	14	1592	1739	4.7%*	8.6%*	–	–	1.2%	1.7%	2%	1.2%
Wang 2013	11	745	995	4.7%	7.9%	–	–	–	–	–	–
Zetoune 2010	5	396	1264	2%	3.9%	1.9%	1.7%	–	–	–	–

*Significant differences

the rate of recurrence with TT occurred with equal frequency in the lateral and central neck (3.4% vs. 3.3%) [49]. Wang et al. found no significant difference in recurrence or long-term complications, but a trend toward lower recurrence with TT with pCND, with a NNT of 31 patients to prevent one recurrence [51].

Limitations of meta-analyses that evaluate the role of pCND in the treatment of cN0 PTC are reflective of the quality of the studies included. Most studies were retrospective, with significant selection bias and differences in patient age, tumor size, ETE, and multifocality. In addition, the studies lacked standardized definitions of recurrence. Many studies did not analyze the dosages of RAI used, which may have an effect on recurrence rates. Overall follow-up was <5 years in the majority of studies included in the six meta-analyses, and very few of them reported overall or disease-free survival. The extent of pCND was also different among the studies.

Summary of Evidence-Based Recommendations for Management of Clinically N0 Disease in a Patient with a 3-cm PTC

The current literature comparing TT with pCND to TT alone for cN0 PTC consists of a predominance of retrospective single-institution studies with only modest follow-up duration and as a result, levels of evidence are weak. Despite this, some conclusions and recommendations can be made based on the available data. Rates of temporary and permanent hypoparathyroidism are higher with TT and pCND compared to TT alone, whereas the rate of RLN dysfunction is similar. When pCND is performed, approximately 50% of patients will have occult microscopic LN metastases [4]. This may result in changes in postoperative management with the potential for overtreatment with radioiodine and an unnecessary increase in the intensity of surveillance. However, the impact of pCND on overall recurrence and survival rates is minimal in contrast to macroscopic metastasis [4, 11]. Most studies do not show a significant reduction in overall recurrence or central neck recurrence with pCND (Table 11.1). Studies have shown that the NNT with a pCND to prevent one recurrence ranges from 20 to 31 patients [45, 51]. Thus, one must weigh the increased risk of complications to prevent one recurrence. In experienced hands, central neck reoperation for recurrent disease can be performed with similar rates of complications compared to CND performed during initial operation [52]. In our view, the potential small decrease in recurrence rate compared to the increased rate of complications after pCND does not justify performing routine pCND for low-risk cN0 PTC.

The patient in the clinical scenario at the beginning of the chapter has a 3-cm PTC in the right lobe of the thyroid gland and a 1.3-cm isoechoic nodule in the left lobe. Preoperative ultrasound and intraoperative assessment do not reveal abnormal lymph nodes. The recommended surgical treatment for this patient is a total thyroidectomy without pCND.

References

1. Zaydfudim V, Feurer ID, Griffin MR, Phay JE. The impact of lymph node involvement on survival in patients with papillary and follicular thyroid carcinoma. Surgery. 2008;144(6):1070–7. discussion 7-8
2. Lundgren CI, Hall P, Dickman PW, Zedenius J. Clinically significant prognostic factors for differentiated thyroid carcinoma: a population-based, nested case-control study. Cancer. 2006;106(3):524–31.
3. Leboulleux S, Rubino C, Baudin E, Caillou B, Hartl DM, Bidart JM, et al. Prognostic factors for persistent or recurrent disease of papillary thyroid carcinoma with neck lymph node metastases and/or tumor extension beyond the thyroid capsule at initial diagnosis. J Clin Endocrinol Metab. 2005;90(10):5723–9.
4. Hughes DT, Rosen JE, Evans DB, Grubbs E, Wang TS, Solórzano CC. Prophylactic central compartment neck dissection in papillary thyroid cancer and effect on locoregional recurrence. Ann Surg Oncol. 2018;25(9):2526–34.
5. Patel KN, Yip L, Lubitz CC, Grubbs EG, Miller BS, Shen W, et al. The American Association of Endocrine Surgeons Guidelines for the definitive surgical management of thyroid disease in adults. Ann Surg. 2020;271(3):e21–93.
6. Haugen BR, Alexander EK, Bible KC, Doherty GM, Mandel SJ, Nikiforov YE, et al. 2015 American Thyroid Association management guidelines for adult patients with thyroid nodules and differentiated thyroid cancer: the American Thyroid Association guidelines task force on thyroid nodules and differentiated thyroid cancer. Thyroid. 2016;26(1):1–133.
7. Viola D, Materazzi G, Valerio L, Molinaro E, Agate L, Faviana P, et al. Prophylactic central compartment lymph node dissection in papillary thyroid carcinoma: clinical implications derived from the first prospective randomized controlled single institution study. J Clin Endocrinol Metab. 2015;100(4):1316–24.
8. Sippel RS, Robbins SE, Poehls JL, Pitt SC, Chen H, Leverson G, et al. A randomized controlled clinical trial: no clear benefit to prophylactic central neck dissection in patients with clinically node negative papillary thyroid cancer. Ann Surg. 2020;272(3):496–503.
9. Kim SK, Woo JW, Lee JH, Park I, Choe JH, Kim JH, et al. Prophylactic central neck dissection might not be necessary in papillary thyroid carcinoma: analysis of 11,569 cases from a single institution. J Am Coll Surg. 2016;222(5):853–64.
10. Zetoune T, Keutgen X, Buitrago D, Aldailami H, Shao H, Mazumdar M, et al. Prophylactic central neck dissection and local recurrence in papillary thyroid cancer: a meta-analysis. Ann Surg Oncol. 2010;17(12):3287–93.
11. Carty SE, Cooper DS, Doherty GM, Duh QY, Kloos RT, Mandel SJ, et al. Consensus statement on the terminology and classification of central neck dissection for thyroid cancer. Thyroid. 2009;19(11):1153–8.
12. Pereira JA, Jimeno J, Miquel J, Iglesias M, Munné A, Sancho JJ, et al. Nodal yield, morbidity, and recurrence after central neck dissection for papillary thyroid carcinoma. Surgery. 2005;138(6):1095–100. discussion 100-1
13. Yazıcı D, Çolakoğlu B, Sağlam B, Sezer H, Kapran Y, Aydın Ö, et al. Effect of prophylactic central neck dissection on the surgical outcomes in papillary thyroid cancer: experience in a single center. Eur Arch Otorhinolaryngol. 2020;277(5):1491–7.
14. Carling T, Carty SE, Ciarleglio MM, Cooper DS, Doherty GM, Kim LT, et al. American Thyroid Association design and feasibility of a prospective randomized controlled trial of prophylactic central lymph node dissection for papillary thyroid carcinoma. Thyroid. 2012;22(3):237–44.
15. O'Connell K, Yen TW, Quiroz F, Evans DB, Wang TS. The utility of routine preoperative cervical ultrasonography in patients undergoing thyroidectomy for differentiated thyroid cancer. Surgery. 2013;154(4):697–701. discussion -3
16. Oltmann SC, Schneider DF, Chen H, Sippel RS. All thyroid ultrasound evaluations are not equal: sonographers specialized in thyroid cancer correctly label clinical N0 disease in well differentiated thyroid cancer. Ann Surg Oncol. 2015;22(2):422–8.

17. Stulak JM, Grant CS, Farley DR, Thompson GB, van Heerden JA, Hay ID, et al. Value of preoperative ultrasonography in the surgical management of initial and reoperative papillary thyroid cancer. Arch Surg. 2006;141(5):489–94. discussion 94-6
18. Kouvaraki MA, Shapiro SE, Fornage BD, Edeiken-Monro BS, Sherman SI, Vassilopoulou-Sellin R, et al. Role of preoperative ultrasonography in the surgical management of patients with thyroid cancer. Surgery. 2003;134(6):946–54. discussion 54-5
19. Network NCC. Thyroid Carcinoma (Version 1.2021) 2021. Available from: https://www.nccn.org/professionals/physician_gls/pdf/thyroid.pdf.
20. Agrawal N, Evasovich MR, Kandil E, Noureldine SI, Felger EA, Tufano RP, et al. Indications and extent of central neck dissection for papillary thyroid cancer: an American Head and Neck Society Consensus Statement. Head Neck. 2017;39(7):1269–79.
21. Pak K, Suh S, Hong H, Cheon GJ, Hahn SK, Kang KW, et al. Diagnostic values of thyroglobulin measurement in fine-needle aspiration of lymph nodes in patients with thyroid cancer. Endocrine. 2015;49(1):70–7.
22. Nixon IJ, Shaha AR. Management of regional nodes in thyroid cancer. Oral Oncol. 2013;49(7):671–5.
23. Leboulleux S, Girard E, Rose M, Travagli JP, Sabbah N, Caillou B, et al. Ultrasound criteria of malignancy for cervical lymph nodes in patients followed up for differentiated thyroid cancer. J Clin Endocrinol Metab. 2007;92(9):3590–4.
24. Shaha AR. Controversies about the central compartment in thyroid cancer. Editorial regarding the article "Clinical impact of cervical lymph node involvement and central neck dissection in patients with papillary thyroid carcinoma: a retrospective analysis of 368 cases" by Alexandre Bozec et al. Eur Arch Otorhinolaryngol. 2011;268(8):1097–9.
25. Lee YS, Kim SW, Kim SK, Kang HS, Lee ES, Chung KW. Extent of routine central lymph node dissection with small papillary thyroid carcinoma. World J Surg. 2007;31(10):1954–9.
26. Roh JL, Park JY, Park CI. Total thyroidectomy plus neck dissection in differentiated papillary thyroid carcinoma patients: pattern of nodal metastasis, morbidity, recurrence, and postoperative levels of serum parathyroid hormone. Ann Surg. 2007;245(4):604–10.
27. Cavicchi O, Piccin O, Caliceti U, De Cataldis A, Pasquali R, Ceroni AR. Transient hypoparathyroidism following thyroidectomy: a prospective study and multivariate analysis of 604 consecutive patients. Otolaryngol Head Neck Surg. 2007;137(4):654–8.
28. Cooper DS, Doherty GM, Haugen BR, Hauger BR, Kloos RT, Lee SL, et al. Revised American Thyroid Association management guidelines for patients with thyroid nodules and differentiated thyroid cancer. Thyroid. 2009;19(11):1167–214.
29. Barney BM, Hitchcock YJ, Sharma P, Shrieve DC, Tward JD. Overall and cause-specific survival for patients undergoing lobectomy, near-total, or total thyroidectomy for differentiated thyroid cancer. Head Neck. 2011;33(5):645–9.
30. Mendelsohn AH, Elashoff DA, Abemayor E, St John MA. Surgery for papillary thyroid carcinoma: is lobectomy enough? Arch Otolaryngol Head Neck Surg. 2010;136(11):1055–61.
31. Haigh PI, Urbach DR, Rotstein LE. Extent of thyroidectomy is not a major determinant of survival in low- or high-risk papillary thyroid cancer. Ann Surg Oncol. 2005;12(1):81–9.
32. Matsuzu K, Sugino K, Masudo K, Nagahama M, Kitagawa W, Shibuya H, et al. Thyroid lobectomy for papillary thyroid cancer: long-term follow-up study of 1,088 cases. World J Surg. 2014;38(1):68–79.
33. Nixon IJ, Ganly I, Patel SG, Palmer FL, Whitcher MM, Tuttle RM, et al. Thyroid lobectomy for treatment of well differentiated intrathyroid malignancy. Surgery. 2012;151(4):571–9.
34. Vaisman F, Shaha A, Fish S, Michael TR. Initial therapy with either thyroid lobectomy or total thyroidectomy without radioactive iodine remnant ablation is associated with very low rates of structural disease recurrence in properly selected patients with differentiated thyroid cancer. Clin Endocrinol. 2011;75(1):112–9.
35. Adam MA, Pura J, Gu L, Dinan MA, Tyler DS, Reed SD, et al. Extent of surgery for papillary thyroid cancer is not associated with survival: an analysis of 61,775 patients. Ann Surg. 2014;260(4):601–5. discussion 5-7

36. Barczyński M, Konturek A, Stopa M, Nowak W. Prophylactic central neck dissection for papillary thyroid cancer. Br J Surg. 2013;100(3):410–8.
37. Calò PG, Pisano G, Medas F, Marcialis J, Gordini L, Erdas E, et al. Total thyroidectomy without prophylactic central neck dissection in clinically node-negative papillary thyroid cancer: is it an adequate treatment? World J Surg Oncol. 2014;12:152.
38. Conzo G, Calò PG, Sinisi AA, De Bellis A, Pasquali D, Iorio S, et al. Impact of prophylactic central compartment neck dissection on locoregional recurrence of differentiated thyroid cancer in clinically node-negative patients: a retrospective study of a large clinical series. Surgery. 2014;155(6):998–1005.
39. Dobrinja C, Troian M, Cipolat Mis T, Rebez G, Bernardi S, Fabris B, et al. Rationality in prophylactic central neck dissection in clinically node-negative (cN0) papillary thyroid carcinoma: is there anything more to say? A decade experience in a single-center. Int J Surg. 2017;41(Suppl 1):S40–S7.
40. Lang BH, Wong KP, Wan KY, Lo CY. Impact of routine unilateral central neck dissection on preablative and postablative stimulated thyroglobulin levels after total thyroidectomy in papillary thyroid carcinoma. Ann Surg Oncol. 2012;19(1):60–7.
41. Perrino M, Vannucchi G, Vicentini L, Cantoni G, Dazzi D, Colombo C, et al. Outcome predictors and impact of central node dissection and radiometabolic treatments in papillary thyroid cancers < or =2 cm. Endocr Relat Cancer. 2009;16(1):201–10.
42. Sadowski BM, Snyder SK, Lairmore TC. Routine bilateral central lymph node clearance for papillary thyroid cancer. Surgery. 2009;146(4):696–703. discussion -5
43. Sywak M, Cornford L, Roach P, Stalberg P, Sidhu S, Delbridge L. Routine ipsilateral level VI lymphadenectomy reduces postoperative thyroglobulin levels in papillary thyroid cancer. Surgery. 2006;140(6):1000–5. discussion 5-7
44. Ywata de Carvalho A, Chulam TC, Kowalski LP. Long-term results of observation vs prophylactic selective level VI neck dissection for papillary thyroid carcinoma at a cancer Center. JAMA Otolaryngol Head Neck Surg. 2015;141(7):599–606.
45. Popadich A, Levin O, Lee JC, Smooke-Praw S, Ro K, Fazel M, et al. A multicenter cohort study of total thyroidectomy and routine central lymph node dissection for cN0 papillary thyroid cancer. Surgery. 2011;150(6):1048–57.
46. Raffaelli M, De Crea C, Sessa L, Giustacchini P, Revelli L, Bellantone C, et al. Prospective evaluation of total thyroidectomy versus ipsilateral versus bilateral central neck dissection in patients with clinically node-negative papillary thyroid carcinoma. Surgery. 2012;152(6):957–64.
47. Liu H, Li Y, Mao Y. Local lymph node recurrence after central neck dissection in papillary thyroid cancers: a meta analysis. Eur Ann Otorhinolaryngol Head Neck Dis. 2019;136(6):481–7.
48. Chen L, Wu YH, Lee CH, Chen HA, Loh EW, Tam KW. Prophylactic central neck dissection for papillary thyroid carcinoma with clinically uninvolved central neck lymph nodes: a systematic review and meta-analysis. World J Surg. 2018;42(9):2846–57.
49. Zhao W, You L, Hou X, Chen S, Ren X, Chen G, et al. The effect of prophylactic central neck dissection on locoregional recurrence in papillary thyroid cancer after Total thyroidectomy: a systematic review and meta-analysis : pCND for the locoregional recurrence of papillary thyroid cancer. Ann Surg Oncol. 2017;24(8):2189–98.
50. Lang BH, Ng SH, Lau LL, Cowling BJ, Wong KP, Wan KY. A systematic review and meta-analysis of prophylactic central neck dissection on short-term locoregional recurrence in papillary thyroid carcinoma after total thyroidectomy. Thyroid. 2013;23(9):1087–98.
51. Wang TS, Cheung K, Farrokhyar F, Roman SA, Sosa JA. A meta-analysis of the effect of prophylactic central compartment neck dissection on locoregional recurrence rates in patients with papillary thyroid cancer. Ann Surg Oncol. 2013;20(11):3477–83.
52. Shen WT, Ogawa L, Ruan D, Suh I, Kebebew E, Duh QY, et al. Central neck lymph node dissection for papillary thyroid cancer: comparison of complication and recurrence rates in 295 initial dissections and reoperations. Arch Surg. 2010;145(3):272–5.

Chapter 12
Impact of Surgeon Volume in Thyroid Operations

Fernanda Romero-Hernandez and Mohamed Abdelgadir Adam

Case

A 60-year-old morbidly obese woman with a history of left carotid endarterectomy 5 years ago presents with a 2.5-cm right papillary thyroid cancer with a metastatic lymph node in the ipsilateral central compartment. The patient lives in a rural area and presents to the only surgeon in town who has been in practice for 20 years but performs about one thyroidectomy per year. The patient decides to undergo total thyroidectomy and ipsilateral central lymph node dissection locally to avoid traveling >100 miles to the nearest surgeon specialist. Surgery is complicated by stridor requiring tracheostomy. Workup postoperatively is significant for bilateral vocal cord paralysis.

Background and Discussion of Salient Points Relating to the Controversy

Papillary thyroid cancer (PTC) is the most common type of differentiated thyroid cancer (DTC), with an incidence of approximately 13.5 per 100,000 [1]. In general, prognosis is excellent when appropriate treatment is employed. Complete surgical resection is the mainstay of treatment; however, extent of surgical resection is determined by a guidelines-based risk stratification system: (1) low-risk DTC includes intrathyroidal tumors with no lymph node metastases or vascular invasion; (2) intermediate-risk DTC includes tumors with microscopic extrathyroidal extension, cervical lymph node metastases, vascular invasion, or radioactive iodine-avid extrathyroidal neck disease; (3) high-risk DTC defined by gross extrathyroidal extension,

F. Romero-Hernandez · M. A. Adam (✉)
Department of Surgery, University of California San Francisco, San Francisco, CA, USA
e-mail: maria.romerohernandez@ucsf.edu; mohamed.adam@ucsf.edu

S. A. Roman et al. (eds.), *Controversies in Thyroid Nodules and Differentiated Thyroid Cancer*, https://doi.org/10.1007/978-3-031-37135-6_12

incomplete tumor resection, distant metastases, or inappropriate postoperative serum thyroglobulin levels [2]. Generally, thyroid lobectomy or total thyroidectomy is offered for patients with low-risk DTC. In contrast, total thyroidectomy with or without cervical lymph node dissection is employed for intermediate- or high-risk tumors. Presence of cervical lymph node metastases is common (20–50% of patients) and can potentially alter treatment in as many as 20% of cases. Thus, accurate preoperative cervical lymph node staging is critical. Central (level VI) or modified radical lateral-neck dissection is typically performed (in addition to total thyroidectomy) for patients with cervical lymph node metastases or high-risk features (Table 12.1) [2].

Thyroidectomy is one of the most commonly performed procedures in the United States, with nearly 200,000 operations performed annually [3]. Overall, thyroidectomy is considered a relatively safe procedure; nevertheless, the incidence of complications, including transient and life threatening, has been reported to be up to 8% [4]. Factors associated with outcomes include a cancer diagnosis, extent of surgery, and, more importantly, surgeon experience [5, 6]. The impact of surgeon experience, defined as annual surgeon volume (number of thyroidectomies performed by a surgeon per year), on clinical and oncologic outcomes has been well documented [7–10]. Two decades ago, Sosa et al. reported a multicenter retrospective study that showed the incidence of operative complications after total thyroidectomy was related to the individual surgeon volume rather than institutional volume [5]. Since then, published data comparing surgeon volume and outcomes have grown exponentially. Implementing high-volume care has transformed thyroidectomy into a safer procedure with fewer complications, shorter hospital stays [5, 8, 11], and lower costs [7, 12, 13]. Thus, high-volume surgical care has become a proxy for quality of care [2, 14, 15].

Table 12.1 Extent of surgical resection by American Thyroid Association guidelines based on risk stratification system for differentiated thyroid cancer

Risk	Definition	Extent of surgical resection
Low risk	Intrathyroidal tumors with no lymph node metastases, or vascular invasion	Thyroid lobectomy or total thyroidectomy
Intermediate risk	Tumors with microscopic extrathyroidal extension, cervical lymph node metastases, vascular invasion, radioactive iodine-avid extrathyroidal neck disease, or vascular invasion	Total thyroidectomy with or without cervical lymph node dissection
High risk	Gross extrathyroidal extension, incomplete tumor resection, distant metastases, or inappropriate postoperative serum thyroglobulin levels	Total thyroidectomy with cervical lymph node dissection

Compiled from the 2015 American Thyroid Association Management Guidelines for Adult Patients with Thyroid Nodules and Differentiated Thyroid Cancer [2]

Surgeon Volume and Clinical Outcomes

Surgical outcomes vary significantly by surgeon volume. In a large cohort of 16,954 patients who underwent total thyroidectomy, Adam et al. reported that patients had an 87% increased likelihood of having a complication if the operating surgeon performs 1 case/year, 68% for 2–5 cases/year, 42% for 6–10 cases/year, 22% for 11–15 cases/year, 10% for 16–20 cases/year, and 3% for 21–25 cases/year [5]. In another study, high-volume surgeons (>100 cases/year) had the lowest rate of complications from total thyroidectomy for cancer (7.5%) compared with 13.4% for intermediate-volume surgeons (10–100 cases/year) and 18.9% for low-volume surgeons [11]. When considering endocrine-specific complications such as hypoparathyroidism and/or recurrent laryngeal nerve (RLN) injury, the same pattern exists with a doubling of the risk of these complications when the operation is performed by low-volume surgeons (Table 12.2) [5].

Surgeon Volume and Oncologic Outcomes

Surgeon volume has also been shown to influence oncologic outcomes. Kim et al. examined the association of surgeon volume (>100 cases/year) with long-term oncologic outcomes in PTC. In their study of 1103 PTC with lateral lymph node metastasis, high-volume surgeons had a significantly higher likelihood of complete surgical resection and recurrence-free survival [16]. In another retrospective study that included 1246 patients who underwent lobectomy or total thyroidectomy, high-volume surgeons (>30 cases) were more likely to perform the correct initial treatment (total thyroidectomy) and have more complete initial resections, translating into better oncologic outcomes [17]. Park et al. found that low-/intermediate-volume surgeons (<99 cases per year) had a higher likelihood of recurrence and significantly shorter disease-free survival in 194 patients with medullary thyroid cancer [18].

Surgeon Volume Versus Years in Practice

Another controversy is the importance of surgeon volume versus surgeon experience (overall years in practice), as these two metrics may not always be synonymous. For example, a surgeon who has been in practice for years may occasionally perform specific procedures such as thyroidectomy, whereas a junior surgeon may perform more thyroidectomies. In a study that examined the interaction between surgeon volume and surgeon experience (years in practice) in high-risk PTC, there was no difference in recurrence-free survival between patients treated by experienced and less experienced high-volume surgeons. However, low-volume

Table 12.2 Risk of thyroid surgery complications by surgeon volume

Author	Cohort	Surgeon volume threshold	Low volume		High volume	
Sosa et al. [7]	5860 patients who underwent thyroid procedures	Four different surgeon volumes: – 1–9 cases/year – 10–29 cases/year – 30–100 cases/year – >100 cases/year.	**1–9 cases/year** Nerve injury: 1.5% Wound: 1.4% Overall: 10.1%	**10–29 cases/year** Nerve injury: 0.5% Wound: 0.5% Overall: 6.7%	**30–100 cases/year** Nerve injury: 0.8% Wound: 0.7% Overall: 6.9%	**>100 cases/year** Nerve injury: 0.4% Wound: 0.7% Overall: 5.9%
Kandil et al. [11]	46,261 patients who underwent thyroid procedures	– Low volume: ≤10 cases/year – Intermediate 10–99 cases/year – High volume > 100 cases/year	**Low volume** Nerve injury: 1.5% Bleeding: 0.5% Hypocalcemia: 12.1% Overall:19.7%	**Intermediate volume** Nerve injury: 1.2% Bleeding: 0.2% Hypocalcemia: 9.4% Overall:13.9%	**High volume** Nerve injury: 0.8% Bleeding: 0.1% Hypocalcemia: 4.7% Overall:8.1%	

Al-Qurayshi et al. [13]	77,863 patients who underwent thyroid procedures	– Low volume: ≤3 cases/year – Intermediate 14–29 cases/year – High volume > 30 cases/year	**Low volume** Nerve injury: 1.2% Bleeding: 2.4% Hypocalcemia: 6.9%	**Intermediate volume** Nerve injury: 0.8% Bleeding: 1.5% Hypocalcemia: 6.3%	**High volume** Nerve injury: 0.7% Bleeding: 1.0% Hypocalcemia: 4.1%	
Adam et al. [5]	16,954 patients who underwent total thyroidectomy.	– Low-volume: ≤25 cases/year – High-volume > 26 cases/year	Endocrine related: 2.3% Bleeding: 1.6% Wound: 1.1% Overall: 6.4%		Endocrine related: 1.6% Bleeding: 1.0% Wound: 0.7% Overall: 4.1%	
Sharma et al. [3]	3808 patients who underwent neck dissections	– Central neck 7.0 cases/year – Lateral neck 3.3 cases/year	**Central-neck dissection** Vocal cord paralysis 1.9% Hypocalcemia 1.5% Any complication 6.0%	**Lateral-neck dissection** Vocal cord paralysis 3.8% Hypocalcemia 1.3% Any complication 8.0%	**Central-neck dissection** Vocal cord paralysis 0.9% Hypocalcemia 0.5% Any complication 2.6%	**Lateral-neck dissection** Vocal cord paralysis 1.3% Hypocalcemia 0.9% Any complication 3.6%

surgeons with more and less experience had a higher hazard ratio of recurrence when compared to experienced high-volume surgeons. The authors concluded that annual surgeon volume is more critical for the risk of PTC recurrence than years of experience [16]. Some data from Europe suggest surgeon age may be associated with improved outcomes [19]. However, annual surgeon volume may be a more specific and representative metric to capture surgeons' experience for a specific procedure.

Surgeon Volume Threshold

While the literature has been consistent regarding the association between increasing surgeon volume and improved outcomes [7, 10–12, 20], the definition of a high-volume thyroid surgeon is controversial. Studies have proposed a variable minimum number of cases defining a high-volume thyroid surgeon, ranging from 20 to 100 cases per year [7, 9, 10, 21, 22]. It has been argued that the reported variation in the definitions of a high-volume thyroid surgeon is the result of how surgeon volume was analyzed in these studies, with most of the studies arbitrarily dividing their cohorts into low- and high-volume groups. A significant difference between the lowest- and highest-volume groups may not necessarily identify the threshold due to the expected effect of outliers and the loss of data between the lowest- and highest-volume points [5, 6]. In a cut point analysis that utilized multivariable restricted cubic splines, Adam et al. identified a thyroid surgeon volume threshold of >25 thyroidectomy cases per year to define a high-volume thyroid surgeon [5]. However, this study was limited to annual surgeon volume and could not account for overall (accumulated) surgeon experience. Some societies have adopted the definition of 25 thyroidectomies per year [15].

Surgeon Volume and Lymph Node Dissection

Lymph node dissection for cervical thyroid metastases is less common but more technically challenging than thyroidectomy alone. Lymph node dissection is an independent risk factor for complications such as RLN injury [23, 24]. Low surgeon volume for lateral-neck dissection has also been related to worse complications and oncologic outcomes. In a retrospective analysis that included 3808 patients, Sharma et al. determined that surgeons who performed >7 lateral-neck dissections had lower rates of overall complications, vocal cord paralysis, and hypocalcemia [3]. Sui et al. also showed that surgeons with less lateral-neck dissections experience (<20 cases/year) had higher rates of recurrence [25].

Surgeon Volume, Quality of Life, and Costs

There is a clear association between high-volume surgical care, improved patient quality of life and satisfaction, and lower healthcare costs. Low-volume care-related complications can negatively impact patient quality of life and out-of-pocket and payer costs. Published data have consistently demonstrated the association between low-volume surgical care and prolonged hospital stay, frequent laboratory testing, need for expensive medications, invasive procedures (e.g., laryngoscopy, temporary tracheostomy, and reoperations), and more frequent postoperative visits [6, 26]. Quality of life is substantially affected after major complications and should be one of the main factors to consider during decision-making conversations. A study that analyzed the quality of life after tracheostomy found a significant reduction in life satisfaction and body self-image perception [27]. This affects not only the patients and their families but also job performance, translating to more cost-impact.

In a retrospective study that included 13,997 patients who underwent thyroid surgery, Stavrakis et al. found that high-volume surgical care was associated with reduced total costs [10]. Specifically, each unit increase in surgeon volume was associated with a significant decrease of $365, concluding that there is a clear relationship between high-volume surgical care and lower healthcare costs. Analyzing specific complications, such as RLN, surgeon volume also has a significant impact on healthcare costs. A study that examined the impact of RNL injury on costs estimated between €2.860 and €34.320 extra costs from productivity loss secondary to RLN injury [28].

High-Volume Care Versus Access

It is clear that referral of patients to high-volume surgeons is associated, on average, with superior outcomes; however, concerns about access to the relatively limited number of high-volume surgeons and geographic barriers and distance are real issues hindering the implementation of high-volume surgical care. The vast majority (81%) of thyroidectomies in the United States are performed by low-volume surgeons, with 50% of surgeons performing 1 case per year [5]. While it is unclear if this pattern of low-volume care is primarily driven by lack of access to high-volume surgeons, there are situations where access is the main issue, especially for patients from rural areas. Rural patients, on average, are older, poorer, and less mobile than patients in metropolitan areas, limiting their ability to travel for high-volume surgical care [29]. With this, rural general surgeons are often faced with performing specialized procedures. In a survey of rural surgeons, thyroidectomy was the most commonly performed specialty procedure (81%) [30].

Because some patients may strongly prefer local surgical care even at the risk of increased morbidity [31], efforts to offer permanent or intermittent high-volume thyroidectomy care in the rural setting may mitigate the rural disparity of thyroidectomy outcomes. In a series of 150 consecutive thyroid and parathyroid procedures performed by a single rural surgeon over 4 years, only 1.3% of patients experienced RLN injury and 0.8% permanent hypoparathyroidism. The authors concluded that outcomes of thyroidectomy and parathyroidectomy largely depend on surgeon experience and can be performed safely in the community by an experienced surgeon [32].

Another concern is that centralizing high-volume surgical care may widen the access gap among disadvantaged groups. In a study that included 16,878 patients undergoing thyroid procedures, Sosa et al. found that Blacks and Hispanics were likelier to undergo procedures by low-volume surgeons [33]. While centralization of high-volume surgical care may be an issue for these vulnerable groups, the gap in their clinical outcomes would otherwise persist. Based on individual patient and surgeon characteristics, it may be reasonable to refer patients with more extensive disease to high-volume surgeons experienced in managing advanced thyroid cancer [2].

Proper communication between patients and surgeons should also be pursued to choose the best decision for treatment. Effective patient-centered communication could increase awareness of all possible treatment options and empower patients to express concerns and preferences for the best decision-making. Mira et al. found that the majority of patients, despite their willingness to be informed, prefer the doctor to make the decisions [34]. Surgeons should be transparent about their experience, outcomes, and long-term implications and encourage patients to take an active role in their care. Using communication tools may help improve this communication pathway. In a study that included 107 patients, Schumm et al. aimed to assess the communication skills of thyroid surgeons utilizing the Makoul Communication Assessment Tool [35]. The authors found that while communication was perceived as excellent, differences in race and ethnicity were identified as risk factors for poor communication. Similarly, in a qualitative study that analyzed the patient's perceptions of communication and its impact on the financial burden, Slavova-Azmanova et al. found that poor communication significantly impacts the ability to undertake clinical decisions, leading to a substantial out-of-pocket expense [36].

Return to the Case and Provide a Summary of Evidence-Based Recommendations for Management

The patient underwent an emergency tracheostomy and stayed in the hospital for 3 weeks. Bilateral vocal cord paralysis from injury of both RLNs is rare but is the most devastating complication after thyroid surgery. Recognition of risk factors for RLN injury and preoperative workup is paramount. The American Thyroid Association guidelines recommend preoperative voice assessment and laryngeal evaluation for all patients with a history of neck surgery or prior external beam radiation to the neck [2]. The patient's history of contralateral carotid

Area of impact	Rationale	Recommendation
Clinical outcomes	High-volume surgeons have less likelihood of: • RNL* injury • Hypocalcemia from hypoparathyroidism	Refer patients with more extensive disease to high-volume surgeons experienced in the management of advanced thyroid cancer.
Oncologic outcomes	High-volume surgeons have higher likelihood of: • Correct initial treatment • Complete surgical resection • Improved disease-free survival	
Lymph node dissection	High-volume care for lateral and central neck dissection is associated with less likelihood of: • Overall complications • Vocal cord paralysis • Hypocalcemia from hypoparathyroidism	
Years in practice	Surgeon-volume is procedure specific by: • Annual surgeon procedure volume (specific and representative metric. • Cumulative years in practice ≠ high-volume	
Cost and quality of life	High-volume surgeons are associated with: • Improved quality of life and patient satisfaction • Reduced costs	Detailed and transparent discussion about trade-offs between risks and benefits of seeking high-volume surgical care should be pursued.
Access	Rural patients may be: • Older, poorer, and less mobile • Limited ability to travel for high-volume surgical care	

Fig. 12.1 Summary of impact of surgeon volume in thyroid surgery (*Recurrent laryngeal nerve)

endarterectomy should have raised the possibility of a pre-existing vagus nerve injury and prompted formal preoperative voice and laryngeal assessment even in the absence of significant vocal symptoms, as patients with chronic vocal paralysis may not have significant vocal symptoms. The planned operation included central lymph node dissection, which increases the risk of RLN injury. The surgeon should have recognized the patient's risk factors, discussed with the patient the complexity of the planned operation, and disclosed the increased likelihood of such serious complications, especially in the hands of a low-volume surgeon. While the local surgeon has over 20 years of overall surgical experience, the surgeon is considered a low-volume thyroid surgeon. Surgeons who perform a thyroid case per year have the highest risk of complications, including double the risk of RLN injury.

Many patients have a strong preference to receive their care locally even at the risk of increased complications, but a detailed transparent discussion about tradeoffs between risk and benefits of seeking higher-volume surgical care should be pursued (Fig. 12.1).

References

1. Powers AE, Marcadis AR, Lee M, Morris LGT, Marti JL. Changes in trends in thyroid cancer incidence in the United States, 1992 to 2016. JAMA. 2019;322(24):2440–1.
2. Haugen BR, Alexander EK, Bible KC, Doherty GM, Mandel SJ, Nikiforov YE, et al. 2015 American Thyroid Association management guidelines for adult patients with thyroid nodules and differentiated thyroid cancer: the American Thyroid Association guidelines task force on thyroid nodules and differentiated thyroid cancer. Thyroid. 2016;26(1):1–133.
3. Sharma RK, Lee J, Liou R, McManus C, Lee JA, Kuo JH. Optimal surgeon-volume threshold for neck dissections in the setting of primary thyroid malignancies. Surgery. 2022;171(1):172–6.

4. Caulley L, Johnson-Obaseki S, Luo L, Javidnia H. Risk factors for postoperative complications in total thyroidectomy: a retrospective, risk-adjusted analysis from the National Surgical Quality Improvement Program. Medicine (Baltimore). 2017;96(5):e5752.

5. Adam MA, Thomas S, Youngwirth L, Hyslop T, Reed SD, Scheri RP, et al. Is there a minimum number of thyroidectomies a surgeon should perform to optimize patient outcomes? Ann Surg. 2017;265(2):402–7.

6. Adam MA, Thomas S, Youngwirth L, Hyslop T, Reed SD, Scheri RP, et al. Reply to: "Surgeon Volume Threshold for Total Thyroidectomy.". Ann Surg. 2018;267(4):e78–9.

7. Sosa JA, Bowman HM, Tielsch JM, Powe NR, Gordon TA, Udelsman R. The importance of surgeon experience for clinical and economic outcomes from thyroidectomy. Ann Surg. 1998;228(3):320–30.

8. Loyo M, Tufano RP, Gourin CG. National trends in thyroid surgery and the effect of volume on short-term outcomes. Laryngoscope. 2013;123(8):2056–63.

9. Gourin CG, Tufano RP, Forastiere AA, Koch WM, Pawlik TM, Bristow RE. Volume-based trends in thyroid surgery. Arch Otolaryngol Head Neck Surg. 2010;136(12):1191–8.

10. Stavrakis AI, Ituarte PHG, Ko CY, Yeh MW. Surgeon volume as a predictor of outcomes in inpatient and outpatient endocrine surgery. Surgery. 2007;142(6):887–99. discussion 887-899

11. Kandil E, Noureldine SI, Abbas A, Tufano RP. The impact of surgical volume on patient outcomes following thyroid surgery. Surgery. 2013;154(6):1346–52. discussion 1352-1353

12. Chowdhury MM, Dagash H, Pierro A. A systematic review of the impact of volume of surgery and specialization on patient outcome. Br J Surg. 2007;94(2):145–61.

13. Al-Qurayshi Z, Robins R, Hauch A, Randolph GW, Kandil E. Association of Surgeon volume with outcomes and cost savings following thyroidectomy: a national forecast. JAMA Otolaryngol Head Neck Surg. 2016;142(1):32.

14. Patel N, Scott-Coombes D. Impact of surgical volume and surgical outcome assessing registers on the quality of thyroid surgery. Best Pract Res Clin Endocrinol Metab. 2019;33(4):101317.

15. Lorenz K, Raffaeli M, Barczyński M, Lorente-Poch L, Sancho J. Volume, outcomes, and quality standards in thyroid surgery: an evidence-based analysis-European Society of Endocrine Surgeons (ESES) positional statement. Langenbeck's Arch Surg. 2020;405(4):401–25.

16. Kim HI, Kim TH, Choe JH, Kim JH, Kim JS, Kim YN, et al. Surgeon volume and prognosis of patients with advanced papillary thyroid cancer and lateral nodal metastasis. Br J Surg. 2018;105(3):270–8.

17. Adkisson CD, Howell GM, McCoy KL, Armstrong MJ, Kelley ML, Stang MT, et al. Surgeon volume and adequacy of thyroidectomy for differentiated thyroid cancer. Surgery. 2014;156(6):1453–9. discussion 1460

18. Park H, Kim HI, Choe JH, Chung MK, Son YI, Hahn SY, et al. Surgeon volume and long-term oncologic outcomes in patients with medullary thyroid carcinoma. Ann Surg Oncol. 2021;28(13):8863–71.

19. Duclos A, Peix JL, Colin C, Kraimps JL, Menegaux F, Pattou F, et al. Influence of experience on performance of individual surgeons in thyroid surgery: prospective cross sectional multicentre study. BMJ. 2012;344:d8041.

20. Oltmann SC, Holt SA. How do we improve patient access to high-volume thyroid surgeons? Surgery. 2014;156(6):1450–2.

21. Weiss A, Lee KC, Brumund KT, Chang DC, Bouvet M. Risk factors for hematoma after thyroidectomy: results from the nationwide inpatient sample. Surgery. 2014;156(2):399–404.

22. Dehal A, Abbas A, Al-Tememi M, Hussain F, Johna S. Impact of surgeon volume on incidence of neck hematoma after thyroid and parathyroid surgery: ten years' analysis of nationwide inpatient sample database. Am Surg. 2014;80(10):948–52.

23. Giulea C, Enciu O, Toma EA, Martin S, Fica S, Miron A. Total thyroidectomy for malignancy-is central neck dissection a risk factor for recurrent nerve injury and postoperative hypocalcemia? A tertiary center experience in Romania. Acta Endocrinol (Buchar). 2019;5(1):80–5.

24. Lee YS, Nam KH, Chung WY, Chang HS, Park CS. Postoperative complications of thyroid cancer in a single center experience. J Korean Med Sci. 2010;25(4):541–5.

25. Siu J, Griffiths R, Noel CW, Austin PC, Pasternak J, Urbach D, et al. Surgical case volume has an impact on outcomes for patients with lateral neck disease in thyroid cancer. Ann Surg Oncol. 2022;29(2):1141–50.
26. Mirallié E, Borel F, Tresallet C, Hamy A, Mathonnet M, Lifante JC, et al. Impact of total thyroidectomy on quality of life at 6 months: the prospective ThyrQoL multicentre trial. Eur J Endocrinol. 2020;182(2):195–205.
27. Gilony D, Gilboa D, Blumstein T, Murad H, Talmi YP, Kronenberg J, et al. Effects of tracheostomy on well-being and body-image perceptions. Otolaryngol Head Neck Surg. 2005;133(3):366–71.
28. Ferrari CC, Rausei S, Amico F, Boni L, Chiang FY, Wu CW, et al. Recurrent laryngeal nerve injury in thyroid surgery: clinical pathways and resources consumption. Head Neck. 2016;38(11):1657–65.
29. White MG, Applewhite MK, Kaplan EL, Angelos P, Huo D, Grogan RH. A tale of two cancers: traveling to treat pancreatic and thyroid cancer. J Am Coll Surg. 2017;225(1):125–136.e6.
30. Stiles R, Reyes J, Helmer SD, Vincent KB. What procedures are rural general surgeons performing and are they prepared to perform specialty procedures in practice? Am Surg. 2019;85(6):587–94.
31. Molt PL. Rural surgery and the volume dilemma [Internet]. [cited 2022 Jun 29]. Available from: https://bulletin.facs.org/2016/10/rural-surgery-and-the-volume-dilemma/
32. Richmond BK, Eads K, Flaherty S, Belcher M, Runyon D. Complications of thyroidectomy and parathyroidectomy in the rural community hospital setting. Am Surg. 2007;73(4):332–6.
33. Sosa JA, Mehta PJ, Wang TS, Yeo HL, Roman SA. Racial disparities in clinical and economic outcomes from thyroidectomy. Ann Surg. 2007;246(6):1083–91.
34. Mira JJ, Guilabert M, Pérez-Jover V, Lorenzo S. Barriers for an effective communication around clinical decision making: an analysis of the gaps between doctors' and patients' point of view. Health Expect. 2014;17(6):826–39.
35. Schumm MA, Ohev-Shalom R, Nguyen DT, Kim J, Tseng CH, Zanocco KA. Measuring patient perceptions of surgeon communication performance in the treatment of thyroid nodules and thyroid cancer using the communication assessment tool. Surgery. 2021;169(2):282–8.
36. Slavova-Azmanova N, Newton JC, Hohnen H, Johnson CE, Saunders C. How communication between cancer patients and their specialists affect the quality and cost of cancer care. Support Care Cancer. 2019;27(12):4575–85.

Chapter 13
Intraoperative/Postoperative Calcium Management in Thyroidectomy

Mariam Ali-Mucheru and Rebecca S. Sippel

Case

A 55-year-old woman in previously good health was found to have a palpable right thyroid nodule during a routine checkup. An ultrasound confirmed a 5-cm hypoechoic right thyroid nodule with scattered microcalcifications, possible extracapsular extension, and no concerning lymphadenopathy. An FNA demonstrated papillary thyroid carcinoma. She was scheduled to undergo a total thyroidectomy but was very concerned about the risks of hypoparathyroidism.

Background

Hypoparathyroidism is the most common complication following surgery in the anterior neck including parathyroidectomy, thyroidectomy, and lymph node neck dissection for malignancy [1–3]. Surgical hypoparathyroidism is most likely to occur due to trauma, devascularization, or inadvertent excision of parathyroid glands during surgery. Transient hypoparathyroidism occurs in 20–30% and permanent hypoparathyroidism in 1–3% of patients after a total thyroidectomy [4]. For those patients who suffer from transient hypoparathyroidism, preventative measures, early identification, and appropriate treatment is essential to minimize its impact on patients [5]. Permanent hypoparathyroidism can have significant

M. Ali-Mucheru
Surgical Specialists of Atlanta, Atlanta, GA, USA
e-mail: ali-mucheru.mariam@mayo.edu

R. S. Sippel (✉)
Department of Surgery, University of Wisconsin-Madison, Madison, WI, USA
e-mail: sippel@surgery.wisc.edu

S. A. Roman et al. (eds.), *Controversies in Thyroid Nodules and Differentiated Thyroid Cancer*, https://doi.org/10.1007/978-3-031-37135-6_13

consequences on health and quality of life of patients. Identification and meticulous dissection and preservation of blood supply to the parathyroid glands are key steps to minimizing the risk of postoperative hypoparathyroidism.

Definition

Hypoparathyroidism is a condition of impaired or inadequate parathyroid hormone (PTH) secretion leading to hypocalcemia and hyperphosphatemia [6]. There is variability in the definition of surgical hypoparathyroidism: certain studies use clinical criteria (symptomatic vs asymptomatic hypocalcemia), biochemical criteria (serum PTH and/or calcium and/or ionized calcium levels), and/or treatment criteria (requirement of calcium and or vitamin D supplementation) [4, 7].

Measuring the serum PTH immediately after surgery is the most sensitive and specific method of assessing the function of the parathyroid glands and for identifying patients at risk of hypoparathyroidism and hypocalcemia [8–12]. Postoperative hypoparathyroidism may be transient or permanent. Permanent hypoparathyroidism is defined as failure of the parathyroid glands to regain normal function 6 months after surgery [2, 6, 11]. While 6 months is the commonly applied definition of permanent hypoparathyroidism, parathyroid gland recovery has been seen in some patients between 6 and 12 months, or even longer after surgery [11].

Risk Factors

Risk factors of postoperative hypoparathyroidism are listed in Table 13.1 [6, 7, 13]. The type and extent of surgery, operative technique, surgeon expertise, and underlying disease process all contribute to the risk of postoperative hypoparathyroidism [2, 6].

Table 13.1 Risk factors for hypoparathyroidism

- Bilateral thyroid procedures (simultaneous or staged)
- Central neck dissection
- Autoimmune thyroid disease (Graves' disease, Hashimoto's thyroiditis)
- Malignancy
- Concurrent thyroidectomy and parathyroidectomy
- Malabsorption (e.g., Gastric bypass)
- Substernal goiter
- Low-volume thyroid surgeon
- Substernal goiter
- Prior neck surgery
- Pediatric patient

Symptoms and Signs

Clinical manifestations of hypocalcemia range from asymptomatic to life threatening, depending on the severity of calcium deficiency [3]. Hypocalcemia is characterized by neuromuscular irritability [14]. The most common mild symptoms include perioral and acral paresthesias, muscle cramps, and stiffness. Severe symptoms include laryngospasm and seizures [15]. Neuropsychiatric symptoms include confusion, anger, depression, lightheadedness, and irritability [7].

Bedside maneuvers such as Chvostek's and Trousseau's sign can be performed in order to assess for tetany. Chvostek's sign is facial muscle twitching upon tapping the preauricular region over the facial nerve (present at baseline in up to 25% of people). Trousseau's sign is flexion of the wrist, thumb, and metacarpophalangeal joints and hyperextension of the fingers upon brachial artery occlusion by inflation of a blood pressure cuff above systolic blood pressure [7, 14]. Cardiovascular signs observed with progressive hypocalcemia include prolongation of the QT interval that can result in Torsades de Pointes, a form of ventricular tachycardia that may degenerate into ventricular fibrillation [7].

Case

Given that the patient will need a total thyroidectomy, how would you manage her parathyroid glands during surgery and her calcium in the perioperative period to minimize complications of hypoparathyroidism?

Perioperative Care

It is helpful to obtain routine baseline labs including serum calcium and PTH prior to a total thyroidectomy. If the baseline calcium is low or below normal, the risk of hypoparathyroidism is increased and studies have shown the benefit of initiating scheduled oral calcium supplementation [15–17]. When the calcium is elevated, checking the PTH helps rule out occult hyperparathyroidism which can be treated concurrently during total thyroidectomy. If the PTH level is elevated, we obtain a 25-hydroxy vitamin D level to identify preexisting vitamin D deficiency, which is a common cause of secondary hyperparathyroidism. Vitamin D facilitates the absorption of calcium from the intestinal tract, increases bone resorption, and decreases renal excretion of calcium and phosphate [7]. Vitamin D deficiency can be mild (20–30 ng/mL), moderate (10 to <20 ng/mL), or severe (below the lowest recordable level, <10 ng/mL). Mild disease can be treated with over-the-counter supplementation; however, moderate-to-severe disease is best treated with high-dose ergocalciferol. Treating vitamin D deficiency using established guidelines prior to surgery optimizes postoperative oral calcium supplementation and can reduce the risk of symptomatic postoperative hypocalcemia [17, 18].

Surgical Considerations

Surgeon experience is imperative in minimizing the risk of surgical hypoparathyroidism: many studies show that high-volume surgeons and centers have lower overall rates of postoperative complications [6]. Parathyroid gland preservation is the best way to reduce the risk of hypoparathyroidism. Visual intraoperative identification of parathyroid glands can be difficult, as the glands are small and can have similar coloration compared to thyroid, fat and lymph nodes [7]. Most surgeons rely on visual cues and landmarks. Parathyroid tissue fluorescence in the presence of a contrast agent or photosensitizer, and detection with infrared fluorescence imaging are promising new techniques to improve intraoperative parathyroid identification [7]. Parathyroid autofluorescence with near-infrared spectroscopy is also helpful in identifying parathyroid tissue [19]. Indocyanine green fluorescence angiography is a new adjunct that may improve the assessment of parathyroid gland blood flow compared to visual inspection and can assess the viability of the glands and the need for possible autotransplantation [20].

Meticulous dissection to preserve the parathyroid glands and their blood supply is the key to minimizing trauma or injury to the glands. If the parathyroid (s) cannot be identified, dissection should be maintained right on the thyroid capsule, and the inferior thyroid artery should be ligated very close to the thyroid gland. The inferior thyroid artery supplies the inferior and superior parathyroid glands in most patients. In order to preserve the venous drainage of the parathyroid glands it is best to take the middle thyroid vein branches as they insert into the thyroid gland. It is not necessary to visualize all four parathyroid glands during thyroidectomy in order to reduce the risk of postoperative hypocalcemia [7]. The inferior parathyroid glands may be located in the thymus, which should be preserved whenever feasible to minimize injury. Attempts to identify parathyroid glands that are not seen during the dissection will likely increase the risk of injury or devascularization.

Any parathyroid glands that appear devascularized or are inadvertently removed should be inspected to ensure the tissue is normal and then autotransplanted into the strap or sternocleidomastoid muscles. If the patient is undergoing surgery for thyroid malignancy, it is best to obtain a frozen section prior to performing autotransplant to ensure that the tissue is truly parathyroid and not a lymph node. The gland should be minced into 1–2 mm fragments which are then directly implanted into a pocket in well-vascularized muscle and marked with a permanent stitch. The authors typically use the sternocleidomastoid muscle as it is easily reachable from the operative field and has a more robust muscle bed to facilitate neovascularization. We typically put the autotransplant in at least two separate pockets in case neovascularization does not develop in one of the pockets. The purpose of parathyroid autotransplantation is to reduce the risk of hypoparathyroidism. An autotransplant does not typically start functioning for 2–3 months after surgery, so the patient will need to be maintained on calcium and/or calcitriol until parathyroid function returns. Since parathyroid autotransplantation is typically not performed on the last remaining gland, it is difficult to know the true take rate of autotransplantation. If it is done with fresh tissue on the day of surgery (as opposed to cryopreserved tissue), the take rate is reported to be 90–95% [21, 22].

Venous congestion of the parathyroid glands can be relieved by sharply scoring the parathyroid gland capsule, which will usually result in an immediate improvement in color. If the arterial blood supply is impaired by venous congestion, the gland can often develop new venous channels and regain function. It is also important to make a habit of inspecting the resected thyroid specimen for parathyroid tissue prior to sending it to pathology. Inadvertent parathyroidectomy or the identification of parathyroid tissue in the surgical specimen is a common finding and occurs in 20–28% of patients undergoing thyroidectomy and/or central neck dissection [6].

Intraoperative PTH, Serum Calcium Testing

Intraoperative PTH (IOPTH) refers to rapid processing of blood specimens drawn during or shortly after thyroid or central neck surgery to determine PTH levels and can influence surgical or postoperative management [7]. In many institutions, IOPTH provides a rapid result compared to standard intact PTH assay. PTH has a short half-life (3–5 min); therefore, the results can be used to influence perioperative decision-making. Serum calcium requires trending over 12–24 h and can be confounded by prophylactic calcium and calcitriol administration or vitamin D deficiency; as a result, most surgeons favor using IOPTH over calcium to predict hypocalcemia and hypoparathyroidism [7].

Multiple studies have examined the utility of using IOPTH for predicting hypoparathyroidism and hypocalcemia, but the optimal strategy for monitoring has been debated and ranges from utilizing a PTH level from 10 min to 24 h after surgery [9–12, 23–27]. The authors recommend obtaining a PTH in the postoperative recovery area after total thyroidectomy. We define a low PTH as a PTH measurement <10 pg/mL as this cut-off best predicts symptomatic hypocalcemia [10, 12, 25].

Postoperative Management

The goal of managing hypoparathyroidism is to avoid the complications of hypocalcemia. The authors utilize the attached algorithm for management based on the PTH level drawn in the recovery room (Table 13.2). It usually takes 24–72 h for the calcium levels to nadir after surgery, so empiric treatment started immediately

Table 13.2 Management of adults with hypoparathyroidism after total thyroidectomy

Postoperative PTH (pg/mL)	Therapy
>20	No scheduled calcium carbonate unless patient has Graves' disease, patients with Graves' disease get Calcium carbonate 1000 mg × TID prophylactically
10–20	Calcium carbonate 1000 mg × TID
4–9	Calcium carbonate 1000 mg × TID Calcitriol 0.25 mcg × BID
>4 (or undetectable)	Calcium carbonate 1000 mg × TID Calcitriol 0.50 mcg × BID

BID twice a day, *TID* three times a day, *PTH* parathyroid hormone

following surgery can minimize the severity of hypocalcemia. The American Thyroid Association guidelines recommend treatment with oral calcium and calcitriol and/or serial calcium measurements until stability is confirmed for anyone with a PTH <15 pg/mL [7]. Ritter et al. studied 1054 total thyroidectomy patients, in which 18% had PTH < 10 pg/mL, 70% resolved within 2 months, 5% resolved within 6–12 months, and 1.9% had permanent hypoparathyroidism after 1 year. Of note, 50% of patients who were labeled as having permanent hypoparathyroidism had recovery of some PTH function but still required supplementation to avoid symptoms of hypocalcemia.

Case

Our patient had a PTH of 9 in the recovery room. What would be the best management to minimize hypocalcemia?

Prophylactic Management

The authors recommend prophylactic treatment with oral calcium carbonate in all postoperative total thyroidectomy patients with a low PTH or at a high risk of hypocalcemia, which is the most widely available and affordable option. We typically start at 1000 mg three times a day but can increase to 2000 mg three times a day if needed. A meta-analysis by Xing et al. found ten randomized controlled trials with 1620 patients who had total thyroidectomy or neck dissection. Calcium supplementation was effective in preventing postoperative hypocalcemia. Calcium plus vitamin D was more effective than calcium alone [15]. Calcitriol is the active form of vitamin D and increases intestinal absorption of calcium and mobilization from the bones [7, 10, 14]. Calcitriol is started at a dose of 0.25–1.0 mcg/day. Routine supplementation of calcium and vitamin D after thyroidectomy is less expensive, results in higher patient utility and incremental gain in quality-adjusted life years compared to selective supplementation [28, 29]. Prophylactic replacement can result in hypercalcemia, so it is important to monitor serum calcium and iPTH levels and taper medications as tolerated. The authors' preference is to utilize a 0.25-mcg tablet prescription of calcitriol so that the dosage can easily be titrated up or down as needed to control symptoms.

Case

Our patient presented to the emergency department 3 days after total thyroidectomy and was complaining of perioral and acral paresthesias and muscle spasms. She reported that she occasionally forgot to take her medications over the last 2 days and did not like their taste. She had taken 8 g of TUMS but was still symptomatic and getting uncomfortable, so she came to the emergency department. What is the next step in management?

Clinically significant surgical hypoparathyroidism ultimately manifests with symptoms of hypocalcemia [6, 7]. The first step is to verify the diagnosis by checking laboratory tests such as serum calcium, phosphorus, magnesium, albumin, ionized calcium, and iPTH. The severity of the hypocalcemia determines the severity of the symptoms. The diagnosis would be confirmed with normal or low albumin-corrected calcium, low ionized calcium, elevated serum phosphorus, and low iPTH [6].

Mild to Moderate Hypoparathyroidism/Mild Hypocalcemia (7.5–8 mg/dL)

The patient's symptoms of perioral and acral paresthesia and muscle spasms are typical for mild to moderate hypocalcemia. A patient with a PTH <15 pg/mL, serum calcium <8.5 mg/dL, or ionized Ca < 1.1 mmol/L, should be on oral supplementation with 2–6 g of calcium carbonate per day or the equivalent dose of calcium citrate [7]. Calcium carbonate (40% elemental calcium) and calcium citrate (20% elemental calcium) are the most common oral calcium supplements and should be taken with meals [7]. Calcium carbonate requires an acidic environment to dissolve so it is important to review if the patient is on proton pump inhibitors. Patients with potential malabsorption (gastric bypass, inflammatory bowel disease, celiac disease) can be switched to calcium citrate which does not require an acidic environment for optimal absorption. Patients should be advised to space out oral calcium and oral thyroid hormone replacement because calcium inhibits levothyroxine absorption [7]. If serial calcium continues to drop and the patient continues to be symptomatic then calcitriol 0.25–0.50 mcg twice a day is started. The authors recommend checking serum calcium every 8–24 h if the patient must be admitted or 1–2 times a week if managed as an outpatient.

Concurrent Hypomagnesemia

Hypomagnesemia is a common cause of hypocalcemia, both by inducing resistance to PTH and by diminishing its secretion [14]. If a patient has hypomagnesemia, hypocalcemia is difficult to correct without first normalizing the serum magnesium concentration. If the magnesium is <1.6 mg/dL in a patient with normal renal function, replace it with 400 mg of magnesium oxide once or twice daily. Oral magnesium also helps with constipation, which is a common side effect of taking high doses of oral calcium. If a patient is hospitalized with hypocalcemia and is found to have a low magnesium level, it is best to correct this while an inpatient with intravenous supplementation as oral supplementation alone can take weeks to normalize magnesium levels.

Severe Hypoparathyroidism/Hypocalcemia (<7.5 mg/dL)

Patients with severe hypocalcemia can present with carpopedal spasm, tetany, seizures, and prolonged QT interval. If patients are progressing despite oral calcium supplements and calcitriol, it is best to admit them for inpatient treatment. If calcium is <7.5 mg/dL the authors recommend obtaining an EKG and starting intravenous calcium. First, the patient should be given a bolus of 1–2 g of calcium gluconate (equivalent to 90 or 180 mg elemental calcium, in 50 mL of 5% dextrose or normal saline) which can be infused over 10–20 min. Intravenous dosing is either 10% calcium gluconate (90 mg of elemental calcium per 10 mL) or 10% calcium chloride (270 mg of elemental calcium per 10 mL). Calcium gluconate is preferred over calcium chloride, which causes phlebitis and local tissue necrosis if delivered through a peripheral intravenous line. In rare cases, if the patient is not responding to intermittent intravenous calcium boluses, a calcium drip can be started. This is typically done by putting 10 g of calcium gluconate in 1 L of normal saline and it can be infused at 100 mL/hr. The patient should stay on a cardiac monitor while receiving the calcium drip. Serial serum calcium levels would be obtained and the drip adjusted as needed to keep the calcium level at a low normal range. The authors also recommend continuing the oral calcium supplements and calcitriol and even titrating the dose up as the drip is weaned.

Thiazide diuretics should be considered if calcium control remains difficult despite previous measures. These improve renal tubular calcium reabsorption and retention. If there are no contraindications, start hydrochlorothiazide 12.5–50 mg daily [7]. Electrolytes should be monitored since thiazide diuretics can also cause hypokalemia and hyponatremia. Loop diuretics should be avoided since they promote urinary calcium loss.

Hungry Bone Syndrome

Patients undergoing thyroidectomy for Graves' disease or a history of prolonged hyperthyroidism are at increased risk for severe symptomatic hypocalcemia and may require treatment for weeks to months before parameters normalize [14]. This is caused by high bone turnover as demineralized bone becomes recalcified.

Permanent Surgical Hypoparathyroidism

The goal of long-term management of hypoparathyroidism is to maintain serum calcium within an asymptomatic range and to preserve bone health. These patients will require lifelong supplementation and their care is best managed in a multidisciplinary fashion with clear communication of goals and expectations between the patient, surgeon, and endocrinologist [6].

Unfortunately, chronic hypoparathyroidism has many devastating effects on health and quality of life. Patients can develop nephrolithiasis, cataracts, soft tissue calcification, nephrocalcinosis, basal ganglia calcification, and renal failure. It is recommended to check a routine renal ultrasound and 24 hour urine studies [6, 7].

The FDA approved recombinant human PTH (1-84) (rhPTH 1-84) in 2015 for treatment of refractory hypoparathyroidism as a second-line therapy. Teriparatide (PTH 1-34) and rhPTH 1-84 are both administered subcutaneously. Randomized trials have shown synthetic PTH 1-34 controlled hypocalcemia and lowered hypercalciuria when compared to calcitriol [30]. rhPTH significantly reduced supplemental calcium and calcitriol requirements without altering serum or urinary calcium concentrations [31].

Case Conclusion

Our patient had a serum calcium of 7.5 mg/dL PO4 5.5 mg/dL, Cr 1.1 mg/dL, Albumin 4.5 g/dL, and PTH 5 pg/mL. This clearly demonstrated hypocalcemia. Her electrocardiogram was normal.

The patient was admitted and treated with intravenous calcium gluconate and continued on oral calcium supplements and calcitriol. Her symptoms resolved over the next 8 hours, and she was discharged home on oral supplements the following day, which were slowly titrated as her PTH recovered and she remained asymptomatic over several weeks.

Take Home Points

- Identification and meticulous dissection are key to avoiding removal of or injury to the parathyroid glands during thyroid surgery.
- Inspect the thyroid specimen for any inadvertently removed parathyroid glands.
- Autotransplant devascularized or inadvertently removed normal parathyroid glands.
- Consider checking a serum iPTH level in the recovery room after surgery which may help predict risk of development of symptomatic hypocalcemia and initiate preventative treatment for patients at risk for symptomatic hypocalcemia.
- Treat hypocalcemia with calcium (oral or intravenous) and/or activated vitamin D depending on severity of symptoms and/or biochemical tests. The addition of low-dose oral hydrochlorothiazide in patients with normal renal function and normal blood pressure may reduce renal calcium excretion and can be used as an adjunct to raising the serum calcium level.

References

1. Clarke BL, Brown EM, Collins MT, et al. Epidemiology and diagnosis of hypoparathyroidism. J Clin Endocrinol Metab. 2016;101(6):2284–99. https://doi.org/10.1210/jc.2015-3908.
2. Bilezikian JP, Khan A, Potts JT, et al. Hypoparathyroidism in the adult: epidemiology, diagnosis, pathophysiology, target-organ involvement, treatment, and challenges for future research. J Bone Miner Res. 2011;26(10):2317–37. https://doi.org/10.1002/jbmr.483.
3. Brandi ML, Bilezikian JP, Shoback D, et al. Management of hypoparathyroidism: summary statement and guidelines. J Clin Endocrinol Metab. 2016;101(6):2273–83. https://doi.org/10.1210/jc.2015-3907.
4. Mehanna HM, Jain A, Randeva H, Watkinson J, Shaha A. Postoperative hypocalcemia-the difference a definition makes. Head Neck. 2009:NA–NA. https://doi.org/10.1002/hed.21175.
5. Doubleday AR, Robbins SE, Macdonald CL, Elfenbein DM, Connor NP, Sippel RS. What is the experience of our patients with transient hypoparathyroidism after total thyroidectomy? Surgery. 2021;169(1):70–6. https://doi.org/10.1016/j.surg.2020.04.029.
6. Kazaure HS, Sosa JA. Surgical hypoparathyroidism. Endocrinol Metab Clin N Am. 2018;47(4):783–96. https://doi.org/10.1016/j.ecl.2018.07.005.
7. Orloff LA, Wiseman SM, Bernet VJ, et al. American Thyroid Association statement on postoperative hypoparathyroidism: diagnosis, prevention, and management in adults. Thyroid. 2018;28(7):830–41. https://doi.org/10.1089/thy.2017.0309.
8. Fahad Al-Dhahri S, Al-Ghonaim YA, Sulieman TA. Accuracy of postthyroidectomy parathyroid hormone and corrected calcium levels as early predictors of clinical hypocalcemia. J Otolaryngol Head Neck Surg. 2010;39(4):342–8. doi:20642997
9. Rivere AE, Brooks AJ, Hayek GA, Wang H, Corsetti RL, Fuhrman GM. Parathyroid hormone levels predict posttotal thyroidectomy hypoparathyroidism. Am Surg. 2014;80(8):817–20. http://www.ncbi.nlm.nih.gov/pubmed/25105405
10. Carter Y, Chen H, Sippel RS. An intact parathyroid hormone-based protocol for the prevention and treatment of symptomatic hypocalcemia after thyroidectomy. J Surg Res. 2014;186(1):23–8. https://doi.org/10.1016/j.jss.2013.09.026.
11. Ritter K, Elfenbein D, Schneider DF, Chen H, Sippel RS. Hypoparathyroidism after total thyroidectomy: incidence and resolution. J Surg Res. 2015;197(2):348–53. https://doi.org/10.1016/j.jss.2015.04.059.

12. Youngwirth L, Benavidez J, Sippel R, Chen H. Parathyroid hormone deficiency after total thyroidectomy: incidence and time. J Surg Res. 2010;163(1):69–71. https://doi.org/10.1016/j.jss.2010.03.059.
13. Schepers A, van de Velde C, Kievit J. Occurrence and prevention of complications in thyroid surgery. In: Clark O, Duh Q-Y, Kebebew E, Gosnell J, Shen W, editors. Textbook of endocrine surgery. 3rd ed. San Francisco: Jaypee Brothers Medical Publishers; 2016. p. 444–5.
14. Cisco RM. Hypoparathyroidism and pseudohypoparathyroidism. In: Clark O, Duh Q-Y, Kebebew E, Gosnell J, Shen W, editors. Textbook of endocrine surgery. 3rd ed. San Francisco: Jaypee Brothers Medical Publishers; 2016. p. 901–4.
15. Xing T, Hu Y, Wang B, Zhu J. Role of oral calcium supplementation alone or with vitamin D in preventing post-thyroidectomy hypocalcaemia; a meta-analysis. Medicine (United States). 2019;98:8. https://doi.org/10.1097/MD.0000000000014455.
16. Seo ST, Chang JW, Jin J, Lim YC, Rha K-S, Koo BS. Transient and permanent hypocalcemia after total thyroidectomy: early predictive factors and long-term follow-up results. Surgery. 2015;158(6):1492–9. https://doi.org/10.1016/j.surg.2015.04.041.
17. Oltmann SC, Brekke AV, Schneider DF, Schaefer SC, Chen H, Sippel RS. Preventing postoperative hypocalcemia in patients with graves disease: a prospective study. Ann Surg Oncol. 2015;22(3):952–8. https://doi.org/10.1245/s10434-014-4077-8.
18. Ramouz A, Hosseini M, Hosseinzadeh SS, Rasihashemi SZ. Preoperative vitamin D supplementation in patients with vitamin D deficiency undergoing total thyroidectomy. Am J Med Sci. 2020;360(2):146–52. https://doi.org/10.1016/j.amjms.2020.04.036.
19. Kose E, Rudin AV, Kahramangil B, et al. Autofluorescence imaging of parathyroid glands: an assessment of potential indications. Surgery. 2020;167:1. https://doi.org/10.1016/j.surg.2019.04.072.
20. Rudin AV, McKenzie TJ, Thompson GB, Farley DR, Lyden ML. Evaluation of parathyroid glands with indocyanine green fluorescence angiography after thyroidectomy. World J Surg. 2019;43:6. https://doi.org/10.1007/s00268-019-04909-z.
21. D'Avanzo A, Parangi S, Morita E, Duh Q-Y, Siperstein AE, Clark OH. Hyperparathyroidism after thyroid surgery and autotransplantation of histologically normal parathyroid glands11No competing interests declared. J Am Coll Surg. 2000;190(5):546–52. https://doi.org/10.1016/S1072-7515(00)00242-8.
22. Moffett JM, Suliburk J. Parathyroid autotransplantation. Endocr Pract. 2011;17:83–9. https://doi.org/10.4158/EP10377.RA.
23. Selberherr A, Scheuba C, Riss P, Niederle B. Postoperative hypoparathyroidism after thyroidectomy: efficient and cost-effective diagnosis and treatment. Surgery. 2015;157(2):349–53. https://doi.org/10.1016/j.surg.2014.09.007.
24. Richards ML. An optimal algorithm for intraoperative parathyroid hormone monitoring. Arch Surg. 2011;146(3):280. https://doi.org/10.1001/archsurg.2011.5.
25. McLeod IK, Arciero C, Noordzij JP, et al. The use of rapid parathyroid hormone assay in predicting postoperative hypocalcemia after total or completion thyroidectomy. Thyroid. 2006;16:3. https://doi.org/10.1089/thy.2006.16.259.
26. McCullough M, Weber C, Leong C, Sharma J. Safety, efficacy, and cost savings of single parathyroid hormone measurement for risk stratification after total thyroidectomy. Am Surg. 2013;79(8):768–74. http://www.ncbi.nlm.nih.gov/pubmed/23896242
27. Mercante G, Anelli A, Giannarelli D, et al. Cost-effectiveness in transient hypocalcemia postthyroidectomy. Head Neck. 2019;41(11):3940–7. https://doi.org/10.1002/hed.25934.
28. Wang TS, Cheung K, Roman SA, Sosa JA. To supplement or not to supplement: a cost-utility analysis of calcium and vitamin D repletion in patients after thyroidectomy. Ann Surg Oncol. 2011;18(5):1293–9. https://doi.org/10.1245/s10434-010-1437-x.
29. Nicholson KJ, Smith KJ, McCoy KL, Carty SE, Yip L. A comparative cost-utility analysis of postoperative calcium supplementation strategies used in the current management of hypocalcemia. Surgery (United States). 2020;167(1):137–43. https://doi.org/10.1016/j.surg.2019.05.077.

30. Winer KK. Synthetic human parathyroid hormone 1-34 vs calcitriol and calcium in the treatment of hypoparathyroidism. JAMA. 1996;276(8):631. https://doi.org/10.1001/jama.1996.03540080053029.
31. Mannstadt M, Clarke BL, Vokes T, et al. Efficacy and safety of recombinant human parathyroid hormone (1–84) in hypoparathyroidism (REPLACE): a double-blind, placebo-controlled, randomised, phase 3 study. Lancet Diabetes Endocrinol. 2013;1(4):275–83. https://doi.org/10.1016/S2213-8587(13)70106-2.

Chapter 14
Indications for Radioactive Iodine

Sara H. Duffus and Lindsay A. Bischoff

Case

A 23-year-old female presented for evaluation of an incidentally discovered thyroid nodule that was found on imaging obtained during an evaluation for headaches. She denied any compressive symptoms, family history of thyroid cancer, or exposure to external beam radiation. Thyroid and neck ultrasound revealed a solitary 3.2 cm hypoechoic right thyroid nodule with irregular margins and macrocalcifications but no evidence of extrathyroidal extension. No suspicious lymph nodes were identified. Thyroid function testing was normal (serum TSH 2.1 mU/L). Fine-needle aspiration revealed cytological findings consistent with papillary thyroid cancer (PTC) (Bethesda VI). The patient underwent a total thyroidectomy with selective central neck dissection. Final surgical pathology revealed a 2.9-cm classic PTC with microscopic extrathyroidal extension but no lymphovascular invasion. Two out of three central neck lymph nodes (level VI) were positive for PTC (metastatic foci were 6 and 7 mm in the greatest dimension) without evidence of extranodal extension. The tumor was classified as pT2 N1a, stage 1 according to the AJCC/TNM VIII Edition [1]. Given the presence of microscopic invasion into the perithyroidal soft tissues and lymph node metastases measuring larger than 2 mm, the patient was classified as intermediate risk for recurrence according to the 2015 ATA initial risk stratification system [2].

At her 6-week postoperative follow-up visit, unstimulated serum thyroglobulin (Tg) level was 0.2 ng/mL with negative antithyroglobulin antibodies (TgAb). The

S. H. Duffus
Department of Pediatrics, University of North Carolina Chapel Hill, Chapel Hill, NC, USA
e-mail: sara_duffus@med.unc.edu

L. A. Bischoff (✉)
Department of Medicine, Vanderbilt University, Nashville, TN, USA
e-mail: lindsay.bischoff@vumc.org

S. A. Roman et al. (eds.), *Controversies in Thyroid Nodules and Differentiated Thyroid Cancer*, https://doi.org/10.1007/978-3-031-37135-6_14

physician and patient engaged in a discussion to weigh the risks and benefits of radioiodine (RAI) administration.

What Is Intermediate Risk?

In order to strike the balance of reducing the risk of persistent or recurrent disease while minimizing treatment-related morbidity and unnecessary treatment in the initial management of patients with DTC, risk stratification is of the utmost importance [2]. The 2015 ATA guidelines include a three-tiered risk stratification system designed to aid clinicians in predicting risk of disease recurrence [2]. This risk stratification system is based on initial surgical pathology and can be used to help guide decisions regarding the use of RAI following initial surgical management. While it is clear which patients are at low and high risk for disease recurrence, the rates for recurrence in the intermediate group are heterogenous and vary from 6% to 30% [2] (Table 14.1). Therefore, it remains important to assess clinical and

Table 14.1 Reported locoregional recurrence risk for given disease characteristics in patients who are classified as intermediate risk by the 2015 ATA Guidelines

Characteristic	Reported locoregional recurrence risk	Citation
<5 Metastatic LN	3–8%	Leboulleux 2005 [8] Sugitani 2004 [60]
Minor extrathyroidal extension	3–9%	Riemann 2010 [13] Jukkola 2004 [14] Ito 2006 [15]
All metastatic LN < 0.2 cm	5%	Cranshaw 2008 [7]
6–10 metastatic LN	7%	Leboulleux 2005 [8]
Vascular invasion	16–30%	Gardner 2000 [17] Nishida 2002 [18] Falvo 2005 [19]
>10 metastatic LN	21%	Leboulleux 2005 [8]
Histologic variant (tall cell, hobnail, columnar cell)	25–27%	Nath 2018 [22] Ambrosi 2017 [23]
Any metastatic LN > 3 cm	27%	Sugitani 2004 [61]
Clinical N1, age < 45 years	28%	Wada 2008 [10]

pathologic disease features as well as patient circumstances within this group when determining if RAI may be appropriate.

For ATA low- and high-risk patients, recommendations are relatively clear regarding the use of RAI. Low-risk patients, including those with intrathyroidal DTC with no evidence of ETE, vascular invasion, or metastases, have low rates of structural disease recurrence in the absence of RAI therapy (0.5%–1% at 5–10 year follow-up), and RAI after surgery is not routinely recommended [3–5]. For high-risk patients, rates of persistent structural disease or recurrence are as high as 68% even after RAI administration, and RAI is generally recommended [6]. Recommendations for intermediate-risk patients, however, are less clear likely because this group reflects a broad range of clinical and pathologic features for which the risk of structural disease recurrence and likelihood of response to RAI treatment varies widely. Individualized assessment of not only disease features, but also the impact of initial treatment (including lobectomy vs total thyroidectomy and extent of lymph node dissection) is key, particularly in this intermediate-risk group. Other factors that may influence the decision to use RAI include age, other comorbidities, pregnancy, breast-feeding plans, and postoperative thyroglobulin and ultrasound findings.

Patients with intermediate-risk disease represent a broad range of clinical and pathologic features with recurrence risk varying widely based on extent of lymph node involvement, persistence of lymph node metastases after RAI, degree of extrathyroidal extension, histology type, and mutation status. Lymph node involvement in this group includes any nodal disease measuring from 0.3 to 3 cm with a risk of recurrence ranging from 7% to 30% [7–9]. However, described rates of recurrence in older patients (over 45 years) with clinical N1 disease have been as high as 42% [10]. While 2015 ATA guidelines do not currently differentiate between N1a (central neck lymph node metastases) and N1b (lateral neck lymph node metastases) disease, some studies have suggested that N1b involvement is associated with increased recurrence risk [11, 12]. Overall, consideration of size and location of involved lymph nodes are important considerations in this group.

The intermediate-risk category also includes minor extrathyroidal extension into the perithyroidal soft tissues with reported recurrence rates of 3–9% [13–16] and PTC with vascular invasion with reported recurrence rates of up to 16–30% [17–19]. More recently, data indicate that minimal extrathyroidal extension only slightly impacts the risk of recurrence (by about 1%) and has no impact on disease-related mortality [20]. Accordingly, the eighth edition of the AJCC TNM staging system removed minor ETE as a factor to upstage a tumor [1, 21].

Microscopic variants of PTC classified within the intermediate-risk group include tall cell variant (reported 27% recurrence) [22], hobnail variant (reported 25% recurrence rate) [23], and columnar cell variant. Additionally, BRAFV600E mutations have been associated with recurrence rates ranging from 11% to 40% [24]. While it appears that BRAFV600E mutations may not substantially increase the risk of recurrence in very low-risk patients, for those with other risk factors such as multifocality and extrathyroidal extension, BRAFV600E mutation has been associated with increased recurrence rates [25]. Although mutational testing is not routinely recommended for risk stratification, patients with multifocal papillary thyroid microcarcinoma (PTMC) with extrathyroidal extension who are known to have BRAFV600E should be considered in the intermediate-risk category [2].

It should be noted that many of the disease features in the intermediate-risk category are often linked. For example, the histopathologic variants listed above are associated with lymph node metastases and extrathyroidal extension [22]. Similarly, BRAFV600E mutations may be associated with aggressive histologic variants, lymph node metastases, and extrathyroidal extension [24]. ATA guidelines recommend considering these features to be on a continuum of risk for recurrent disease and emphasize the importance of individualized care [2], Table 14.1.

Given that the recurrence risk varies substantially in the intermediate category, the ATA guidelines recommend that RAI "should be considered" for this group [2]. The decision to administer RAI should be highly individualized based on the combination of clinical and pathological features. Both recurrence risks and response rates to RAI should be discussed with the patient to help facilitate shared decision-making for optimal care. Additionally, dynamic reevaluation of these disease features over time based on response of the tumor to initial therapy remains critical in appropriately escalating or deescalating monitoring and treatment over the patient's lifetime.

Indications for RAI for Intermediate-Risk Patients

There are three potential reasons to administer RAI, each with a different goal. The most common, RAI adjuvant therapy, is aimed at reducing the risk of recurrence in patients with high and some intermediate-risk cases. Another reason for RAI aims at treating known disease, either structural or biochemical. A third reason to give RAI is aimed at ablating remnant thyroid tissue in patients with low risk for recurrence in order to achieve an undetectable thyroglobulin. The dose of RAI administered differs for each of these three purposes. This chapter will focus on the use of RAI with the goal of reducing risk of recurrence.

The three-tiered system predicting risk for recurrence as described by the 2015 ATA guidelines has been validated in several studies [26, 27] and appears to be a good predictor of recurrence. The benefit of RAI in patients with intermediate risk for recurrence, however, remains unclear [28–31]. This is in part due to the heterogeneity of this risk category as well as lack of clear evidence that RAI reduces thyroid cancer recurrence in these specific pathologic presentations. As a result, the clinical management of these patients varies widely and is largely determined by the practice culture of an institution or an individual provider.

Strategies to aid the clinician's recommendation for or against RAI may include assessing specific features of the pathology that may be concerning, postoperative thyroglobulin, neck ultrasound, or iodine radioisotope whole-body scanning (Fig. 14.1). While this category is heterogeneous, there are patients who are more clearly high-intermediate risk (for example, a 2.9-cm lymph node metastasis) or

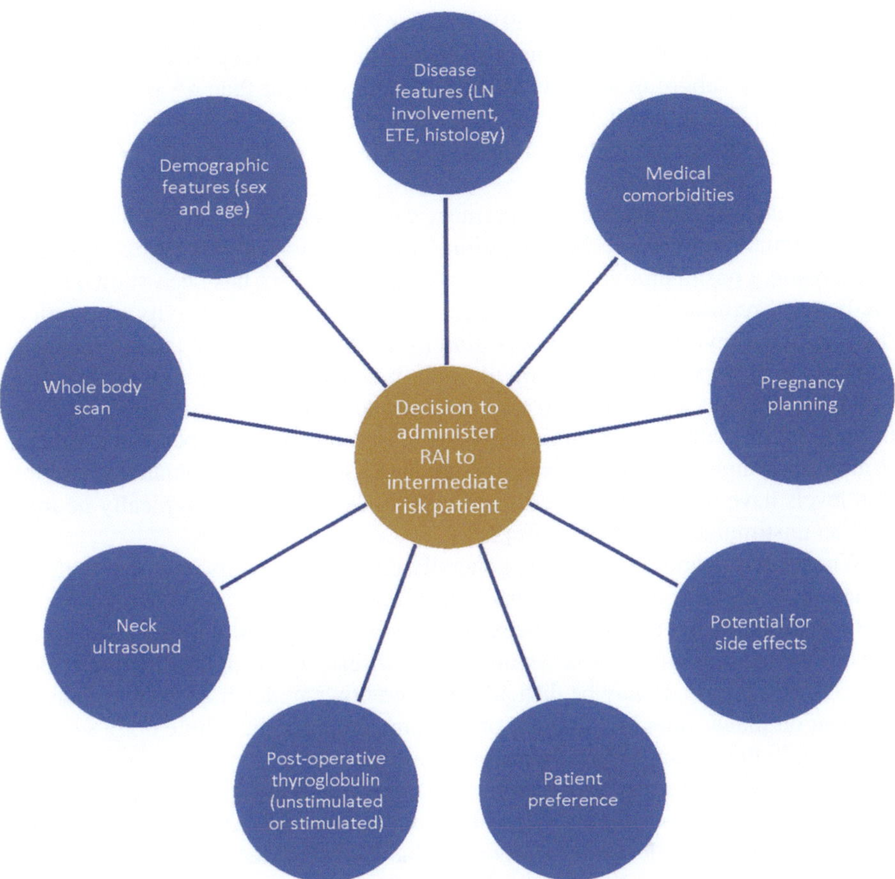

Fig. 14.1 Factors that contribute to decision regarding RAI administration in intermediate-risk patients

low-intermediate risk (a single 0.3 cm lymph node metastasis). The high-intermediate-risk patients are more likely to benefit from RAI to help decrease their risk for recurrence, but those with lower-intermediate risk may not.

The controversy regarding RAI use for intermediate-risk patients is highlighted by a systematic review that describes 11 studies in which improvements in recurrence rates were reported, while 13 other studies found no benefit [30]. Several studies have attempted to define subgroups within the intermediate-risk population for whom RAI ablation is associated with improved survival and recurrence. One Surveillance, Epidemiology, and End Results (SEER) database study demonstrated that RAI ablation was only associated with improved disease-specific survival in patients with male gender, age $\geq$ 45 years, and primary tumor size $\geq$2 cm [28]. A similar National Cancer Database (NCDB) and SEER study identified intermediate-risk subgroups with lymph node metastases and T $\geq$ 3 disease as experiencing a mortality benefit with RAI use [29]. Another NCDB study found an association with improved overall survival in all intermediate-risk patients who received RAI, as well as in a subgroup analysis among patients younger than 45 years and older than 65 years [32]. Overall, these clinical features can aid clinicians in further stratifying intermediate-risk patients into lower and higher likelihoods of benefiting from RAI.

Postoperative thyroglobulin assessment can be helpful in determining if there may be remaining disease, thereby aiding in the decision of whether to administer RAI. While a postoperative stimulated thyroglobulin of <1 has been shown to be a predictor of remission [33, 34], the degree of thyroglobulin positivity also reflects the size of the thyroid remnant left behind [35]. This complicates the interpretation and use of postoperative thyroglobulin as a tumor marker. Combining the serum thyroglobulin measurement with neck ultrasound is useful to evaluate if elevated thyroglobulin is due to a benign remnant or is concerning for persistent disease. With recent improvements in thyroglobulin assay sensitivity, stimulated thyroglobulin levels have become less useful and clinical assessment can typically be made with an unstimulated measurement [36].

Whole body scanning (WBS) is generally reserved for cases in which high thyroglobulin levels are detected but neck ultrasonography does not identify disease. WBS is generally not utilized in the setting of low thyroglobulin levels given its low sensitivity and potential to miss small-volume disease in the neck when used alone [37–39]. In addition, it may be difficult to differentiate nodal disease from a thyroid remnant on planar imaging, making pre-treatment diagnostic whole body scanning unhelpful in the setting of low thyroglobulin.

Other important factors that must be considered include patient preference, pregnancy planning, comorbidities, living situation, and age. Given the excellent overall prognosis of thyroid cancer, it is important that the use of RAI therapy is not at the expense of patients' quality of life. Ultimately, shared decision-making with the patient is paramount when determining the use of RAI in intermediate-risk patients (Fig. 14.1).

Side Effects of RAI on Young Patients

Side effects of RAI therapy, while overall low, should be considered against its benefits (Table 14.2). Early, dose-related side effects such as nausea, decreased taste and smell, salivary gland damage (sialadenitis), lacrimal duct obstruction, and increase in dental caries should be considered. While sour candies and parotid message have been suggested to help prevent sialadenitis, there is conflicting evidence regarding their usefulness and guidelines have not supported any modality for prevention of any of these early side effects [2, 40]. While the rates are low and often self-limited, permanent epiphora, xerostomia, and dysphagia can occur [41–43].

More concerning side effects such as transient bone marrow suppression and gonadal toxicity are rare but increase in frequency with higher lifetime cumulative

Table 14.2 Side effects of RAI in young patients classified by timing after RAI administration

Timing after RAI administration	Side effects
Early (within 7–10 days)	• Nausea and vomiting. • Decreased taste and smell. • Salivary gland damage (sialadenitis). • Increase in dental caries.
Intermediate (10 days–1 year)	• Nasolacrimal duct obstruction. • Bone marrow suppression. • Gonadal toxicity.
Late (after 1 year)	• Secondary malignancy. • Pulmonary fibrosis.

doses of RAI (600mci or higher) [44, 45]. Bone marrow suppression after a single empiric dose of RAI is rare overall, with most occurring in the elderly [46].

When considering RAI in a patient of child-bearing age, the potential for gonadal toxicity should be taken into account. In women, several studies have demonstrated a decrease in anti-mullerian hormone after empiric RAI, however, there is currently no evidence that fertility is reduced [47–51]. In addition, there does not appear to be any increase in obstetrical complications or congenital abnormalities if pregnancy occurs 6 months or more after administration of RAI [52]. In men, empiric doses of RAI are associated with a rise in FSH but similarly no study has demonstrated decreased fertility. While it has been postulated that lifelong cumulative doses of 400 mci and higher may be enough to cause permanent damage to the germinal epithelium in men, and while higher doses do appear to result in persistent elevations of FSH, no decline in fertility has been reported [53, 54].

Second primary malignancy rates appear to increase after RAI therapy and are dose dependent. In a SEER database study, thyroid cancer survivors who received RAI had an elevated observed over expected (O/E) ratio, indicating they are more likely to experience another non-thyroid primary malignancy as compared to both the general population (O/E = 1.20) and unirradiated thyroid cancer patients (O/E = 1.05) [55]. Other studies have similarly reported an increased risk of a second primary malignancy ranging from 14% to 84% as compared to those who did not receive RAI for their thyroid cancer [56, 57]. The dose at which this risk increases is not clear. In a study of patients who received high lifetime cumulative doses of RAI (600–2200 mci), 1.1% developed a secondary primary malignancy after a mean f/u of 6.9 years (±3.5) [44]. Another study found the risk to increase at 200mci [56]. These data highlight the importance of weighing the use of RAI as well as the dose chosen, particularly in a population where disease-specific mortality is low and recurrence risk is intermediate.

Pulmonary fibrosis is an uncommon side effect of RAI and is felt to be a risk primarily in pediatric patients after multiple consecutive RAI therapies in the setting of lung metastasis. Radiation pneumonitis with high dose RAI in the setting of large pulmonary tumor burden is a concern, particularly with high doses at one time; subsequent pulmonary fibrosis may also develop [58, 59]. In some cases, dosimetry may be helpful to allow the highest dose that can be safely administered.

Although the risk of side effects from RAI is low, they should be weighed against the risk of thyroid cancer recurrence in each patient. Postoperative tumor assessment can be helpful to guide the use of RAI in intermediate-risk patients. Additional factors that should be considered include life expectancy, comorbidities, pregnancy planning, and patient preference.

Case Follow-Up

The 23-year-old female with intermediate-risk disease (pT2 N1a, stage 1) and her physician engaged in a discussion regarding the risks and benefits of receiving RAI. Given the presence of microscopic invasion into the perithyroidal soft tissues and 2 lymph node metastases measuring between 0.2 and 3 cm, her risk of recurrence was estimated to be between 3% and 9% [9, 13–16]. Specifically, the potential need for reoperation in the setting of disease recurrence and the possibility of perioperative complications was discussed. Her low unstimulated TG levels (0.2 ng/mL), young age, lack of aggressive histology, and lack of metastatic lymph node disease outside the central neck were reassuring clinical features. Her desires for future pregnancies, long life expectancy, and potential for side effects with RAI were also taken into consideration. Ultimately, a shared decision-making model was used to tailor the decision regarding RAI administration to the patient's particular clinical features and preferences.

References

1. Tuttle MML, Haugen B, Shah J, Sosa JA, Rohren E, Subramaniam RM, Hunt JL, Perrier ND. In: Amin MBES, Greene F, Byrd D, Brookland RK, Washington MK, Gershenwald JE, Compton CC, Hess KR, Sullivan DC, Jessup JM, Brierley J, Gaspar LE, Schilsky RL, Balch CM, Winchester DP, Asare EA, Madera M, Gress DM, Meyer L, editors. Thyroid-differentiated and anaplastic carcinoma. New York, NY: Springer International Publishing; 2017.
2. Haugen BR, Alexander EK, Bible KC, Doherty GM, Mandel SJ, Nikiforov YE, et al. 2015 American Thyroid Association management guidelines for adult patients with thyroid nodules and differentiated thyroid cancer: the American Thyroid Association guidelines task force on thyroid nodules and differentiated thyroid cancer. Thyroid. 2016;26(1):1–133.
3. Vaisman F, Shaha A, Fish S, Michael TR. Initial therapy with either thyroid lobectomy or total thyroidectomy without radioactive iodine remnant ablation is associated with very low rates of structural disease recurrence in properly selected patients with differentiated thyroid cancer. Clin Endocrinol. 2011;75(1):112–9.
4. Schvartz C, Bonnetain F, Dabakuyo S, Gauthier M, Cueff A, Fieffe S, et al. Impact on overall survival of radioactive iodine in low-risk differentiated thyroid cancer patients. J Clin Endocrinol Metab. 2012;97(5):1526–35.
5. Durante C, Montesano T, Attard M, Torlontano M, Monzani F, Costante G, et al. Long-term surveillance of papillary thyroid cancer patients who do not undergo postoperative radioiodine remnant ablation: is there a role for serum thyroglobulin measurement? J Clin Endocrinol Metab. 2012;97(8):2748–53.

6. Tuttle RM, Tala H, Shah J, Leboeuf R, Ghossein R, Gonen M, et al. Estimating risk of recurrence in differentiated thyroid cancer after total thyroidectomy and radioactive iodine remnant ablation: using response to therapy variables to modify the initial risk estimates predicted by the new American Thyroid Association staging system. Thyroid. 2010;20(12):1341–9.
7. Cranshaw IM, Carnaille B. Micrometastases in thyroid cancer. An important finding? Surg Oncol. 2008;17(3):253–8.
8. Leboulleux S, Rubino C, Baudin E, Caillou B, Hartl DM, Bidart JM, et al. Prognostic factors for persistent or recurrent disease of papillary thyroid carcinoma with neck lymph node metastases and/or tumor extension beyond the thyroid capsule at initial diagnosis. J Clin Endocrinol Metab. 2005;90(10):5723–9.
9. Randolph GW, Duh QY, Heller KS, LiVolsi VA, Mandel SJ, Steward DL, et al. The prognostic significance of nodal metastases from papillary thyroid carcinoma can be stratified based on the size and number of metastatic lymph nodes, as well as the presence of extranodal extension. Thyroid. 2012;22(11):1144–52.
10. Wada N, Masudo K, Nakayama H, Suganuma N, Matsuzu K, Hirakawa S, et al. Clinical outcomes in older or younger patients with papillary thyroid carcinoma: impact of lymphadenopathy and patient age. Eur J Surg Oncol. 2008;34(2):202–7.
11. de Meer SG, Dauwan M, de Keizer B, Valk GD, Borel Rinkes IH, Vriens MR. Not the number but the location of lymph nodes matters for recurrence rate and disease-free survival in patients with differentiated thyroid cancer. World J Surg. 2012;36(6):1262–7.
12. Llamas-Olier AE, Cuellar DI, Buitrago G. Intermediate-risk papillary thyroid cancer: risk factors for early recurrence in patients with excellent response to initial therapy. Thyroid. 2018;28(10):1311–7.
13. Riemann B, Kramer JA, Schmid KW, Dralle H, Dietlein M, Schicha H, et al. Risk stratification of patients with locally aggressive differentiated thyroid cancer. Results of the MSDS trial. Nuklearmedizin. 2010;49(3):79–84.
14. Jukkola A, Bloigu R, Ebeling T, Salmela P, Blanco G. Prognostic factors in differentiated thyroid carcinomas and their implications for current staging classifications. Endocr Relat Cancer. 2004;11(3):571–9.
15. Ito Y, Tomoda C, Uruno T, Takamura Y, Miya A, Kobayashi K, et al. Prognostic significance of extrathyroid extension of papillary thyroid carcinoma: massive but not minimal extension affects the relapse-free survival. World J Surg. 2006;30(5):780–6.
16. Radowsky JS, Howard RS, Burch HB, Stojadinovic A. Impact of degree of extrathyroidal extension of disease on papillary thyroid cancer outcome. Thyroid. 2014;24(2):241–4.
17. Gardner RE, Tuttle RM, Burman KD, Haddady S, Truman C, Sparling YH, et al. Prognostic importance of vascular invasion in papillary thyroid carcinoma. Arch Otolaryngol Head Neck Surg. 2000;126(3):309–12.
18. Nishida T, Katayama S, Tsujimoto M. The clinicopathological significance of histologic vascular invasion in differentiated thyroid carcinoma. Am J Surg. 2002;183(1):80–6.
19. Falvo L, Catania A, D'Andrea V, Marzullo A, Giustiniani MC, De Antoni E. Prognostic importance of histologic vascular invasion in papillary thyroid carcinoma. Ann Surg. 2005;241(4):640–6.
20. Diker-Cohen T, Hirsch D, Shimon I, Bachar G, Akirov A, Duskin-Bitan H, et al. Impact of minimal extra-thyroid extension in differentiated thyroid cancer: systematic review and meta-analysis. J Clin Endocrinol Metab. 2018;
21. Tuttle RM, Haugen B, Perrier ND. Updated American Joint Committee on Cancer/Tumor-Node-Metastasis staging system for differentiated and anaplastic thyroid cancer (eighth edition): what changed and why? Thyroid. 2017;27(6):751–6.
22. Nath MC, Erickson LA. Aggressive variants of papillary thyroid carcinoma: hobnail, tall cell, columnar, and solid. Adv Anat Pathol. 2018;25(3):172–9.
23. Ambrosi F, Righi A, Ricci C, Erickson LA, Lloyd RV, Asioli S. Hobnail variant of papillary thyroid carcinoma: a literature review. Endocr Pathol. 2017;28(4):293–301.

24. Tufano RP, Teixeira GV, Bishop J, Carson KA, Xing M. BRAF mutation in papillary thyroid cancer and its value in tailoring initial treatment: a systematic review and meta-analysis. Medicine (Baltimore). 2012;91(5):274–86.
25. Niemeier LA, Kuffner Akatsu H, Song C, Carty SE, Hodak SP, Yip L, et al. A combined molecular-pathologic score improves risk stratification of thyroid papillary microcarcinoma. Cancer. 2012;118(8):2069–77.
26. Grani G, Zatelli MC, Alfo M, Montesano T, Torlontano M, Morelli S, et al. Real-world performance of the American Thyroid Association risk estimates in predicting 1-year differentiated thyroid cancer outcomes: a prospective multicenter study of 2000 patients. Thyroid. 2021;31(2):264–71.
27. Park S, Kim WG, Song E, Oh HS, Kim M, Kwon H, et al. Dynamic risk stratification for predicting recurrence in patients with differentiated thyroid cancer treated without radioactive iodine remnant ablation therapy. Thyroid. 2017;27(4):524–30.
28. Wang X, Zhu J, Li Z, Wei T. The benefits of radioactive iodine ablation for patients with intermediate-risk papillary thyroid cancer. PLoS One. 2020;15(6):e0234843.
29. Orosco RK, Hussain T, Noel JE, Chang DC, Dosiou C, Mittra E, et al. Radioactive iodine in differentiated thyroid cancer: a national database perspective. Endocr Relat Cancer. 2019;26(10):795–802.
30. Lamartina L, Durante C, Filetti S, Cooper DS. Low-risk differentiated thyroid cancer and radioiodine remnant ablation: a systematic review of the literature. J Clin Endocrinol Metab. 2015;100(5):1748–61.
31. Kim SK, Woo JW, Lee JH, Park I, Choe JH, Kim JH, et al. Radioactive iodine ablation may not decrease the risk of recurrence in intermediate-risk papillary thyroid carcinoma. Endocr Relat Cancer. 2016;23(5):367–76.
32. Ruel E, Thomas S, Dinan M, Perkins JM, Roman SA, Sosa JA. Adjuvant radioactive iodine therapy is associated with improved survival for patients with intermediate-risk papillary thyroid cancer. J Clin Endocrinol Metab. 2015;100(4):1529–36.
33. Kim TY, Kim WB, Kim ES, Ryu JS, Yeo JS, Kim SC, et al. Serum thyroglobulin levels at the time of 131I remnant ablation just after thyroidectomy are useful for early prediction of clinical recurrence in low-risk patients with differentiated thyroid carcinoma. J Clin Endocrinol Metab. 2005;90(3):1440–5.
34. Piccardo A, Arecco F, Puntoni M, Foppiani L, Cabria M, Corvisieri S, et al. Focus on high-risk DTC patients: high postoperative serum thyroglobulin level is a strong predictor of disease persistence and is associated to progression-free survival and overall survival. Clin Nucl Med. 2013;38(1):18–24.
35. Yang SP, Bach AM, Tuttle RM, Fish SA. Serial neck ultrasound is more likely to identify false-positive abnormalities than clinically significant disease in low-risk papillary thyroid cancer patients. Endocr Pract. 2015;21(12):1372–9.
36. Dominguez JM, Nilo F, Contreras T, Carmona R, Droppelmann N, Gonzalez H, et al. Neck sonography and suppressed thyroglobulin have high sensitivity for identifying recurrent/persistent disease in patients with low-risk thyroid cancer treated with total thyroidectomy and radioactive iodine ablation, making stimulated thyroglobulin unnecessary. J Ultrasound Med. 2017;36(11):2299–307.
37. Prabhu M, Samson S, Reddy A, Venkataramanarao SH, Chandrasekhar NH, Pillai V, et al. Role of preablative stimulated thyroglobulin in prediction of nodal and distant metastasis on iodine whole-body scan. Indian J Nucl Med. 2018;33(2):93–8.
38. Pacini F, Capezzone M, Elisei R, Ceccarelli C, Taddei D, Pinchera A. Diagnostic 131-iodine whole-body scan may be avoided in thyroid cancer patients who have undetectable stimulated serum Tg levels after initial treatment. J Clin Endocrinol Metab. 2002;87(4):1499–501.
39. Mazzaferri EL, Robbins RJ, Spencer CA, Braverman LE, Pacini F, Wartofsky L, et al. A consensus report of the role of serum thyroglobulin as a monitoring method for low-risk patients with papillary thyroid carcinoma. J Clin Endocrinol Metab. 2003;88(4):1433–41.

40. Son SH, Lee CH, Jung JH, Kim DH, Hong CM, Jeong JH, et al. The preventive effect of parotid gland massage on salivary gland dysfunction during high-dose radioactive iodine therapy for differentiated thyroid cancer: a randomized clinical trial. Clin Nucl Med. 2019;44(8):625–33.
41. Kloos RT, Duvuuri V, Jhiang SM, Cahill KV, Foster JA, Burns JA. Nasolacrimal drainage system obstruction from radioactive iodine therapy for thyroid carcinoma. J Clin Endocrinol Metab. 2002;87(12):5817–20.
42. Almeida JP, Sanabria AE, Lima EN, Kowalski LP. Late side effects of radioactive iodine on salivary gland function in patients with thyroid cancer. Head Neck. 2011;33(5):686–90.
43. Suat B, Deniz Tuna E, Ozgur Y, Muhammet Y, Tevfik FC. The effects of radioactive iodine therapy on olfactory function. Am J Rhinol Allergy. 2016;30(6):206–10.
44. Kaewput C, Pusuwan P. Outcomes following I-131 treatment with cumulative dose exceeding or equal to 600 mCi in differentiated thyroid carcinoma patients. World J Nucl Med. 2021;20(1):54–60.
45. Probst S, Abikhzer G, Chausse G, Tamilia M. I-131 radiation-induced myelosuppression in differentiated thyroid cancer therapy. Mol Imaging Radionucl Ther. 2018;27(2):84–7.
46. Duskin-Bitan H, Leibner A, Amitai O, Diker-Cohen T, Hirsch D, Benbassat C, et al. Bone-marrow suppression in elderly patients following empiric radioiodine therapy: real-life data. Thyroid. 2019;29(5):683–91.
47. Piek MW, Postma EL, van Leeuwaarde R, de Boer JP, Bos AME, Lok C, et al. The effect of radioactive iodine therapy on ovarian function and fertility in female thyroid cancer patients: a systematic review and meta-analysis. Thyroid. 2021;31(4):658–68.
48. Evranos B, Faki S, Polat SB, Bestepe N, Ersoy R, Cakir B. Effects of radioactive iodine therapy on ovarian reserve: a prospective pilot study. Thyroid. 2018;28(12):1702–7.
49. van Velsen EFS, Visser WE, van den Berg SAA, Kam BLR, van Ginhoven TM, Massolt ET, et al. Longitudinal analysis of the effect of radioiodine therapy on ovarian reserve in females with differentiated thyroid cancer. Thyroid. 2020;30(4):580–7.
50. Acibucu F, Acibucu DO, Akkar OB, Dokmetas HS. Evaluation of ovarian reserve with AMH level in patients with well-differentiated thyroid cancer receiving radioactive iodine ablation treatment. Exp Clin Endocrinol Diabetes. 2016;124(10):593–6.
51. Anderson C, Engel SM, Weaver MA, Zevallos JP, Nichols HB. Birth rates after radioactive iodine treatment for differentiated thyroid cancer. Int J Cancer. 2017;141(11):2291–5.
52. Kim HO, Lee K, Lee SM, Seo GH. Association between pregnancy outcomes and radioactive iodine treatment after thyroidectomy among women with thyroid cancer. JAMA Intern Med. 2020;180(1):54–61.
53. Hyer S, Vini L, O'Connell M, Pratt B, Harmer C. Testicular dose and fertility in men following I(131) therapy for thyroid cancer. Clin Endocrinol. 2002;56(6):755–8.
54. Ceccarelli C, Canale D, Battisti P, Caglieresi C, Moschini C, Fiore E, et al. Testicular function after 131I therapy for hyperthyroidism. Clin Endocrinol. 2006;65(4):446–52.
55. Brown AP, Chen J, Hitchcock YJ, Szabo A, Shrieve DC, Tward JD. The risk of second primary malignancies up to three decades after the treatment of differentiated thyroid cancer. J Clin Endocrinol Metab. 2008;93(2):504–15.
56. Silva-Vieira M, Carrilho Vaz S, Esteves S, Ferreira TC, Limbert E, Salgado L, et al. Second primary cancer in patients with differentiated thyroid cancer: does radioiodine play a role? Thyroid. 2017;27(8):1068–76.
57. Sawka AM, Thabane L, Parlea L, Ibrahim-Zada I, Tsang RW, Brierley JD, et al. Second primary malignancy risk after radioactive iodine treatment for thyroid cancer: a systematic review and meta-analysis. Thyroid. 2009;19(5):451–7.
58. Chen L, Shen Y, Luo Q, Yu Y, Lu H, Zhu R. Pulmonary fibrosis following radioiodine therapy of pulmonary metastases from differentiated thyroid carcinoma. Thyroid. 2010;20(3):337–40.
59. Rall JE, Alpers JB, Lewallen CG, Sonenberg M, Berman M, Rawson RW. Radiation pneumonitis and fibrosis: a complication of radioiodine treatment of pulmonary metastases from cancer of the thyroid. J Clin Endocrinol Metab. 1957;17(11):1263–76.

60. Sugitani I, Kasai N, Fujimoto Y, Yanagisawa A. A novel classification system for patients with PTC: addition of the new variables of large (3 cm or greater) nodal metastases and reclassification during the follow-up period. Surgery. 2004;135(2):139–48.
61. Sugita H, Osaka S, Toriyama M, Osaka E, Yoshida Y, Ryu J, et al. Correlation between the histological grade of chondrosarcoma and the expression of MMPs, ADAMTSs and TIMPs. Anticancer Res. 2004;24(6):4079–84.

Chapter 15
Recurrent Nodal Metastases of Papillary Thyroid Cancer

Ray Wang and Julie A. Miller

Case

A 61-year-old woman presented for follow-up 5 years after having undergone a total thyroidectomy and central lymph node dissection followed by radioactive iodine ablation for intermediate-risk stage II (T2 N1a M0) papillary thyroid cancer (PTC). Post-radioactive iodine surveillance ultrasounds (US) demonstrated no sonographically suspicious nodes and basal serum thyroglobulin had remained undetectable in the absence of thyroglobulin antibodies over 5 years. She was taking 100 mcg of levothyroxine daily, and her thyroid stimulating hormone (TSH) was 0.4 mU/L. The patient's most recent surveillance ultrasound revealed a 6-mm level VI lymph node (Fig. 15.1), suspicious for possible recurrence. However, serum thyroglobulin (Tg) remained 0.1 ug/L and Tg antibody was <10 kIU/L.

What is the best management strategy for this patient?

R. Wang
Department of Diabetes and Endocrinology, Royal Melbourne Hospital, Parkville, VIC, Australia

J. A. Miller (✉)
Department of Endocrine Surgery, Royal Melbourne Hospital, Parkville, VIC, Australia
e-mail: Julie.miller@mh.org.au

S. A. Roman et al. (eds.), *Controversies in Thyroid Nodules and Differentiated Thyroid Cancer*, https://doi.org/10.1007/978-3-031-37135-6_15

Fig. 15.1 Surveillance neck ultrasound demonstrating a 6-mm level VI lymph node with a small cystic component

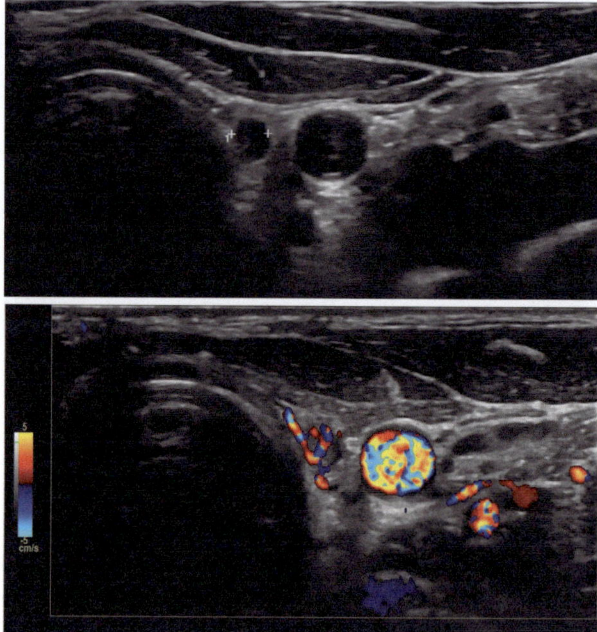

DTC Nodal Recurrence: Epidemiology

Locoregional cervical lymph node recurrence occurs in 4–30% of patients with differentiated thyroid cancer (DTC), and may present as late as 30 years after initial cancer diagnosis [1–3]. In contemporary studies, the mean time to recurrence is usually within 5 years [4, 5] likely reflecting changes in surveillance protocols as well as sensitivity of imaging modalities. Using the American Thyroid Association (ATA) risk stratification system, the risk of structural disease recurrence of DTC is on a continuum that ranges from <6% in low-risk patients, 8–32% in intermediate-risk patients, and up to 30–55% in high-risk patients [6].

DTC has an excellent overall long-term survival even with locoregional recurrence (LR), with some series reporting 90% survival at 8 years [7]. Lymph node metastases confer a small but definite increase in mortality [8, 9], and 8–10% of patients with LR will die from their malignancy [3, 10]. Patients with recurrent regional disease have far better disease-specific survival than those with distant metastases [6], but not as long as those who harbour recurrences localized to the thyroid bed alone or those who have no recurrence [1].

Identifying which subset of patients with LR are at higher risk of morbidity and mortality is key to deciding which of these patients will benefit from intervention. Small volume subclinical nodal involvement confers a vastly different prognostic impact compared with bulky macroscopic nodal disease [11]. It is well established that bulky or invasive nodal disease should be resected surgically if possible [6, 12, 13]. However, with increasing sensitivity of thyroglobulin assays and high-resolution ultrasound, very low-volume recurrences are now detectable. Whether resection of small volume locoregional nodal recurrence improves mortality is unclear, and there is a lack of high-quality prospective data in this area. It is likely that many small, subclinical lymph nodes would previously never have been detected, and may not progress or contribute to morbidity or mortality. It is worth remembering, however, that if left untreated for a prolonged period, even small volume tracheo-esophageal groove disease potentially confers a risk of aerodigestive tract invasion with high morbidity and mortality if progression occurs [14]. Local invasion also makes surgical re-intervention more challenging and potentially dangerous [15, 16].

Nodal Recurrence Management

Distinguishing between nodal recurrences that are likely to progress and should therefore be resected or treated, versus recurrences that are likely to be indolent and can be safely monitored, is a critical but challenging task in the management of DTC patients with LR. Patient preference is also an important factor in decision-making. Selecting the optimal intervention for cervical nodal recurrence involves balancing the competing interests of improving disease-related patient outcomes whilst minimizing treatment-related complications and morbidity. Any suspicious nodal disease seen on imaging should be selected for either active surveillance or intervention. If intervention is being considered, fine needle aspiration (FNA) is indicated to confirm the presence of malignant cells. If a positive cytology result would not alter management, then surveillance is appropriate, and FNA can be delayed until it may influence management decisions.

All patients with structural recurrence should be managed with TSH suppression whenever possible. The options for treatment for patients with clinically significant locoregional disease, in order of preference, are surgical resection; I-131 therapy for radioactive iodine (RAI) responsive disease; and directed therapy modalities such as non-surgical ablation techniques or external beam radiotherapy (EBRT) (Table 15.1) [6]. Systemic therapy options (e.g. kinase inhibitor therapy) can be considered for selected cases if the above modalities are ineffective or unsuitable, but will not be discussed in depth in this chapter.

Regardless of the specific treatment modality selected, a multidisciplinary team approach involving the patient in treatment decisions is highly recommended to optimize outcomes.

TSH Suppression

TSH is a growth factor for DTC and suppressing TSH with exogenous levothyroxine can help reduce tumour growth, progression, and recurrence [15]. A TSH target <0.1 mU/L is recommended in patients with nodal recurrence [6]. Contraindications

Table 15.1 Overview of differing treatment modalities for nodal recurrence

Treatment modality	Benefits	Risks
Active surveillance	Potential to reduce unnecessary intervention	Potential to miss opportunity to treat recurrence at an earlier stage
Reoperation	Highest response rates	Surgical complications including hypoparathyroidism, nerve injury
RAI	Useful as an adjunct to debulking	Response rates lower in bulky disease
RFA	Minimally invasive procedure for medium volume disease	Potential for burns and nerve damage Difficult to target smaller lesions Need for multiple treatment sessions Expertise required
PEI	Minimally invasive procedure for small volume disease	Difficult to adequately treat larger lesions Need for multiple treatment sessions Expertise required
EBRT	Useful in bulky unresectable disease	Irradiated fields make any subsequent operative intervention difficult

RAI radioactive iodine, *RFA* radiofrequency ablation, *PEI* percutaneous ethanol injection, *EBRT* external beam radiotherapy

to TSH-suppression therapy are uncommon but may include poorly controlled rapid atrial fibrillation and intolerance of treatment.

Surgery

Surgical resection of gross macroscopic nodal recurrence has long been the mainstay of therapeutic intervention for LR. According to the 2015 ATA Guidelines, therapeutic compartment-based neck dissection should be performed for persistent or recurrent disease if central neck nodes are ≥8 mm or if lateral neck nodes are ≥10 mm [6]. Suspicious lymph nodes on imaging meeting these size thresholds should undergo FNA and consideration for resection, whilst smaller nodes may be better managed initially with active surveillance [17, 18]. In concordance with these recommendations, the 2016 UK National Multidisciplinary Guidelines state that resecting recurrent nodes <5–8 mm has not been proven to be beneficial [19].

Reoperation in a previously dissected region can be challenging due to altered anatomy from scarring and loss of tissue plane definition [20]. Reoperation is associated with higher surgical risks compared with initial surgery. Risks are higher still with bilateral neck dissection compared with unilateral dissection. Potential complications of reoperative central lymph node dissection include recurrent laryngeal nerve (RLN) injury with resultant vocal cord paralysis, hypoparathyroidism with hypocalcaemia, bleeding, and oesophageal or tracheal injury [20, 21]. Lateral lymph node dissection complications include chyle leak, spinal accessory nerve damage/shoulder dysfunction and, less commonly, injury to the marginal mandibular nerve, sympathetic trunk, phrenic, hypoglossal, or vagus nerves [22]. In general, reoperative thyroid surgery is associated with a 1–1.7% risk of permanent RLN injury, a 1–2.6% risk of transient RLN injury, a 3–5.2% risk of transient hypoparathyroidism, and a 1.7–2.5% risk of permanent hypoparathyroidism [23–25]. Furthermore, these risks may be higher than reported due to publication bias. The higher complication risks of reoperation must be weighed against the benefits of controlling macroscopic nodal disease [6]. An experienced high-volume thyroid cancer surgeon is recommended for revision surgery. Surgical expertise in performing revision thyroid cancer surgery is a "discrete surgical skill set" [6], and the skill and experience of the surgeon are key to reducing reoperative risk.

After compartment-based nodal dissection for recurrent disease, 51–100% of patients will have no evidence of persistent structural disease [18], basal Tg is reduced by 60–98%, and 20–70% of patients will go on to have an unmeasurable Tg postoperatively [6, 26–30]. Results after repeat resection of recurrent/persistent PTC demonstrate diminishing returns with further subsequent reoperations. In a retrospective case series of 70 patients with median follow-up over 13.1 years, an ATA excellent response was achieved in 44.3% after first reoperation for nodal recurrence, 27.1% after second reoperation, 37.9% after third reoperation, and this reduced to 16.7% after fourth reoperation [31]. In another series of 86 patients with a mean follow-up of 59.4 months, 46.5% biochemical cure after first reoperation for recurrence; of those undergoing second reoperation 33.3% achieve biochemical cure; of those undergoing third reoperation 16.6% [5]. Compartmental resection should be considered for the first structural recurrence if feasible, but a more limited or selective dissection should be considered in subsequent recurrences to minimize treatment-related complications given the worsening disease biology and subsequent reduced chance of cure [17]. The survival benefit of resecting involved lymph nodes remains unclear, however; even if there is no survival benefit in reoperation for structural disease, achieving an excellent response can reduce follow-up frequency and degree of TSH suppression required [31]. Peace of mind for the patient and treating team is also a potentially valuable benefit of achieving an excellent treatment response.

The decision to surgically intervene on cervical nodal recurrence must take into account whether distant metastatic disease is present but can still be offered, even in the presence of known distant metastases, in order to prevent subsequent aerodigestive tract obstruction [6, 32]. In addition, resection of iodine-avid disease in the neck may increase delivery of iodine to distant metastases.

Active Surveillance

Reoperation is associated with increased risk of peri-operative complications, as well as increased medical costs to patients and the healthcare system [33]. Surgical intervention is recommended when the benefits of surgery outweigh the risks. In low-risk cases, active surveillance with serial radiological imaging combined with biochemical Tg and Tg antibody monitoring should be considered. Active surveillance is appropriate for patients with low-volume cervical recurrence with small, non-palpable lymph nodes where the risk of progression or the probable effectiveness of reoperation to achieve a biochemical response is low [28]. This is especially pertinent when balancing the higher risks of reoperation in previously dissected compartments, and when the biology of the disease is believed to be indolent, as frequently observed in classic PTC with a long disease-free interval.

In a cohort of 107 patients who underwent reoperation for histologically confirmed locoregional nodal disease, a retrospective review of serial pre-operative computed tomography (CT) imaging revealed that 56% were stable cases of persistent disease, 15% had progressive persistent disease and 29% had true nodal recurrence [34]. Though limited significantly by selection bias, this study suggested that most patients with nodal disease may have radiologically stable disease, at least over the 1.9 years median follow-up interval between serial CT scans. Another retrospective study of 89 patients selected for active surveillance of biopsy-confirmed lymph node metastases, followed up for 3 years, found 36% of those under active surveillance developed new lymph node metastases [35]. A retrospective analysis of 166 patients (mostly intermediate risk) with US features suspicious for nodal recurrence without FNA followed for a median 3.5 years, with median 13 mm nodes (nearly all in the lateral compartments), found 20% of patients showed progression by 3 mm or more [36]. In the absence of biopsy confirmation of malignancy, a portion of these sonographically suspicious nodes may not have represented true nodal recurrence. Finally, another study of 83 patients [37] with FNA-confirmed nodal recurrence with median 13 mm nodes, found that only 20.5% of patients had an increase of 3 mm or more when followed-up for a median 86 months. Even within this biopsy-confirmed cohort, 39.7% of nodes resolved during follow-up imaging.

Therefore, in the carefully selected patient with small volume LN recurrence and favourable biological features, active surveillance with serial radiological and biochemical monitoring is a feasible management option. Many such patients can be monitored with minimal risk of progression and the subgroup of patients that demonstrate progressive disease would then warrant intervention. The decision-making process must consider a multitude of factors [6, 17, 18, 38] (Table 15.2). Certain tumour biology factors may predispose the patient to a greater likelihood of aggressive disease and therefore weigh in favour of earlier intervention; these include histology from the primary surgery demonstrating presence of extrathyroidal extension or extranodal extension, as well as original tumour size and presence of specific molecular markers such as *BRAF* mutations. Other factors to consider include time from primary surgery to recurrence, size of the recurrence, rate of growth, iodine vs FDG avidity, as well as location and proximity to critical anatomical structures in the neck. Additional factors to consider include whether reoperation will be in a previously dissected compartment, whether contralateral vocal cord paralysis is present, and whether the recurrence is in a central or lateral compartment. Finally, patient factors that can impact decision-making include a patient's comorbidities, anaesthetic risk, overall long-term prognosis as well as personal preferences.

Table 15.2 Factors influencing decision between active surveillance vs intervention for nodal recurrence

Characteristics	Favours active surveillance	Favours intervention
Original tumour biology	Absence of *BRAF* mutation	>4 cm primary tumour Extrathyroidal extension Extranodal extension Presence of *BRAF* mutation
Nodal recurrence	<8 mm central node (short axis) <10 mm lateral node (short axis) Long disease-free interval Iodine-avid disease	≥8 mm central node (short axis) ≥10 mm lateral node (short axis) Short duration between primary surgery and recurrence FDG avid disease
Surgery	Presence of contralateral vocal cord paralysis Central compartment recurrence	Recurrence in a previously undissected compartment Lateral compartment recurrence
Patient	Poor overall prognosis High anaesthetic risk Extensive comorbidities Reduced expected long-term survival for non-PTC-related reasons	Patient anxiety regarding persistent disease

Radioactive Iodine

Radioactive Iodine (RAI) may be used as an adjunct to surgery for nodal recurrence if residual RAI-avid disease remains [6], but is not generally recommended as the primary modality of treatment for LR. In a study of 103 patients with residual locoregional DTC after initial surgery and RAI, 50 underwent reoperation followed by a second RAI treatment whilst 53 underwent a second RAI treatment without reoperation [39]. In the group who underwent reoperation, there was ongoing evidence of locoregional disease on imaging in 47.7% of patients, compared to 93.6% in those without reoperation, suggesting RAI is more effective as an adjunct to surgical clearance or debulking procedures rather than as the primary treatment modality.

RAI is often insufficient in treating bulky nodal recurrence [40] and even with high-dose radiation, RAI is successful in treating only around 80% of iodine-avid lymph node metastases [41]. This oft-quoted ablation rate comes from a 1992 study before the availability of high resolution US and serum Tg, such that the successful treatment rate in the era of more sensitive surveillance techniques is likely to be significantly lower. In a more modern retrospective study of 118 post-thyroidectomy patients with PTC and suspicious LN on post-operative imaging, with RAI treatment 28% achieved an excellent response [42]. In those who responded, mean LN size was 5.15 mm, compared to 9.65 mm in those who did not respond to RAI.

RAI complications include secondary malignancy, sialadenitis, nausea, and vomiting [38].

External Beam Radiotherapy

External Beam Radiotherapy (EBRT) is associated with significant morbidity and poor overall efficacy [6] but is a therapeutic option for critical unresectable or non-iodine-avid disease. As repeat surgery in an irradiated field is incredibly difficult, EBRT is generally recommended only in patients with recurrent/persistent disease who are not surgical candidates and in whom RAI is no longer appropriate (due to reaching maximum RAI doses or in cases of non-RAI-avid disease) [20].

EBRT to the neck is associated with significant morbidity and adverse events, and toxicity includes mucositis, dermatitis, dysphagia, and oesophagitis [20, 43], with 12–20% experiencing grade three toxicity in one series [43]. Therefore, when EBRT is used for unresectable locoregional disease, intensity modulated radiation therapy (IMRT) techniques or stereotactic radiotherapy techniques have been recommended to deliver precision high-dose radiation to target regions [6, 44, 45].

Non-Surgical Ablative Techniques

Radiofrequency Ablation

Radiofrequency Ablation (RFA) involves real-time ultrasound-guided percutaneous insertion of an electrode with an active tip into tumour nodules under local anaesthetic [46]. Application of radiofrequency energy induces focal tumour necrosis [47].

A 2012 Consensus Statement from the Korean Society of Thyroid Radiology acknowledges RFA as an accepted treatment modality for nodal recurrence and is indicated in patients who are deemed high-risk surgical candidates or in those who decline repeat surgery [48].

It is worth noting that it can take months to years for ablated nodules to complete their reduction in size. Ongoing volume reduction can be seen 18–24 months after treatment [48, 49], and this must be borne in mind during surveillance imaging post-RFA. The RFA electrode is often too large to insert into small lesions (<10 mm) [50]. If the lesion is close to major nerves, application of RFA in closer proximity is associated with a risk of thermal nerve injury [50].

Percutaneous Ethanol Injection

PEI therapy involves injection of 99% ethanol solution into cervical lymph node metastases without the need for general anaesthesia [51]. PEI can be performed at the bedside or in the office and does not require the space or resources of an operating theatre with general anaesthesia [52]. Studies to date are limited by small numbers, short follow-up, and inclusion of many small lymph nodes <8 mm [51, 53, 54].

Available data suggests larger lymph nodes >20 mm may be difficult to treat effectively with PEI [6]. Complications of PEI include discomfort, skin necrosis, and RLN damage [51].

Compared to reoperation, PEI is less effective at treating LR, with a systematic review finding that reoperation was successful in 94.8% of cases compared to 87.5% with PEI ($p < 0.001$) [52].

Compared to RFA, PEI is likely less effective at treating LR (especially larger lymph nodes), and requires a greater number of treatment sessions (mean 1.2 vs 2.1 sessions), but is associated with a lower complication rate [55, 56].

Other local ablation techniques, such as laser, microwave, and high-frequency ultrasound (HIFU) ablation, have also been reported in the literature but are less widely used.

Case Discussion

Let us return to the case scenario: the 61-year-old woman with a 6-mm level VI lymph node recurrence, low basal thyroglobulin, with a history of intermediate-risk PTC and previous total thyroidectomy, central lymph node dissection, and RAI. Given the small size of the nodal recurrence and absence of elevated basal thyroglobulin, as well as the location of recurrence in a previously dissected compartment, we recommend active surveillance. Serial ultrasounds may demonstrate that the lymph node remains stable in size and requires no intervention. If surveillance with serial monitoring detects an increase in lymph node size with concerning ultrasound features, then intervention may be undertaken. The options of surgical resection vs local ablation techniques could then be considered depending on local expertise and reoperative risk.

Summary

Management of patients with nodal recurrence of PTC must consider multiple tumour- and patient-related factors (Fig. 15.2). The optimal management strategy should provide the greatest benefit to the patient whilst minimizing the risk of harm and must balance the generally excellent prognosis of most PTCs with the potential risks of intervention. The decision-making process should involve a multidisciplinary team and always in consultation with an appropriately informed patient. The first decision to make is whether intervention is necessary, or whether active surveillance is preferred. If intervention is recommended, surgical resection, where feasible, is the treatment of choice. If surgery is not feasible, the options of RAI, EBRT, and non-surgical ablation techniques may be considered.

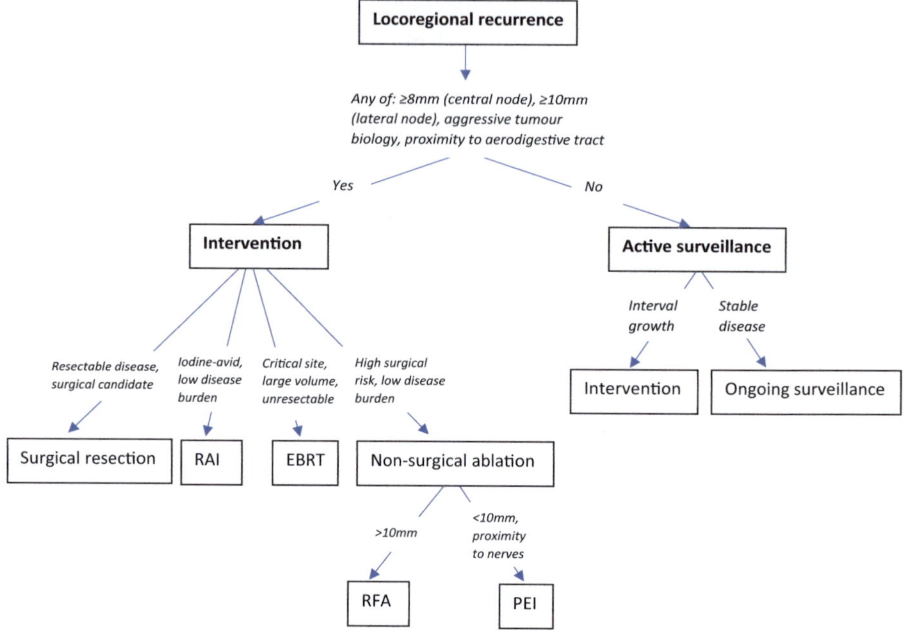

Fig. 15.2 Locoregional recurrence management decision-making algorithm

References

1. Grant CS, Hay ID, Gough IR, Bergstrahl EJ, Goellner JR, McConahey WM. Local recurrence in papillary thyroid carcinoma: is extent of surgical resection important? Surgery. 1988;104(6):954–62.
2. Mazzaferri EL, Jhiang SM. Long-term impact of initial surgical and medical therapy on papillary and follicular thyroid cancer. Am J Med. 1994;97(5):418–28. https://doi.org/10.1016/0002-9343(94)90321-2. Erratum in: Am J Med 1995 Feb;98(2):215
3. Stokkel MP, Duchateau CS, Dragoiescu C. The value of FDG-PET in the follow-up of differentiated thyroid cancer: a review of the literature. Q J Nucl Med Mol Imaging. 2006;50(1):78–87.
4. Lamartina L, Handkiewicz-Junak D. Follow-up of low risk thyroid cancer patients: can we stop follow-up after 5 years of complete remission? Eur J Endocrinol. 2020;182(5):D1–D16. https://doi.org/10.1530/EJE-19-0960.
5. Rivera-Robledo CG, Velázquez-Fernández D, Pantoja JP, Sierra M, Pérez-Enriquez B, Rivera-Moscoso R, Chapa M, Herrera MF. Recurrent papillary thyroid carcinoma to the cervical lymph nodes: outcomes of compartment-oriented lymph node resection. World J Surg. 2019;43(11):2842–9. https://doi.org/10.1007/s00268-019-05094-9.
6. Haugen BR, Alexander EK, Bible KC, Doherty GM, Mandel SJ, Nikiforov YE, Pacini F, Randolph GW, Sawka AM, Schlumberger M, Schuff KG, Sherman SI, Sosa JA, Steward DL, Tuttle RM, Wartofsky L. 2015 American Thyroid Association management guidelines for adult patients with thyroid nodules and differentiated thyroid cancer: the American Thyroid Association guidelines task force on thyroid nodules and differentiated thyroid cancer. Thyroid. 2016;26(1):1–133. https://doi.org/10.1089/thy.2015.0020.
7. Robbins RJ, Wan Q, Grewal RK, Reibke R, Gonen M, Strauss HW, Tuttle RM, Drucker W, Larson SM. Real-time prognosis for metastatic thyroid carcinoma based on 2-[18F]fluoro-2-

deoxy-D-glucose-positron emission tomography scanning. J Clin Endocrinol Metab. 2006;91(2):498–505. https://doi.org/10.1210/jc.2005-1534.
8. Adam MA, Pura J, Goffredo P, Dinan MA, Reed SD, Scheri RP, Hyslop T, Roman SA, Sosa JA. Presence and number of lymph node metastases are associated with compromised survival for patients younger than age 45 years with papillary thyroid cancer. J Clin Oncol. 2015;33(21):2370–5. https://doi.org/10.1200/JCO.2014.59.8391.
9. Asimakopoulos P, Nixon IJ, Shaha AR. Differentiated and medullary thyroid cancer: surgical management of cervical lymph nodes. Clin Oncol (R Coll Radiol). 2017;29(5):283–9. https://doi.org/10.1016/j.clon.2017.01.001.
10. Chéreau N, Buffet C, Trésallet C, Tissier F, Leenhardt L, Menegaux F. Recurrence of papillary thyroid carcinoma with lateral cervical node metastases: predictive factors and operative management. Surgery. 2016;159(3):755–62. https://doi.org/10.1016/j.surg.2015.08.033.
11. Randolph GW, Duh QY, Heller KS, LiVolsi VA, Mandel SJ, Steward DL, Tufano RP, Tuttle RM, American Thyroid Association Surgical Affairs Committee's Taskforce on Thyroid Cancer Nodal Surgery. The prognostic significance of nodal metastases from papillary thyroid carcinoma can be stratified based on the size and number of metastatic lymph nodes, as well as the presence of extranodal extension. Thyroid. 2012;22(11):1144–52. https://doi.org/10.1089/thy.2012.0043.
12. Ito Y, Higashiyama T, Takamura Y, Kobayashi K, Miya A, Miyauchi A. Prognosis of patients with papillary thyroid carcinoma showing postoperative recurrence to the central neck. World J Surg. 2011;35(4):767–72. https://doi.org/10.1007/s00268-010-0924-3.
13. Uchida H, Imai T, Kikumori T, Hayashi H, Sato S, Noda S, Idota A, Kiuchi T. Long-term results of surgery for papillary thyroid carcinoma with local recurrence. Surg Today. 2013;43(8):848–53. https://doi.org/10.1007/s00595-012-0353-z.
14. Sugitani I, Fujimoto Y, Yamamoto N. Papillary thyroid carcinoma with distant metastases: survival predictors and the importance of local control. Surgery. 2008;143(1):35–42. https://doi.org/10.1016/j.surg.2007.06.011.
15. Caron NR, Clark OH. Well differentiated thyroid cancer. Scand J Surg. 2004;93(4):261–71. https://doi.org/10.1177/145749690409300403.
16. Machens A, Hinze R, Lautenschläger C, Thomusch O, Dralle H. Thyroid carcinoma invading the cervicovisceral axis: routes of invasion and clinical implications. Surgery. 2001;129(1):23–8. https://doi.org/10.1067/msy.2001.108699.
17. Tufano RP, Clayman G, Heller KS, Inabnet WB, Kebebew E, Shaha A, Steward DL, Tuttle RM, American Thyroid Association Surgical Affairs Committee Writing Task Force. Management of recurrent/persistent nodal disease in patients with differentiated thyroid cancer: a critical review of the risks and benefits of surgical intervention versus active surveillance. Thyroid. 2015;25(1):15–27. https://doi.org/10.1089/thy.2014.0098.
18. Urken ML, Milas M, Randolph GW, Tufano R, Bergman D, Bernet V, Brett EM, Brierley JD, Cobin R, Doherty G, Klopper J, Lee S, Machac J, Mechanick JI, Orloff LA, Ross D, Smallridge RC, Terris DJ, Clain JB, Tuttle M. Management of recurrent and persistent metastatic lymph nodes in well-differentiated thyroid cancer: a multifactorial decision-making guide for the Thyroid Cancer Care Collaborative. Head Neck. 2015;37(4):605–14. https://doi.org/10.1002/hed.23615.
19. Mitchell AL, Gandhi A, Scott-Coombes D, Perros P. Management of thyroid cancer: United Kingdom National Multidisciplinary Guidelines. J Laryngol Otol. 2016;130(S2):S150–60. https://doi.org/10.1017/S0022215116000578.
20. Caron NR, Clark OH. Papillary thyroid cancer: surgical management of lymph node metastases. Curr Treat Options in Oncol. 2005;6(4):311–22. https://doi.org/10.1007/s11864-005-0035-9.
21. Mittendorf EA, Wang X, Perrier ND, Francis AM, Edeiken BS, Shapiro SE, Lee JE, Evans DB. Followup of patients with papillary thyroid cancer: in search of the optimal algorithm. J Am Coll Surg. 2007;205(2):239–47. https://doi.org/10.1016/j.jamcollsurg.2007.02.079.

22. Dralle H, Machens A. Surgical management of the lateral neck compartment for metastatic thyroid cancer. Curr Opin Oncol. 2013;25(1):20–6. https://doi.org/10.1097/CCO.0b013e328359ff1f.

23. Chao TC, Jeng LB, Lin JD, Chen MF. Reoperative thyroid surgery. World J Surg. 1997;21(6):644–7. https://doi.org/10.1007/s002689900287.

24. Lefevre JH, Tresallet C, Leenhardt L, Jublanc C, Chigot JP, Menegaux F. Reoperative surgery for thyroid disease. Langenbeck's Arch Surg. 2007;392(6):685–91. https://doi.org/10.1007/s00423-007-0201-6.

25. Levin KE, Clark AH, Duh QY, Demeure M, Siperstein AE, Clark OH. Reoperative thyroid surgery. Surgery. 1992;111(6):604–9.

26. Al-Saif O, Farrar WB, Bloomston M, Porter K, Ringel MD, Kloos RT. Long-term efficacy of lymph node reoperation for persistent papillary thyroid cancer. J Clin Endocrinol Metab. 2010;95(5):2187–94. https://doi.org/10.1210/jc.2010-0063.

27. Clayman GL, Shellenberger TD, Ginsberg LE, Edeiken BS, El-Naggar AK, Sellin RV, Waguespack SG, Roberts DB, Mishra A, Sherman SI. Approach and safety of comprehensive central compartment dissection in patients with recurrent papillary thyroid carcinoma. Head Neck. 2009;31(9):1152–63. https://doi.org/10.1002/hed.21079.

28. Hughes DT, Laird AM, Miller BS, Gauger PG, Doherty GM. Reoperative lymph node dissection for recurrent papillary thyroid cancer and effect on serum thyroglobulin. Ann Surg Oncol. 2012;19(9):2951–7. https://doi.org/10.1245/s10434-012-2380-9.

29. Schuff KG, Weber SM, Givi B, Samuels MH, Andersen PE, Cohen JI. Efficacy of nodal dissection for treatment of persistent/recurrent papillary thyroid cancer. Laryngoscope. 2008;118(5):768–75. https://doi.org/10.1097/MLG.0b013e318162cae9.

30. Yim JH, Kim WB, Kim EY, Kim WG, Kim TY, Ryu JS, Gong G, Hong SJ, Shong YK. The outcomes of first reoperation for locoregionally recurrent/persistent papillary thyroid carcinoma in patients who initially underwent total thyroidectomy and remnant ablation. J Clin Endocrinol Metab. 2011;96(7):2049–56. https://doi.org/10.1210/jc.2010-2298.

31. Onuma AE, Beal EW, Nabhan F, Hughes T, Farrar WB, Phay J, Ringel MD, Kloos RT, Shirley LA. Long-term efficacy of lymph node reoperation for persistent papillary thyroid cancer: 13-year follow-up. Ann Surg Oncol. 2019;26(6):1737–43. https://doi.org/10.1245/s10434-019-07263-5.

32. Dralle H, Machens A. Surgical approaches in thyroid cancer and lymph-node metastases. Best Pract Res Clin Endocrinol Metab. 2008;22(6):971–87. https://doi.org/10.1016/j.beem.2008.09.018.

33. Lim YC, Koo BS. Predictive factors of skip metastases to lateral neck compartment leaping central neck compartment in papillary thyroid carcinoma. Oral Oncol. 2012;48(3):262–5. https://doi.org/10.1016/j.oraloncology.2011.10.006.

34. Kim TM, Kim JH, Yoo RE, Kim SC, Chung EJ, Hong EK, Jo S, Kang KM, Choi SH, Sohn CH, Rhim JH, Park SW, Park YJ. Persistent/recurrent differentiated thyroid cancer: clinical and radiological characteristics of persistent disease and clinical recurrence based on computed tomography analysis. Thyroid. 2018;28(11):1490–9. https://doi.org/10.1089/thy.2018.0151.

35. Maciel J, Donato S, Simões H, Leite V. Clinical outcomes of a conservative approach in cervical lymph node metastases of thyroid cancer. Clin Endocrinol. 2020; https://doi.org/10.1111/cen.14306.

36. Robenshtok E, Fish S, Bach A, Domínguez JM, Shaha A, Tuttle RM. Suspicious cervical lymph nodes detected after thyroidectomy for papillary thyroid cancer usually remain stable over years in properly selected patients. J Clin Endocrinol Metab. 2012;97(8):2706–13. https://doi.org/10.1210/jc.2012-1553.

37. Tomoda C, Sugino K, Matsuzu K, Uruno T, Ohkuwa K, Kitagawa W, Nagahama M, Ito K. Cervical lymph node metastases after thyroidectomy for papillary thyroid carcinoma usually remain stable for years. Thyroid. 2016;26(12):1706–11. https://doi.org/10.1089/thy.2016.0225.

38. Goyal RM, Jonklaas J, Burman KD. Management of recurrent cervical papillary thyroid cancer. Endocrinol Metab Clin N Am. 2014;43(2):565–72. https://doi.org/10.1016/j.ecl.2014.02.014.
39. Hirsch D, Gorshtein A, Robenshtok E, Masri-Iraqi H, Akirov A, Duskin Bitan H, Shimon I, Benbassat C. Second radioiodine treatment: limited benefit for differentiated thyroid cancer with locoregional persistent disease. J Clin Endocrinol Metab. 2018;103(2):469–76. https://doi.org/10.1210/jc.2017-01790.
40. Grebe SK, Hay ID. Thyroid cancer nodal metastases: biologic significance and therapeutic considerations. Surg Oncol Clin N Am. 1996;5(1):43–63.
41. Maxon HR 3rd, Englaro EE, Thomas SR, Hertzberg VS, Hinnefeld JD, Chen LS, Smith H, Cummings D, Aden MD. Radioiodine-131 therapy for well-differentiated thyroid cancer—a quantitative radiation dosimetric approach: outcome and validation in 85 patients. J Nucl Med. 1992;33(6):1132–6.
42. Wu X, Gu H, Gao Y, Li B, Fan R. Clinical outcomes and prognostic factors of radioiodine ablation therapy for lymph node metastases from papillary thyroid carcinoma. Nucl Med Commun. 2018;39(1):22–7. https://doi.org/10.1097/MNM.0000000000000777.
43. Romesser PB, Sherman EJ, Shaha AR, Lian M, Wong RJ, Sabra M, Rao SS, Fagin JA, Tuttle RM, Lee NY. External beam radiotherapy with or without concurrent chemotherapy in advanced or recurrent non-anaplastic non-medullary thyroid cancer. J Surg Oncol. 2014;110(4):375–82. https://doi.org/10.1002/jso.23656.
44. Brierley JD, Giuliani ME. Chapter 14: external radiation in differentiated thyroid cancer in the era of IMRT and modern radiation planning techniques. In: Mallick UK, Harmer C, Mazzaferri EL, Kendall-Taylor P, editors. Practical Management of Thyroid Cancer: a multidisciplinary approach. 2nd ed. Switzerland: Springer Nature; 2018. p. 147–52.
45. Kawabe J, Higashiyama S, Sougawa M, Yoshida A, Kotani K, Shiomi S. Usefulness of stereotactic radiotherapy using CyberKnife for recurrent lymph node metastasis of differentiated thyroid cancer. Case Rep Endocrinol. 2017;2017:7956726. https://doi.org/10.1155/2017/7956726.
46. Baek JH, Kim YS, Sung JY, Choi H, Lee JH. Locoregional control of metastatic well-differentiated thyroid cancer by ultrasound-guided radiofrequency ablation. AJR Am J Roentgenol. 2011;197(2):W331–6. https://doi.org/10.2214/AJR.10.5345.
47. Monchik JM, Donatini G, Iannuccilli J, Dupuy DE. Radiofrequency ablation and percutaneous ethanol injection treatment for recurrent local and distant well-differentiated thyroid carcinoma. Ann Surg. 2006;244(2):296–304. https://doi.org/10.1097/01.sla.0000217685.85467.2d.
48. Na DG, Lee JH, Jung SL, Kim JH, Sung JY, Shin JH, Kim EK, Lee JH, Kim DW, Park JS, Kim KS, Baek SM, Lee Y, Chong S, Sim JS, Huh JY, Bae JI, Kim KT, Han SY, Bae MY, Kim YS, Baek JH. Korean Society of Thyroid Radiology (KSThR); Korean Society of Radiology. Radiofrequency ablation of benign thyroid nodules and recurrent thyroid cancers: consensus statement and recommendations. Korean J Radiol. 2012;13(2):117–25. https://doi.org/10.3348/kjr.2012.13.2.117.
49. Guang Y, Luo Y, Zhang Y, Zhang M, Li N, Zhang Y, Tang J. Efficacy and safety of percutaneous ultrasound guided radiofrequency ablation for treating cervical metastatic lymph nodes from papillary thyroid carcinoma. J Cancer Res Clin Oncol. 2017;143(8):1555–62. https://doi.org/10.1007/s00432-017-2386-6.
50. Guenette JP, Monchik JM, Dupuy DE. Image-guided ablation of postsurgical locoregional recurrence of biopsy-proven well-differentiated thyroid carcinoma. J Vasc Interv Radiol. 2013;24(5):672–9. https://doi.org/10.1016/j.jvir.2013.02.001.
51. Kim SY, Kim SM, Chang H, Kim BW, Lim CY, Lee YS, Chang HS, Park CS. Long-term outcomes of ethanol injection therapy for locally recurrent papillary thyroid cancer. Eur Arch Otorhinolaryngol. 2017;274(9):3497–501. https://doi.org/10.1007/s00405-017-4660-2.
52. Fontenot TE, Deniwar A, Bhatia P, Al-Qurayshi Z, Randolph GW, Kandil E. Percutaneous ethanol injection vs reoperation for locally recurrent papillary thyroid cancer: a systematic review and pooled analysis. JAMA Otolaryngol Head Neck Surg. 2015;141(6):512–8. https://doi.org/10.1001/jamaoto.2015.0596. Erratum in: JAMA Otolaryngol Head Neck Surg. 2015 Aug;141(8):760

53. Hay ID, Lee RA, Davidge-Pitts C, Reading CC, Charboneau JW. Long-term outcome of ultrasound-guided percutaneous ethanol ablation of selected "recurrent" neck nodal metastases in 25 patients with TNM stages III or IVA papillary thyroid carcinoma previously treated by surgery and 131I therapy. Surgery. 2013;154(6):1448–54.; discussion 1454-5. https://doi.org/10.1016/j.surg.2013.07.007.
54. Heilo A, Sigstad E, Fagerlid KH, Håskjold OI, Grøholt KK, Berner A, Bjøro T, Jørgensen LH. Efficacy of ultrasound-guided percutaneous ethanol injection treatment in patients with a limited number of metastatic cervical lymph nodes from papillary thyroid carcinoma. J Clin Endocrinol Metab. 2011;96(9):2750–5. https://doi.org/10.1210/jc.2010-2952.
55. Lee SJ, Jung SL, Kim BS, Ahn KJ, Choi HS, Lim DJ, Kim MH, Bae JS, Kim MS, Jung CK, Chong SM. Radiofrequency ablation to treat loco-regional recurrence of well-differentiated thyroid carcinoma. Korean J Radiol. 2014;15(6):817–26. https://doi.org/10.3348/kjr.2014.15.6.817.
56. Shin JE, Baek JH, Lee JH. Radiofrequency and ethanol ablation for the treatment of recurrent thyroid cancers: current status and challenges. Curr Opin Oncol. 2013;25(1):14–9. https://doi.org/10.1097/CCO.0b013e32835a583d.

Chapter 16
Management of Non-Invasive Follicular Thyroid Neoplasm with Papillary-like Features (NIFT-P)

May-Anh Nguyen and Jesse D. Pasternak

Case

A 35-year-old euthyroid female patient without relevant clinical history underwent a right thyroid lobectomy for a 3-cm thyroid nodule. Preoperative work-up of this nodule demonstrated a solid, isoechoic, and well-demarcated smooth-bordered nodule without evidence of microcalcification on ultrasound (TI-RADS 3) and follicular neoplasm (Bethesda category IV) on fine needle aspiration. Surgical pathology after lobectomy reported a completely excised 3 cm non-invasive follicular thyroid neoplasm with papillary-like features (NIFT-P). The patient is now seen in follow-up to discuss the pathology report and next steps.

Background

Definition

Non-invasive follicular thyroid neoplasm with papillary-like features (NIFT-P) is a predominantly non-invasive neoplasm arising from thyroid follicular cells showing follicular growth patterns with nuclear features of papillary thyroid carcinoma.

M.-A. Nguyen · J. D. Pasternak (✉)
Section of Endocrine Surgery, Division of General Surgery, University Health Network, University of Toronto, Toronto, ON, Canada
e-mail: mayanh.nguyen@mail.utoronto.ca; jesse.pasternak@uhn.ca

S. A. Roman et al. (eds.), *Controversies in Thyroid Nodules and Differentiated Thyroid Cancer*, https://doi.org/10.1007/978-3-031-37135-6_16

181

History of Classification

The manuscript by Nikiforov et al. [1] published in 2016 prompted a discussion for a paradigm shift in the management of specific types of non-invasive thyroid lesions, previously classified as encapsulated follicular variant of papillary thyroid carcinoma (FVPTC) which were divided into invasive and non-invasive subtypes [2]. The nomenclature revision highlighted the *indolent* behavior of encapsulated follicular tumors without capsular invasion. The driving force for a change in nomenclature included minimizing overtreatment of these thyroid lesions since they would no longer be classified as a malignancy. Further, de-escalation of treatment and de-stigmatizing these low-risk lesions as "non-cancers" could reduce the psychological and emotional burden of harboring thyroid cancer as well as avoid complications from invasive treatments. (there are a few papers on this) [1].

This study found that among all patients ($n = 109$) with non-invasive encapsulated FVPTC, there were no deaths of disease after median follow-up of 13 years. By comparison, in patients with invasive encapsulated FVPTC, 12% ($n = 101$) had adverse events including distant metastases and mortality [1]. From a pathologic standpoint, these NIFT-P lesions harbor RAS-like properties similar to FVPTC rather than BRAF-like lesions such as classical PTC [1, 3].

Prognosis

NIFT-P has an excellent long-term prognosis. Recent population-based outcomes data with long-term follow-up suggest that NIFT-P is a low-risk thyroid neoplasm with recurrence or metastatic disease from 0% to 9% [4–6]. In contrast, the prognosis of invasive FVPTC has at least 5% risk of recurrence with some data showing a risk approaching 20% of recurrence or metastatic disease [6, 7].

Diagnosis

Histologic Features

NIFT-P is a diagnosis of exclusion that requires histologic evaluation of the nodule capsule in toto for invasion. For this reason, lobectomy is the preferred diagnostic and therapeutic treatment for the majority of these lesions. This recommendation is in keeping with ATA guidelines for other low-risk well-differentiated thyroid cancers [7].

The inclusion and exclusion criteria for NIFT-P diagnosis were initially described by Nikiforov et al. [1]. Recent studies have suggested that a revision may be necessary to exclude NIFT-P diagnosis for presence of any papillae [8]. These criteria are summarized in Fig. 16.1. An example of the microscopic features seen in NIFT-P is depicted in Fig. 16.2.

Diagnostic Controversy

Accurate pathologic reporting is key to the diagnosis of NIFT-P. The incidence of NIFT-P has been reported to be from 2.1% up to 23% of all PTC cases in North American, European, and Asian literature [9]. This suggests that while there may be variability in rates of NIFT-P across populations, center-specific variability of pathologic interpretation plays a crucial role in determining incidence. Availability of specialty-trained endocrine pathology expertise, institutional specimen

Inclusion Criteria	Exclusion Criteria
Encapsulated or partially encapsulated (surrounded by well-formed fibrous connective tissue capsule)	Any invasion (tumour capsule, vascular, extra-thyroidal extension or spread)
Complete absence of tumour capsule and vascular invasion	Presence of PTC variant (ie. tall cell, columnar cell)
Predominantly follicular pattern of growth, colloid easily identified	True papillary structures (fibrovascular core surrounded by neoplastic cells)
Characteristic nuclear features of papillary thyroid carcinoma (PTC) based on: - Nuclear size and shape - Nuclear membrane irregularities - Nuclear chromatic characteristics	Papillary structures and/or psamomma bodies (calcified remnants of papillary structures)
	Tumour necrosis
	Increased mitoses ($\geq$3 mitoses per 10 high-power fields)

Fig. 16.1 NIFT-P histologic diagnosis

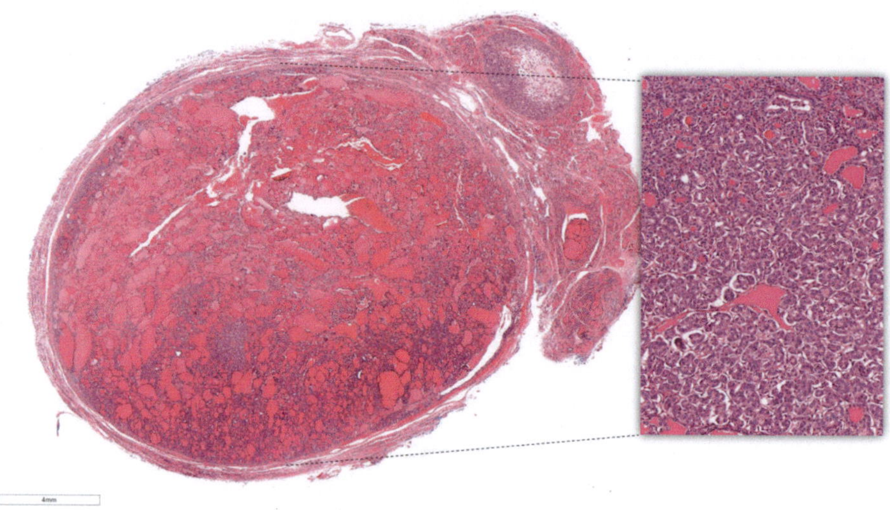

Fig. 16.2 NIFT-P under microscopy; tumor capsule in toto demonstrated. Reference: Dr. Ozgur Mete Library

preparation protocols to evaluate the capsule in toto, and application of the diagnostic criteria of NIFT-P may result in center and regional variability [5, 10, 11].

Previous literature on pathologic reporting of thyroid tumors has demonstrated significant inter-observer variation [10–14]. Even in the expert pathologist group, it has been demonstrated that complete agreement for a tumor to be classified as NIFT-P vs EFVPTC is only seen in 10% of cases [5]. This is reflected in the Nikiforov study where the inter-observer agreement cut-off to classify NIFT-P is 50% [1]. It has been shown that in a high-volume quaternary endocrine pathologist practice, a significant proportion of specimens were not properly handled to optimally assess the entire tumor capsule for invasion [5, 6]. This may lead to potential misclassification of these tumors at both at high- and lower-volume institutions.

Additional studies are currently underway looking at the potential role of molecular testing to aid the diagnosis of NIFT-P using fine needle aspiration preoperatively. Data have suggested that EFVPTC and NIFT-P are tumors from the *RAS-like* mutation pathway rather than *BRAF* mutation pathways seen in classical variant PTC [3, 14]. This has resulted in further studies looking at molecular markers for each tumor subtype and further attempts to identify lower-risk tumors preoperatively, specifically NIFT-P.

Molecular characterization may be useful for clinical decision-making when expert endocrine pathologists and optimal specimen preparation may not be available [15]. Furthermore, suspected NIFT-P cases that demonstrate BRAF-like pathway mutations or other more aggressive molecular profiles may warrant additional review, sampling, or follow-up [14–16]. More stringent criteria for NIFT-P are likely to evolve as more data are published.

Surgical Management

Thyroid Lobectomy

Multiple studies have demonstrated excellent oncologic outcomes for thyroid lobectomy in the treatment of low-risk thyroid cancer. Thyroid lobectomy is accepted for the treatment of most patients with NIFT-P. Thyroid lobectomy provides complete resection of the tumor as well as the opportunity for the pathologist to completely assess the tumor capsule and surrounding vessels. Current practice guidelines have supported thyroid lobectomy for NIFT-P.

In patients where NIFT-P is found incidentally on diagnostic thyroid lobectomy, the overall surgical management and decision for completion thyroidectomy should be based on the pathology of the dominant tumor for which surgical management was initially indicated. Having an incidental finding of NIFT-P, possibly in addition to the dominant tumor, should not "upstage" the initial tumor and require additional surgery or RAI therapy.

In order to confidently identify this entity, a review of the entire capsule of the thyroid nodule is essential. This limits the diagnosis to lesions that have already been excised. Surveillance of these lesions while in situ is not practical and therefore surgical management is ubiquitous.

Surveillance

Follow-up of patients who have been diagnosed with NIFT-P after resection of thyroid nodules is variable. One of the benefits of reclassifying these lesions related to their indolent clinical behavior was simplification of follow-up and to minimize further treatment. Unfortunately, there has been a growing literature showing that patients with a diagnosis of NIFT-P may develop recurrence or metastasis (Bongers/Pasternak). Whether this is related to misclassifying this entity as benign or an existent subtype of this entity which is more aggressive, remains unknown. Therefore, completely discharging patients with NIFT-P from any form of surveillance is not supported. Given the very low risk of metastatic disease in these patients, follow-up similar to very low-risk thyroid cancer can be considered. The American Thyroid Association 2015 guidelines suggest periodic ultrasounds (6–12 months) and target TSH ranges of low-normal level (0.5–2) for low-risk thyroid cancer which may be applied to patients with NIFT-P [7]. Thyroglobulin follow-up continues to be studied but some studies have not shown this to be helpful in the short to medium term [17]. Some data have suggested 10 years of follow-up for very low-risk cancers given the potential for a long delay between presentation and metastatic development for some follicular cell tumors [3, 17, 18]. However, ideal surveillance duration for NIFT-P patients remains unclear.

Case: Suggestions for the Patient

For the patient scenario above, the following steps should be considered:

- A pathology review of the slides to confirm diagnosis, ensuring that the tumor capsule is completely examined.
- Counselling on the excellent prognosis with no further treatment necessary.
- Long-term surveillance consisting of ultrasound and TSH suppression has given recent data demonstrating rare instances of recurrence or metastatic disease.

Evidence-Based Recommendations

The evidence-based recommendations for management of NIFT-P are summarized as follows:

1. *NIFT-P is an extremely low-risk neoplasm with excellent prognosis that requires surgical excision for diagnosis.*
2. *Thorough review of pathology slides to distinguish between NIFT-P and FVPTC is necessary, preferably by an endocrine pathologist at a high-volume center, to prevent misclassification due to inter-observer variation and to minimize overtreatment.*
3. *If definitive diagnosis of NIFT-P is made after thyroid lobectomy, there is no requirement for completion thyroidectomy or RAI.*
4. *Surveillance for NIFT-P after lobectomy should be similar to disease monitoring strategies for low-risk well-differentiated thyroid cancers, consisting of periodic physical examination, TSH suppression, and neck ultrasound.*

Acknowledgments We would like to thank Dr. Ozgur Mete for his insight on this topic and for providing the pathology photo of a histological example of NIFT-P.

References

1. Nikiforov YE, Seethala RR, Tallini G, Baloch ZW, Basolo F, Thompson LDR, Barletta J, Wenig BM, Ghuzlan AA, Kakudo K, Giordano TJ, Alves VA, Khanafshar E, Asa SL, El-Naggar AK, Gooding WE, Hodak SP, Lloyd RV, Maytal G, Mete O, Nikiforova MN, Nosé V, Papotti M, Poller DN, Sadow PM, Tischler AS, Tuttle RM, Wall KB, LiVolsi VA, Randolph GW, Ghossein RA. Nomenclature Revision for encapsulated follicular variant of papillary thyroid carcinoma: a paradigm shift to reduce overtreatment of indolent tumors. JAMA Oncol. 2016;2(8):1023–9. https://doi.org/10.1001/jamaoncol.2016.0386. PMC 5539411. PMID 27078145
2. Ganly I, Wang L, Tuttle RM, Katabi N, Ceballos GA, Harach HR, Ghossein R. Invasion rather than nuclear features correlates with outcome in encapsulated follicular tumors: further evidence for the reclassification of the encapsulated papillary thyroid carcinoma follicular variant. Hum Pathol. 2015;46(5):657–64. https://doi.org/10.1016/j.humpath.2015.01.010. PMC 4981329. PMID 25721865

3. Geramizadeh B, Maleki Z. Non-invasive follicular thyroid neoplasm with papillary-like nuclearfeatures (NIFTP): a review and update. Endocrine. 2019;64(3):433–40. https://doi.org/10.1007/s12020-019-01887-z.
4. Zajkowska K, Kopczyński J, Góźdź S, Kowalska A. Noninvasive follicular thyroid neoplasm with papillary-like nuclear features: a problematic entity. Endocr Connect. 2020;9(3):R47–58. Advance online publication. https://doi.org/10.1530/EC-19-0566.
5. Parente DN, Kluijfhout WP, Bongers PJ, Verzijil R, Devon KM, Rotstein LE, Goldstein DP, Asa SL, Mete O, Pasternak JD. Clinical safety of renaming encapsulated follicular variant of papillary thyroid carcinoma: is NIFTP truly benign? World J Surg. 2018;42(2):321–6.
6. Eskander A, Hall SF, Manduch M, Griffiths R, Irish JC. A population-based study on NIFTP incidence and survival: is NIFTP really a "benign" disease? Ann Surg Oncol. 2019;26(5):1376–84.
7. Haugen BR, Alexander EK, Bible KC, Doherty GM, Mandel SJ, Nikiforov YE, Pacini F, Randolph GW, Sawka AM, Schlumberger M, Schuff KG, Sherman SI, Sosa JA, Steward DL, Tuttle RM, Wartofsky L. 2015 American Thyroid Association Management Guidelines for Adult Patients with Thyroid Nodules and Differentiated Thyroid Cancer: The American Thyroid Association Guidelines Task Force on Thyroid Nodules and Differentiated Thyroid Cancer. Thyroid. 2016;26(1):1–133. https://doi.org/10.1089/thy.2015.0020. PMC 4739132. PMID 26462967
8. Cho U, Mete O, Kim MH, Bae JS, Jung CK. Molecular correlates and rate of lymph node metastasis of non-invasive follicular thyroid neoplasm with papillary-like nuclear features and invasive follicular variant papillary thyroid carcinoma: the impact of rigid criteria to distinguish non-invasive follicular thyroid neoplasm with papillary-like nuclear features. Mod Pathol. 2017;30:810–25. https://doi.org/10.1038/modpathol.2017.9.
9. Bychkov A, Jung CK, Liu Z, Kakudo K. Noninvasive follicular thyroid neoplasm with papillary-like nuclear features in Asian practice: perspectives for surgical pathology and cytopathology. Endocr Pathol. 2018;29(3):276–88. https://doi.org/10.1007/s12022-018-9519-6.
10. Saxen E, Franssila K, Bjarnason O, et al. Observer variation in histologic classification of thyroid cancer. Acta Pathol Microbiol Scand Sect A Pathol. 1978;86A:483–6.
11. Elsheikh TM, Asa SL, Chan JK, et al. Interobserver and intraobserver variation among experts in the diagnosis of thyroid follicular lesions with borderline nuclear features of papillary carcinoma. Am J Clin Pathol. 2008;130:736–44.
12. Lloyd RV, Erickson LA, Casey MB, et al. Observer variation in the diagnosis of follicular variant of papillary thyroid carcinoma. Am J Surg Pathol. 2004;28:1336–40.
13. Hirokawa M, Carney JA, Goellner JR, et al. Observer variation of encapsulated follicular lesions of the thyroid gland. Am J Surg Pathol. 2002;26:1508–14.
14. Rivera M, Ricarte-Filho J, Knauf J, et al. Molecular genotyping of papillary thyroid carcinoma, follicular variant according to its histological sub- types (encapsulated vs infiltrative) reveals distinct BRAF and RAS mutation patterns. Mod Pathol. 2010;23:1191–200.
15. Howitt BE, Jia Y, Sholl LM, Barletta JA. Molecular alterations in partially- encapsulated or well-circumscribed follicular variant of papillary thyroid carcinoma. Thyroid. 2013;23:1256–62.
16. Brandler TC, Liu CZ, Cho M, Zhou F, Cangiarella J, Yee-Chang M, Shi Y, Simsir A, Sun W. Does noninvasive follicular thyroid neoplasm with papillary-like nuclear features (NIFTP) have a unique molecular profile? Am J Clin Pathol. 2018;150(5):451–60. https://doi.org/10.1093/ajcp/aqy075.
17. Lloyd RV, Asa SL, LiVolsi VA, Sadow PM, Tischler AS, Ghossein RA, Tuttle RM, Nikiforov YE. The evolving diagnosis of noninvasive follicular thyroid neoplasm with papillary-like nuclear features (NIFTP). Hum Pathol. 2018;74:1–4. https://doi.org/10.1016/j.humpath.2017.12.027.
18. Bongers PJ, Greenberg CA, Hsiao R, Vermeer M, Vriens MR, Lutke Holzik MF, Goldstein DP, Devon K, Rotstein LE, Sawka AM, Pasternak JD. Differences in long-term quality of life between hemithyroidectomy and total thyroidectomy in patients treated for low-risk differentiated thyroid carcinoma. Surgery. 2020;167(1):94–101. https://doi.org/10.1016/j.surg.2019.04.060.

Chapter 17
Timing of Long-Term Postoperative Surveillance for Low-Risk Differentiated Thyroid Cancer

Stephanie Fish

Case

A 52-year-old female presented with a 1.5-cm right thyroid nodule noted incidentally on magnetic resonance imaging (MRI) of the neck. A thyroid ultrasound (US) revealed a solitary 15 × 12 × 12 mm right midpole nodule. The nodule was hypoechoic and solid with slightly irregular margins, but no microcalcifications. There were no nodules in the left lobe and no abnormal lymph nodes (see US Image 17.1). Fine needle aspiration cytology revealed papillary thyroid cancer (PTC). She underwent a right thyroid lobectomy. The final pathology revealed a right 1.3 cm PTC, classic type, with no vascular invasion and no extrathyroidal extension. The surgical margins were negative. Six weeks after surgery, the thyroid stimulating hormone (TSH) level was 1.25 mU/L with free thyroxine (FT4) of 1.2 ng/dL; the thyroglobulin (Tg) level was 4.9 ng/mL with negative thyroglobulin antibodies (TgAb).

She then underwent her first surveillance testing 6 months later. The TSH was 1.32 mU/L with a Tg of 4.2 ng/mL and negative TgAb. The US of the neck showed no right thyroid bed nodules. The left lobe had normal echogenicity without nodules. There were no abnormal lymph nodes. She was not taking thyroid hormone medication.

This is T1N0M0 disease, stage I. The overall prognosis is excellent with a long-term survival of 99% [1]. The risk of recurrence is low as the tumor is small and confined to the thyroid gland. She has had an excellent response to therapy with no suspicious findings on neck ultrasound and a low-normal Tg level. What is the most appropriate long-term surveillance for this patient?

S. Fish (✉)
Endocrinology Division, Memorial Sloan Kettering Cancer Center, New York, NY, USA
e-mail: fishs@mskcc.org

© The Author(s), under exclusive license to Springer Nature Switzerland AG 2023
S. A. Roman et al. (eds.), *Controversies in Thyroid Nodules and Differentiated Thyroid Cancer*, https://doi.org/10.1007/978-3-031-37135-6_17

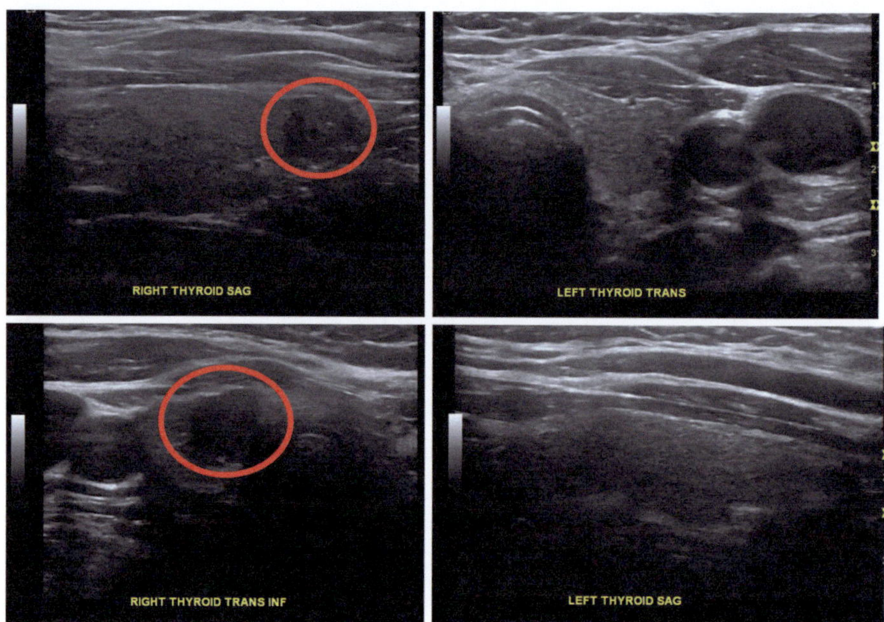

Image 17.1 Ultrasound images of thyroid gland with solitary 1.5 cm solid hypothyroid right thyroid nodule

Background

Approximately 90% of patients with differentiated thyroid cancer (DTC) have low-risk disease. Patients with low-risk thyroid cancer are classified as American Joint Committee on Cancer (AJCC) Tumor, Node, Metastasis (TNM) stage I or stage II. The AJCC TNM staging system utilizes patient age, tumor size, cervical lymph node involvement, and the presence of distant metastasis when predicting risk of death from DTC [1]. This staging system is focused only on predicting overall survival, and it is not intended to predict risk of recurrence, which is more common in patients with DTC.

Among all patients with DTC, 20-30% will experience a recurrence during surveillance while only 4–7% will die of thyroid cancer during the first 10 years of surveillance [2–5]. However, for patients with low-risk DTC, the likelihood of recurrence is just 1–5% and the chance of death from thyroid cancer is nearly 0% [3, 6]. The American Thyroid Association (ATA) Risk Stratification System defines low risk based on the likelihood of recurrence [6, 7]. See Table 17.1 for the ATA criteria for low-risk DTC.

The primary goal of thyroid cancer surveillance is to provide dynamic risk stratification, to identify recurrence early, and to tailor treatment or monitoring to these findings. There are several controversies regarding the long-term surveillance of patients with low-risk DTC. After thyroid surgery, TSH suppression has been a standard treatment in all patients with DTC. However, it is not clear that this is necessary for patients with low-risk DTC. Neck US and serum Tg measurement with

Table 17.1 ATA risk stratification

Low risk	
PTC (with all the following)	No local or distant metastases
	All macroscopic tumor has been resected
	No tumor invasion of locoregional tissues or structures
	The tumor does not have aggressive histology (tall cell, hobnail variant, columnar cell variant)
	If RAI is given, there are no avid metastatic foci outside the thyroid bed on the post-treatment whole-body scan
	No vascular invasion
	Clinical N0 or ≤ 5 pathology N1 micrometastases (<0.2 cm in largest dimension)
Encapsulated follicular variant of PTC	Intrathyroidal
Papillary microcarcinoma (<1 cm)	Intrathyroidal, unifocal, or multifocal, including BRAF V600E mutated (if known)
Follicular thyroid cancer (with the following)	Intrathyroidal, well-differentiated with capsular invasion and no or minimal (<4 foci) vascular invasion

TgAb are the cornerstones of long-term surveillance [8, 9]. However, the timing and frequency of these tests are widely debated, especially because both the risk of recurrence and the risk of death are so low in this patient population.

Thyroid Hormone Treatment

Thyroid hormone supplementation is used to treat postsurgical hypothyroidism. This may not be necessary after thyroid lobectomy if patients are able to maintain the serum TSH within the target range [6]. Suppressive doses of thyroid hormone are used to prevent the growth of DTC and have been shown to improve the overall outcomes in patients with DTC [10–13]. For many years, most patients with low-risk DTC were treated with suppressive doses of thyroid hormone for at least 5 years after diagnosis to prevent tumor growth from TSH stimulation [14]. However, more recent studies show no improvement in overall survival with TSH suppression [15]. Hovens et al. [16] assessed death and recurrence among 366 patients with DTC taking Levothyroxine after total thyroidectomy and radioactive iodine ablation (RAI) with a median follow-up of 8.85 years. They found no difference in the rates of death and recurrence among patients with or without TSH suppression. As a result, less aggressive TSH suppression has been recommended for low-risk DTC patients [17]. Based on the 2015 ATA guidelines [6], low-risk DTC patients with undetectable serum Tg levels after total thyroidectomy may be maintained with a TSH level at the lower end of the reference range (0.5–2.0 mU/L). For low-risk patients who have low, but detectable, serum Tg levels, TSH may be maintained at or slightly below the lower limit of normal (0.1–0.5 mU/L). There is little data on optimal TSH goal after lobectomy. The 2015 ATA guidelines recommend that the TSH is maintained in the mid to lower reference range (0.5–2.0 mU/L) while surveillance is continued [6]. For most patients with low-risk DTC who are being monitored with surveillance, the goal TSH level is in the low-normal range to avoid the risk of long-term TSH suppression on the heart and bones.

Imaging

Cervical lymph node metastases are the most common site of recurrence for DTC, especially PTC. The standard surveillance imaging includes obtaining a US at 6–12 months after thyroid surgery. US is the most sensitive imaging modality for the detection of metastatic cervical lymph nodes as well as recurrent disease in the thyroidectomy bed [18–20]. Other imaging modalities such as diagnostic whole-body scan (WBS) with radioiodine, computed tomography (CT), MRI, and positron emission tomography (PET) are not indicated in low-risk patients.

During long-term surveillance, US is typically performed yearly to assess for disease recurrence. Although there are many benefits to US surveillance, it is important to interpret US findings carefully, especially in low-risk DTC patients with low or undetectable Tg levels as these patients have a very low risk of recurrence [18]. In ATA low-risk patients without structural evidence of disease on initial surveillance testing, routine screening with ultrasound is more likely to identify false-positive results rather than clinically significant structural disease. Yang et al. [21] followed 171 patients with low-risk DTC for a median of 8 years. Small structural recurrence was identified in two (1.2%) patients. False-positive ultrasound findings were noted in 114 (67%) patients. These false-positive findings can lead to increased testing and patient anxiety. See Image 17.2 for some findings that can be seen on surveillance US including nonspecific thyroid bed nodules, nonspecific prominent cervical lymph nodes, and small abnormal cervical lymph nodes.

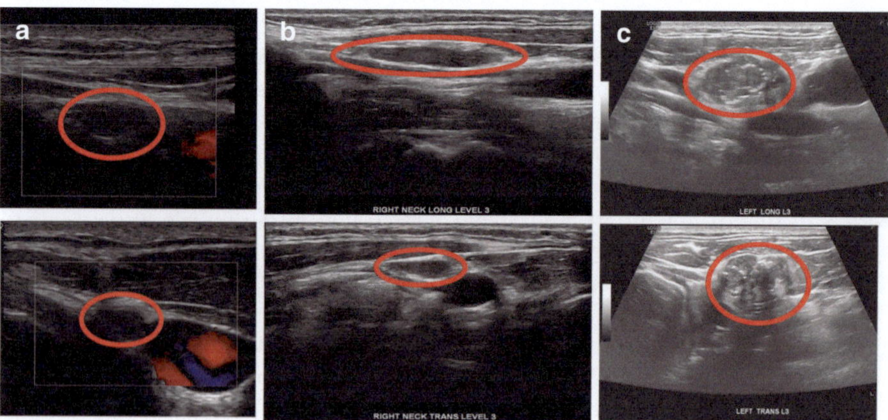

Image 17.2 Ultrasound images (**a**) nonspecific thyroid bed nodule, (**b**) prominent cervical lymph node, and (**c**) abnormal cervical lymph node

If the initial US 6–12 months after surgery is reassuring, then repeating an US is not necessary unless there is a measurable or rising Tg level or if there is a palpable lymph node in the neck [6]. However, in patients treated with thyroid lobectomy, the US is the main tool for surveillance since these patients will have a detectable Tg level due to the residual thyroid lobe. The timing and frequency of US in low-risk DTC patients after lobectomy remains unclear and additional studies are needed to best determine the most appropriate surveillance recommendations.

Thyroglobulin

Tg, a glycoprotein stored in the colloid of thyroid follicles, is a sensitive marker of DTC. A detectable or increasing Tg level is highly indicative of residual or recurrent thyroid cancer [22]. TgAb levels should always be measured when measuring Tg. TgAb are present in 10% of the general population and in approximately 20–25% of patients with DTC [23]. TgAb will interfere with the measurement of Tg in all assays, making the Tg level unreliable.

In the follow-up of low-risk DTC, it is recommended to monitor serum Tg level every 6–12 months during the first year of follow-up. In the absence of TgAb interference, serum Tg levels have a high degree of sensitivity and specificity to detect DTC, especially after total thyroidectomy and RAI ablation. Uncertainty exists over the optimal cutoff level for both stimulated and unstimulated postoperative Tg levels 4–6 weeks after surgery [6]. Most studies have focused on the role of Tg after total thyroidectomy and RAI treatment. Recent studies have evaluated the role of Tg after total thyroidectomy without RAI treatment. There are limited data on the utility of Tg after thyroid lobectomy, but its role appears to be more limited.

Studies have shown a good correlation between low Tg levels and an excellent response to therapy in DTC patients treated with total thyroidectomy and RAI. In a series of 425 patients, Malandrino et al. [24] observed that a basal Tg of <0.15 ng/mL was associated with a low likelihood of residual disease. Brassard et al. [25] looked at the risk of recurrence in 715 patients with DTC treated with a total thyroidectomy and lymph node dissection. Most of the patients were treated with RAI. During a median follow-up of 6.2 years, 32 patients (4.5%) were diagnosed with a recurrence. A thyroglobulin cutoff of <0.27 ng/mL had a maximal sensitivity (72%) and specificity (86%) for recurrence. With this cutoff, 117 (16%) patients had a positive Tg level, and of these, 23 (20%) had recurrent disease. Recurrence was observed among just 9 (1.5%) of the 598 patients with a Tg level below this cutoff [25].

Studies have evaluated the role of Tg in patients who did not undergo RAI remnant ablation after total thyroidectomy. Durante et al. [26] studied 290 low-risk DTC patients who had not undergone RAI treatment and found that the Tg levels were < 1.0 ng/mL within 5 years of surgery in 95% of patients, and the Tg levels were < 0.2 ng/mL in 80% of these patients. Nascimento et al. [27] reported a retrospective review of 76 consecutive low-risk DTC patients treated with total thyroidectomy alone and followed for a median of 2.5 years. They found that an unstimulated Tg of >2 ng/mL was sufficient to detect all patients with disease recurrence.

The value of measuring Tg levels after thyroid lobectomy is less clear. Momesso et al. [28] studied the response to therapy in 187 patients with DTC treated with lobectomy and 320 patients treated with total thyroidectomy without RAI. Four hundred and thirty-three patients (85.4%) had low-risk disease. The median follow-up was 100.5 months. With negative TgAb and negative imaging, none of the patients experienced recurrence if the unstimulated Tg level after total thyroidectomy was <0.2 ng/mL and after lobectomy was <30 ng/mL.

Studies have questioned the 30 ng/mL cutoff and several studies show a limited value of Tg as an independent predictor of thyroid cancer recurrence in patients treated with a thyroid lobectomy [29, 30]. A cohort study by Park et al. [30] evaluated 208 patients with low-risk DTC treated with lobectomy and not requiring thyroid hormone replacement therapy. Nineteen patients (9%) developed recurrent disease during a median follow-up of 6.9 years. Overall, serum Tg increased by about 10% per year, and there was no significant difference in Tg increase or Tg-to-TSH ratio between patients with or without recurrence. Similar findings were reported by Ritter et al. [29] in a cohort study of 167 DTC patients treated with thyroid lobectomy who were followed for a mean of 6.5 years. They observed recurrence in 7.2% of the cohort, but Tg levels, Tg dynamics, and anti-Tg antibody dynamics were not predictive of recurrence.

Recurrence of low-risk DTC after thyroid lobectomy occurs primarily in the contralateral lobe and neck lymph nodes. Based on the current data, periodic imaging of the neck with US is the preferred way to detect structural recurrence after lobectomy. Many clinicians measure Tg and TgAb levels with yearly TSH after thyroid lobectomy. This is reasonable, but the results need to be interpreted while keeping in mind the underlying risk of recurrence and imaging results.

Summary and Conclusion

Now, we return to the 52-year-old female with a right 1.5 cm PTC, classic type, with no vascular invasion and no extrathyroidal extension. She was treated with a right thyroid lobectomy. She had an excellent response to surgery based on the negative neck US performed 6 months after surgery. The serum Tg is normal at 4.2 ng/mL with negative TgAb. The risk of recurrence is very low.

The optimal length and interval of long-term surveillance for this patient with low-risk DTC remains unknown; but it is likely that less frequent testing is appropriate. After surgery, patients typically have laboratory testing for TSH, Tg, and TgAb as well as a neck ultrasound in 6–12 months. If this testing shows an excellent response to treatment with a low Tg level, negative TgAb, and no suspicious findings on neck ultrasound, the patient can be followed with a yearly unstimulated Tg [6]. TSH suppression is not indicated in the treatment of low-risk DTC. Annual US is likely not necessary as it can lead to the identification of false-positive results and increased patient anxiety. Measurement of Tg is useful in the surveillance of patients treated with total thyroidectomy with or without RAI. However, Tg is not consistently predictive of recurrence in patients treated with thyroid lobectomy.

In patients with low-risk DTC, there is no survival benefit from life-long surveillance. Wang et al. [31] looked at the cost of surveillance in 1087 DTC patients after thyroidectomy. The cost of surveillance to identify each recurrence was $147,819 in low-risk patients, six and seven times higher than the cost of surveillance in intermediate and high-risk patients, respectively. Because the risk of recurrence is so low in patients with low-risk DTC, the risk of frequent testing in identifying clinically insignificant recurrences that may lead to unnecessary treatment outweigh the benefits [32]. With sensitive Tg and US technology, one can identify more thyroid cancer recurrences, but in most cases, there is no associated improvement in disease-specific survival [4].

The recommendations for long-term surveillance of patients with low-risk DTC are evolving. Over several years, the approach to the initial treatment of thyroid cancer has changed from a one-size-fits-all approach to an individualized approach based on tumor characteristics. Similarly, the approach to long-term surveillance of patients with DTC needs to be individualized by incorporating our knowledge of the risk of death and the risk of recurrence. Based on the data available, it appears that yearly follow-up is not necessary for low-risk DTC patients, especially after 5 years as most thyroid cancer recurrences occur in the cervical lymph nodes within 5 years of initial treatment. Long-term surveillance of low-risk DTC patients treated with a thyroid lobectomy is even less clear as Tg is a less accurate predictor of recurrence and intermittent imaging with thyroid US is primarily recommended for surveillance. As more patients are treated with thyroid lobectomy, additional studies are necessary to determine the best approach to long-term surveillance.

References

1. AJCC. AJCC cancer staging manual. New York: Springer; 2017.
2. Banerjee M, Muenz DG, Chang JT, Papaleontiou M, Haymart MR. Tree-based model for thyroid cancer prognostication. J Clin Endocrinol Metab. 2014;99(10):3737–45.
3. Tuttle RM, Tala H, Shah J, Leboeuf R, Ghossein R, Gonen M, Brokhin M, Omry G, Fagin JA, Shaha A. Estimating risk of recurrence in differentiated thyroid cancer after total thyroidectomy and radioactive iodine remnant ablation: using response to therapy variables to modify the initial risk estimates predicted by the new American Thyroid Association staging system. Thyroid. 2010;20(12):1341–9.
4. Banerjee M, Wiebel JL, Guo C, Gay B, Haymart MR. Use of imaging tests after primary treatment of thyroid cancer in the United States: population based retrospective cohort study evaluating death and recurrence. BMJ. 2016;354:i3839.
5. Okuyucu K, Ince S, Alagoz E, Emer O, San H, Balkan E, Ayan A, Meric C, Haymana C, Acıkel C, Gunalp B, Karacalioglu AO, Arslan N. Risk factors and stratification for recurrence of patients with differentiated thyroid cancer, elevated thyroglobulin and negative I-131 whole-body scan, by restaging (18)F-FDG PET/CT. Hell J Nucl Med. 2016;19(3):208–17.

6. Haugen BR, Alexander EK, Bible KC, Doherty GM, Mandel SJ, Nikiforov YE, Pacini F, Randolph GW, Sawka AM, Schlumberger M, Schuff KG, Sherman SI, Sosa JA, Steward DL, Tuttle RM, Wartofsky L. 2015 American Thyroid Association management guidelines for adult patients with thyroid nodules and differentiated thyroid cancer: the American Thyroid Association guidelines task force on thyroid nodules and differentiated thyroid cancer. Thyroid. 2016;26(1):1–133.

7. Cooper DS, Doherty GM, Haugen BR, Kloos RT, Lee SL, Mandel SJ, Mazzaferri EL, McIver B, Pacini F, Schlumberger M, Sherman SI, Steward DL, Tuttle RM. American Thyroid Association (ATA) guidelines taskforce on thyroid nodules and differentiated thyroid cancer. Revised American Thyroid Association management guidelines for patients with thyroid nodules and differentiated thyroid cancer. Thyroid. 2009;19(11):1167–214.

8. Schvartz C, Bonnetain F, Dabakuyo S, Gauthier M, Cueff A, Fieffé S, Pochart JM, Cochet I, Crevisy E, Dalac A, Papathanassiou D, Toubeau M. Impact on overall survival of radioactive iodine in low-risk differentiated thyroid cancer patients. J Clin Endocrinol Metab. 2012;97(5):1526–35.

9. Pacini F, Schlumberger M, Dralle H, Elisei R, Smit JW, Wiersinga W, European Thyroid Cancer Taskforce. European consensus for the management of patients with differentiated thyroid carcinoma of the follicular epithelium. Eur J Endocrinol. 2006;154(6):787–803.

10. Mazzaferri EL, Jhiang SM. Long-term impact of initial surgical and medical therapy on papillary and follicular thyroid cancer. Am J Med. 1994;97(5):418–28.

11. Surgery of the thyroid gland (the Lettsomian lectures). BMJ. 1937;1(3973):460–1.

12. Cooper DS. TSH suppressive therapy: an overview of long-term clinical consequences. Hormones (Athens). 2010;9(1):57–9.

13. Pujol P, Daures JP, Nsakala N, Baldet L, Bringer J, Jaffiol C. Degree of thyrotropin suppression as a prognostic determinant in differentiated thyroid cancer. J Clin Endocrinol Metab. 1996;81(12):4318–23.

14. Mazzaferri EL, Young RL, Oertel JE, Kemmerer WT, Page CP. Papillary thyroid carcinoma: the impact of therapy in 576 patients. Medicine (Baltimore). 1977;56(3):171–96.

15. Jonklaas J, Sarlis NJ, Litofsky D, Ain KB, Bigos ST, Brierley JD, Cooper DS, Haugen BR, Ladenson PW, Magner J, Robbins J, Ross DS, Skarulis M, Maxon HR, Sherman SI. Outcomes of patients with differentiated thyroid carcinoma following initial therapy. Thyroid. 2006;16(12):1229–42.

16. Hovens GC, Stokkel MP, Kievit J, Corssmit EP, Pereira AM, Romijn JA, Smit JW. Associations of serum thyrotropin concentrations with recurrence and death in differentiated thyroid cancer. J Clin Endocrinol Metab. 2007;92(7):2610–5.

17. Biondi B, Cooper DS. Benefits of thyrotropin suppression versus the risks of adverse effects in differentiated thyroid cancer. Thyroid. 2010;20(2):135–46.

18. Kobaly K, Mandel SJ, Langer JE. Clinical review: thyroid cancer mimics on surveillance neck sonography. J Clin Endocrinol Metab. 2015;100(2):371–5.

19. Leboulleux S, Girard E, Rose M, Travagli JP, Sabbah N, Caillou B, Hartl DM, Lassau N, Baudin E, Schlumberger M. Ultrasound criteria of malignancy for cervical lymph nodes in patients followed up for differentiated thyroid cancer. J Clin Endocrinol Metab. 2007;92(9):3590–4.

20. Leenhardt L, Erdogan MF, Hegedus L, Mandel SJ, Paschke R, Rago T, Russ G. 2013 European thyroid association guidelines for cervical ultrasound scan and ultrasound-guided techniques in the postoperative management of patients with thyroid cancer. Eur Thyroid J. 2013;2(3):147–59.

21. Yang SP, Bach AM, Tuttle RM, Fish SA. Serial neck ultrasound is more likely to identify false-positive abnormalities than clinically significant disease in low-risk papillary thyroid cancer patients. Endocr Pract. 2015;21(12):1372–9.

22. Baudin E, Do Cao C, Cailleux AF, Leboulleux S, Travagli JP, Schlumberger M. Positive predictive value of serum thyroglobulin levels, measured during the first year of follow-up after thyroid hormone withdrawal, in thyroid cancer patients. J Clin Endocrinol Metab. 2003;88(3):1107–11.

23. Spencer CA, Bergoglio LM, Kazarosyan M, Fatemi S, LoPresti JS. Clinical impact of thyroglobulin (Tg) and Tg autoantibody method differences on the management of patients with differentiated thyroid carcinomas. J Clin Endocrinol Metab. 2005;90(10):5566–75.
24. Malandrino P, Latina A, Marescalco S, Spadaro A, Regalbuto C, Fulco RA, Scollo C, Vigneri R, Pellegriti G. Risk-adapted management of differentiated thyroid cancer assessed by a sensitive measurement of basal serum thyroglobulin. J Clin Endocrinol Metab. 2011;96(6):1703–9.
25. Brassard M, Borget I, Edet-Sanson A, Giraudet AL, Mundler O, Toubeau M, Bonichon F, Borson-Chazot F, Leenhardt L, Schvartz C, Dejax C, Brenot-Rossi I, Toubert ME, Torlontano M, Benhamou E, Schlumberger M, Group TW, THYRDIAG Working Group. Long-term follow-up of patients with papillary and follicular thyroid cancer: a prospective study on 715 patients. J Clin Endocrinol Metab. 2011;96(5):1352–9.
26. Durante C, Montesano T, Attard M, Torlontano M, Monzani F, Costante G, Meringolo D, Ferdeghini M, Tumino S, Lamartina L, Paciaroni A, Massa M, Giacomelli L, Ronga G, Filetti S, PTC Study Group. Long-term surveillance of papillary thyroid cancer patients who do not undergo postoperative radioiodine remnant ablation: is there a role for serum thyroglobulin measurement? J Clin Endocrinol Metab. 2012;97(8):2748–53.
27. Nascimento C, Borget I, Troalen F, Al Ghuzlan A, Deandreis D, Hartl D, Lumbroso J, Chougnet CN, Baudin E, Schlumberger M, Leboulleux S. Ultrasensitive serum thyroglobulin measurement is useful for the follow-up of patients treated with total thyroidectomy without radioactive iodine ablation. Eur J Endocrinol. 2013;169(5):689–93.
28. Momesso DP, Vaisman F, Yang SP, Bulzico DA, Corbo R, Vaisman M, Tuttle RM. Dynamic risk stratification in patients with differentiated thyroid cancer treated without radioactive iodine. J Clin Endocrinol Metab. 2016;101(7):2692–700.
29. Ritter A, Mizrachi A, Bachar G, Vainer I, Shimon I, Hirsch D, Diker-Cohen T, Duskin-Bitan H, Robenshtok E. Detecting recurrence following lobectomy for thyroid cancer: role of thyroglobulin and thyroglobulin antibodies. J Clin Endocrinol Metab. 2020;105:e2145–51.
30. Park S, Jeon MJ, Oh H-S, Lee Y-M, Sung T-Y, Han M, Han JM, Kim T-Y, Chung K-W, Kim EY, et al. Changes in serum thyroglobulin levels after lobectomy in patients with low-risk papillary thyroid cancer. Thyroid. 2018;28:997–1003.
31. Wang LY, Roman BR, Migliacci JC, Palmer FL, Tuttle RM, Shaha AR, Shah JP, Patel SG, Ganly I. Cost-effectiveness analysis of papillary thyroid cancer surveillance. Cancer. 2015;121(23):4132–40.
32. Onkendi EO, McKenzie TJ, Richards ML, Farley DR, Thompson GB, Kasperbauer JL, Hay ID, Grant CS. Reoperative experience with papillary thyroid cancer. World J Surg. 2014;38(3):645–52.

Chapter 18
External-Beam Radiation for Patients with Differentiated Thyroid Cancer: Is There a Role?

Jelena Lukovic and James D. Brierley

Case

A 72-year-old woman presented to her family doctor with symptoms of an upper respiratory tract infection. On examination, she was found to have a right neck mass prompting further investigation with ultrasound and fine needle aspiration. Cytology showed papillary thyroid carcinoma. She was subsequently referred to a thyroid surgeon. On review of systems, she reported hoarseness over the last 4 months, and laryngoscopy demonstrated immobile right vocal cord. Given her clinical presentation, a CT scan was ordered and identified a large thyroid mass with apparent involvement of the trachea and esophagus (Fig. 18.1a, b). In addition, she was found to have enlarged lateral nodes adjacent to the carotid artery with no obvious vascular invasion. Her case was presented at a multidisciplinary tumor board and the consensus recommendation was for surgical resection as the initial treatment.

The patient underwent a total thyroidectomy, central neck node dissection, and right lateral neck dissection. At the time of surgery, the right recurrent laryngeal nerve was found to be encased by tumor and was therefore sacrificed. Extrathyroidal extension of the primary tumor involved the outer muscle layers of the esophagus which were dissected down to the mucosa. The trachea was invaded with full-thickness intraluminal disease and 3.5 cm of the trachea was resected and primarily repaired. She tolerated the surgery well and recovered uneventfully.

Final pathology revealed an infiltrating papillary thyroid carcinoma with focal areas of dedifferentiation and poorly differentiated disease. The mass measured 5.4 cm with angioinvasion and focal tall cell change (up to 10%) with involvement

J. Lukovic · J. D. Brierley (✉)
Department of Radiation Oncology, University of Toronto, Toronto, ON, Canada

Department of Radiation Oncology, Princess Margaret Cancer Centre, Toronto, ON, Canada
e-mail: jelena.lukovic@uhn.ca; james.brierley@uhn.ca

S. A. Roman et al. (eds.), *Controversies in Thyroid Nodules and Differentiated Thyroid Cancer*, https://doi.org/10.1007/978-3-031-37135-6_18

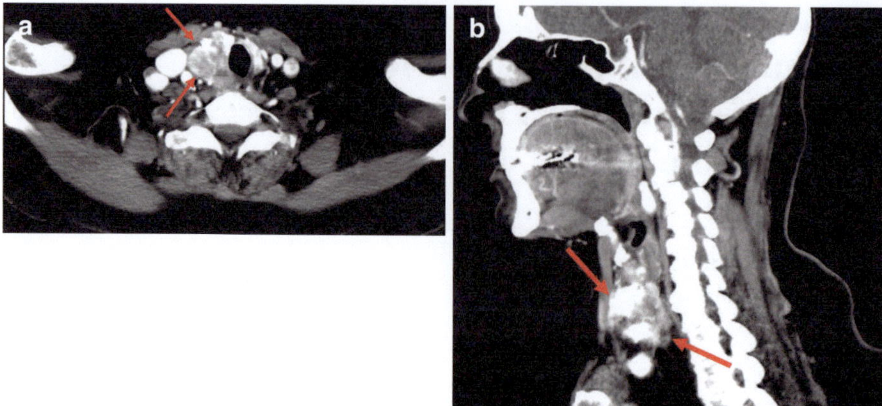

Fig. 18.1 (**a**) Diagnostic CT demonstrated a large thyroid mass with invasion into the trachea; axial view. (**b**) Sagittal view of the diagnostic CT scan demonstrating the large thyroid mass with esophageal invasion

of resected strap muscle. One lymph level IV/V node contained metastatic disease with extranodal extension. Thirty-three additional lymph nodes had no metastatic disease. The primary tumor extended to the painted margin of the tracheal resection and extended to the cauterized edge of the resected esophageal muscle.

She received radioactive iodine (RAI) ^{131}I 200 mCi with thyrotropin alpha stimulation. At the time of treatment, her TSH was suitably elevated, the thyroglobulin was 0.1 ug/l, and her thyroglobulin antibodies were 376 IU/ml. Post-iodine whole body scan showed uptake in the neck but no evidence of iodine-avid metastatic disease. On a follow-up CT scan of the head and neck, however, there were postoperative changes but no evidence of gross residual disease. On chest CT there were several small lung nodules up to 7 mm in size, suspicious for metastases. Her case was discussed again at multidisciplinary tumor board and following the group recommendations, she was referred to Radiation Oncology for consideration of postoperative external beam radiotherapy (EBRT).

She was seen and assessed by a Radiation Oncologist. At the time of her initial consultation, she was not sure if she wished to pursue any further treatment—she felt she was only starting to recover from her extensive surgery and RAI and was additionally concerned about the potential side effects of EBRT.

Background and Discussion

Although the role of postoperative RAI is well-established in patients with moderate- to high-risk differentiated thyroid cancer, the role of EBRT is less well-defined. The rationale for considering EBRT in addition to postoperative RAI is to reduce the risk of locoregional recurrence in patients considered to be at high risk. Such patients tend to be older, with locally advanced disease and significant ETE. Local recurrence in the thyroid bed can be problematic, as uncontrolled cancer in this area can cause obstruction of the esophagus and airway, skin necrosis, and, in rare cases, carotid artery rupture.

A role of EBRT in local control of invasive papillary thyroid cancer was first described in 1966 [1]. Most of the published literature since that point demonstrating the possible benefit of EBRT has consisted of single-institution retrospective studies and are therefore subject to selection bias. Similarly, not all series have included patients who received RAI in addition to EBRT and the method of determining and recording recurrence is inconsistent. Many of these studies include patients we may now consider to be at relatively low risk [2].

Farahati J et al. reported the clinical outcomes of adjuvant radiotherapy for 874 patients with differentiated thyroid cancer. All patients had what was then considered T4 disease (ETE with or without invasion of local structures—in the current classification system, some of these patients may be classified as T3b). All patients had RAI and TSH suppression and the minimum age was 40 years. In this prospective study, the addition of EBRT was a predictive factor for improvement in time to local regional recurrence ($p < 0.004$) and time to distant failure ($p < 0.001$) [3]. Although there was an attempt at a randomized controlled trial, it was not successful because of failure to enroll sufficient patients and because some low-risk patients were included [4].

A retrospective analysis from the Princess Margaret Cancer Centre included 729 patients treated between 1958 and 1998. Within this cohort, for patients over the age of 60 years with gross extrathyroidal extension but no gross residual disease after surgery, there was both a survival (10-year cause-specific survival (EBRT: 81.0% vs. no EBRT: 64.6%; $p = 0.04$) and local control (10-year LRFR 95.9% with EBRT vs. 85.4% with no EBRT, $p = 0.01$) advantage with EBRT. Following this analysis, postoperative EBRT was adopted as the standard treatment for patients with ETE [5].

The limited available retrospective data have been used to create guidelines recommending EBRT for patients with DTCs in certain high-risk situations. For instance, the American Thyroid Association guidelines in 2009 recommended consideration for EBRT in patients older than 45 years with gross extrathyroidal extension and a high likelihood of microscopic residual disease [6]. The recommendation in the 2016 update, however, was less explicit, advising surgery combined with additional therapy such as RAI and/or EBRT for tumors that invade the upper aerodigestive tract [7]. The United Kingdom National Multidisciplinary Guidelines recommend that EBRT should be considered in addition to RAI in patients where there is residual disease after surgery [8]. The American Head and Neck Society (AHNS) issued a statement that EBRT is recommended for patients with gross residual or unresectable locoregional disease, except for patients less than 45 years old with a limited gross disease that is RAI-avid. In addition, after complete resection, EBRT may be considered in select patients over 45 years with high likelihood of microscopic residual disease and low likelihood of responding to RAI [9]. The

AHNS also commented that a higher age cutoff could be appropriate, and that cervical lymph node involvement alone should not be an indication for adjuvant EBRT.

Surgeons are much more likely to obtain clear margins in patients with anterior extension into the strap muscles than in patients with posterior extension into the tracheoesophageal region. This is reflected in the sixth edition TNM staging system, wherein T3 tumors were defined as those measuring more than 4 cm in greatest dimension and limited to the thyroid, or any tumor with minimal extrathyroidal extension (e.g., extension to sternothyroid muscle or perithyroidal soft tissues). T4a tumors were defined as those extending beyond the thyroid capsule and invading any of the following: subcutaneous soft tissues, larynx, trachea, esophagus, and recurrent laryngeal nerve [10, 11]. We recommend EBRT for older patients with T4a tumors and presumed microscopic disease. This recommendation, however, was based on our retrospective data in patients treated between 1958 and 1998 described above. Since that time, surgical specialization and expertise have no doubt reduced the recurrence rate in these high-risk patients. Therefore, it is necessary to define more clearly who may benefit from EBRT in addition to surgery and RAI.

The controversy regarding the benefit of EBRT is illustrated by a population-based study of the National Cancer Database (NCDB), which revealed that patients who received EBRT had significantly higher 5- and 10-year hazard of death whereas the use of RAI was associated with significantly improved survival [12]. It is important to note, however, that the cohort who received EBRT comprised significantly older patients who had more advanced-stage disease, suggesting potential selection bias for patients with worse disease. In addition, the database unfortunately did not include local control rates, which is an essential outcome to consider when reviewing a locoregional therapy such as EBRT.

In a French review of 13 papers, a scoring system was developed to define a cohort of patients who would benefit from EBRT. Any patient who scored 6 or more points would be recommended EBRT. Age over 60 years, ETE, and microscopic residual disease all score two points each giving a total of 6 and thereby supporting the recommendation of EBRT for patients over 60 with microscopic residual and ETE [13]. The recommendation for the use of EBRT from retrospective reviews has been supported by a multi-institutional analysis from France of 254 patients from 18 centers, with T3 or T4 disease, nodal disease, or positive surgical margins. By propensity score analysis although there was no survival advantage there was an improvement in local control with EBRT [14].

Two meta-analyses add additional uncertainty surrounding the role of EBRT. A 2014 meta-analysis reported on 2388 patients from eight studies—the mean recurrence rate in patients receiving EBRT regardless of stage or residual disease status was 8%, compared with 25% in patients who did not receive EBRT (p = 03) [15]. Conversely, a more recent meta-analysis that included nine studies concluded that although locoregional control was improved by EBRT without any significant toxicity, the benefit was small and there was no benefit in survival, progression-free survival, or cancer-specific survival. A panel that reviewed the meta-analysis on behalf of the Italian Association of Radiotherapy and Clinical Oncology judged the harm/benefit balance was uncertain [16].

The heterogeneous, primarily retrospective reviews together demonstrate the difficulty in giving definite evidence-based advice in the absence of a well-structured randomized controlled trial, in an uncommon subset of high-risk patients that may still have relatively indolent disease. The existing evidence is based on small studies that often recruit patients over a prolonged period during which surgical and radiation techniques change and improve. It remains essential to clearly identify patients at high risk for local recurrence with age and local extent being two of the most important prognostic factors. As noted earlier, the definition of T category was revised in the sixth edition TNM and more recently in the eighth edition and the prognostic significance of age was revised and changed from 45 to 55 years.

A recent retrospective review helps to more clearly define patients who benefit from EBRT. Although it presents a relatively small cohort of patients (n = 88), its strengths include detailed information regarding the extent of ETE and the fact that it includes patients who were treated in the modern era of centralized experienced surgery and modern radiation techniques. All patients had RAI and 44 had additional EBRT. All patients had T4a disease and the extent of ETE was classified by extent of tracheal involvement, esophageal involvement, recurrent laryngeal nerve laryngeal involvement, and extent of resection. Patients who received RAI alone had a lower disease-free survival than those who had RAI and EBRT (43% versus 57% at 4 years; effect size 14%, 95% CI: −7%–33%). On subgroup analysis, this effect was seen in patients with minimal tracheal perichondrium or esophageal muscularis involvement but was not seen in the subset of patients who had only RLN involvement. Age and esophageal involvement were additional significant poor prognostic factors [17].

Over time, our own guidelines have evolved—we currently recommend EBRT for patients with gross extrathyroidal extension with T4a disease over the age of 55 but exclude patients with RLN involvement that has been resected off the nerve by an experienced thyroid surgeon. Although not discussed above, we also recommend EBRT for all patients with gross residual disease unless they are young, the extent of disease is minimal, and there appears to be adequate RAI uptake in the area of concern.

After determining that a patient is at potential risk of unsalvageable thyroid bed recurrence and would benefit from EBRT, it is important that careful radiation treatment planning is performed and the potential risk of significant toxicity is kept to a minimum. This is aided by the use of modern radiation treatment planning with Intensity Modulated Radiation Therapy (IMRT) [18], Unfortunately, the most significant acute and possible late toxicities to the esophagus, pharynx, larynx, and trachea cannot be avoided, as these structures are invariably in the greatest area of concern for recurrence and therefore receive high-dose radiation. Other structures of concern include the mandible, parotids, and pharyngeal constrictors. Toxicity can potentially be reduced by restricting the volume irradiated. We tend to restrict the volume treated to the thyroid bed and adjacent nodal volumes rather than routinely treating the whole cervical nodal chain. Our usual radiation volume therefore includes the surgical thyroidectomy bed and nodal levels III, IV, VI, and part of level V, extending from the hyoid bone superiorly to the aortic arch inferiorly. It is our institutional policy to deliver 66–60 Gy in 33–30 fractions to the thyroid bed and areas of surgical dissection if there is a concern for macroscopic or microscopic residual disease (respectively), and 56 Gy in 33 fractions or 54 Gy in 30 fractions to undissected areas at risk for microscopic disease.

Recommendation and Treatment

Given our patient's age and extent of ETE involving the posterior structures of the trachea and esophagus and microscopic residual disease, she meets our institutional guideline criteria for postoperative EBRT. Importantly, in a modern series of patients with T4a disease, Tam et al. reported a local relapse-free rate of 34% with RAI alone and only 3% in patients treated with RAI and EBRT [17]. Our patient is in a similar group of high-risk T4a patients in whom relapse would require ablative surgery; therefore, achieving maximum local control is vital. As there was no gross residual disease on her post-operative CT scan, she was prescribed 60Gy in 30 fractions to the thyroid bed and ipsilateral level IV and partial V. The contralateral neck received 54 Gy in 30 fractions (Fig. 18.2a, b). This was well-tolerated, with expected side effects of esophagitis, tracheal inflammation, and pharyngitis. She required a soft diet during her treatment but fully recovered 4 weeks later. Following treatment completion, she feels well and has returned to work as a travel agent. Her only complaint is of thickened saliva. CT shows no evidence of recurrence in the neck but slow progression of lung nodules. Her thyroglobulin remains undetectable. With the slow growth and small size of her lung metastases, however, she remains on observation, and she has not yet been considered for treatment with targeted agents.

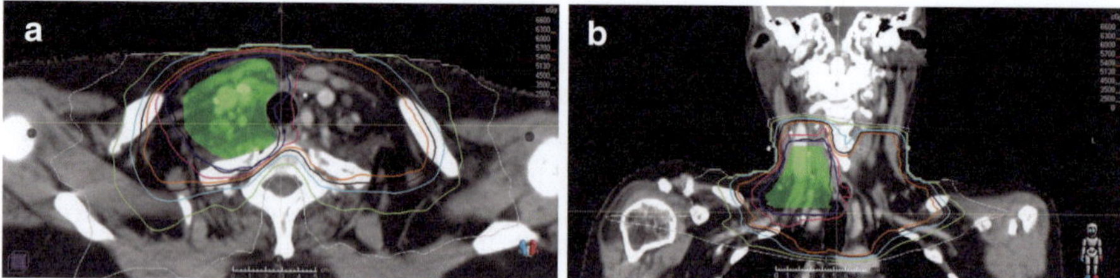

Fig. 18.2 (**a**) Axial slice demonstrating the clinical target volume (CTV—green shading) and isodose distribution for the external beam radiation therapy treatment plan. All tissue within the blue isodose line receives 60 Gy or more and all tissue within the orange isodose line received 54 Gy. (**b**) Coronal CT slice demonstrating the clinical target volume (CTV—green shading) and isodose distribution for the external beam radiation therapy treatment plan. All tissue within the black isodose line receives 60 Gy or more and all tissue within the orange isodose line received 54 Gy

References

1. Sheline GE, Galante M, Lindsay S. Radiation therapy in the control of persistent thyroid cancer. Am J Roentgenol Radium Therapy, Nucl Med. 1966;97(4):923–30.
2. Brierley J, Sherman E. The role of external beam radiation and targeted therapy in thyroid cancer. Semin Radiat Oncol. 2012;22(3):254–62. Epub 2012/06/13
3. Farahati J, Reiners C, Stuschke M, Muller SP, Stuben G, Sauerwein W, et al. Differentiated thyroid cancer. Impact of adjuvant external radiotherapy in patients with perithyroidal tumor infiltration (stage pT4). Cancer. 1996;77(1):172–80.
4. Biermann M, Pixberg M, Riemann B, Schuck A, Heinecke A, Schmid KW, et al. Clinical outcomes of adjuvant external-beam radiotherapy for differentiated thyroid cancer - results after 874 patient-years of follow-up in the MSDS-trial. Nuklearmedizin. 2009;48(3):89–98. quiz N15. Epub 2009/03/27
5. Brierley J, Tsang R, Panzarella T, Bana N. Prognostic factors and the effect of treatment with radioactive iodine and external beam radiation on patients with differentiated thyroid cancer seen at a single institution over 40 years. Clin Endocrinol. 2005;63(4):418–27.
6. Cooper DS, Doherty GM, Haugen BR, Kloos RT, Lee SL, Mandel SJ, et al. Revised American Thyroid Association management guidelines for patients with thyroid nodules and differentiated thyroid cancer. Thyroid. 2009;19(11):1167–214. Epub 2009/10/29
7. Haugen BR, Alexander EK, Bible KC, Doherty GM, Mandel SJ, Nikiforov YE, et al. 2015 American Thyroid Association management guidelines for adult patients with thyroid nodules and differentiated thyroid cancer: the American Thyroid Association guidelines task force on thyroid nodules and differentiated thyroid cancer. Thyroid. 2016;26(1):1–133. Epub 2015/10/16
8. Mitchell AL, Gandhi A, Scott-Coombes D, Perros P. Management of thyroid cancer: United Kingdom National Multidisciplinary Guidelines. J Laryngol Otol. 2016;130(S2):S150–S60. Epub 2016/11/15
9. Kiess AP, Agrawal N, Brierley JD, Duvvuri U, Ferris RL, Genden E, et al. External-beam radiotherapy for differentiated thyroid cancer locoregional control: a statement of the American Head and Neck Society. Head Neck. 2016;38(4):493–8. Epub 2015/12/31
10. Sobin LH, Wittekind C, editors. TNM classification of malignant tumours. 6th ed. New York: John Wiley & Sons; 2002.
11. Greene FL, Page DL, Flemming ID, Fritz AG, Balch CM, Haller DG, et al. AJCC cancer staging manual. 6th ed. New York: Springer-Verlag; 2002.
12. Yang Z, Flores J, Katz S, Nathan CA, Mehta V. Comparison of survival outcomes following postsurgical radioactive iodine versus external beam radiation in stage IV differentiated thyroid carcinoma. Thyroid. 2017;27(7):944–52. Epub 2017/04/28
13. Sun XS, Sun SR, Guevara N, Marcy PY, Peyrottes I, Lassalle S, et al. Indications of external beam radiation therapy in non-anaplastic thyroid cancer and impact of innovative radiation techniques. Crit Rev Oncol Hematol. 2013;86(1):52–68. Epub 2012/10/24
14. Servagi Vernat S, Khalifa J, Sun XS, Kammerer E, Blais E, Faivre JC, et al. 10-year Locoregional control with postoperative external beam radiotherapy in patients with locally advanced high-risk non-anaplastic thyroid carcinoma De novo or at relapse, a propensity score analysis. Cancers. 2019;11:6. Epub 2019/06/30
15. Fussey JM, Crunkhorn R, Tedla M, Weickert MO, Mehanna H. External beam radiotherapy in differentiated thyroid carcinoma: a systematic review. Head Neck. 2016;38(Suppl 1):E2297–305. Epub 2015/09/04
16. Dicuonzo S, Pedretti S, Mangoni M, Monari F, Fanetti G, Borsatti E, et al. Adjuvant radiotherapy and radioiodine treatment for locally advanced differentiated thyroid cancer: systematic review and meta-analysis. Tumori. 2021;Epub 2021/03/17:300891621996817.
17. Tam S, Amit M, Boonsripitayanon M, Cabanillas ME, Busaidy NL, Gunn GB, et al. Adjuvant external beam radiotherapy in locally advanced differentiated thyroid cancer. JAMA Otolaryngol Head Neck Surg. 2017;143(12):1244–51. Epub 2017/11/04

18. Schwartz DL, Lobo MJ, Ang KK, Morrison WH, Rosenthal DI, Ahamad A, et al. Postoperative external beam radiotherapy for differentiated thyroid cancer: outcomes and morbidity with conformal treatment. Int J Radiat Oncol Biol Phys. 2009;74(4):1083–91. Epub 2008/12/20

Index

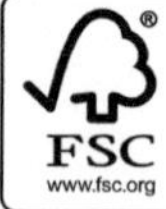